AF594019

The Science We Have Loved and Taught

The Science We Have Loved and Taught

Dartmouth Medical School's First Two Centuries

CONSTANCE E. PUTNAM

Foreword by James E. Wright

University Press of New England / Hanover and London

Published by University Press of New England,
One Court Street, Lebanon, NH 03766
www.upne.com

Printed in the United States of America
5 4 3 2 1

CIP data appear at the end of the book

Publication of this history has been made possible through the generosity of Katharine Swift, M.D., and the late Thomas P. Almy, M.D.; Ernest J. Moorhead; and Gilbert R. Tanis and the late Frances H. Tanis.

Most of the documents essential to the writing of this book are found in the Dartmouth College Archives. Permission was granted to quote from letters, memoranda, special reports, faculty minutes, provosts' and presidents' papers, trustees' minutes, and numerous other documents (such as items from the alumni files) and is gratefully acknowledged. This permission also extended to the reprinting of documents found in Appendix B, Appendix C, and Appendix D.

Permission to quote from documents owned by three other libraries is also gratefully acknowledged: the Beinecke Rare Book and Manuscript Library at Yale University Library, and the Massachusetts Historical Society.

For Dartmouth Doctors:
quondam nunc et futuris

Contents

Illustrations

Foreword

JAMES E. WRIGHT

President, Dartmouth College

James Wright, the 16th president of Dartmouth College, has held that office since 1998 and has been a member of the Dartmouth faculty since 1969. A noted historian, he specializes in American political history and is a member of the American Academy of Arts and Sciences.

DARTMOUTH COLLEGE TOOK its first step as a pioneer in the establishment of professional schools with the 1797 founding of Dartmouth Medical School. It was the fourth medical school in the country and the first in a rural area. Founder Nathan Smith, a Harvard-educated doctor, had begun his medical practice in 1787 in Cornish, New Hampshire, just down the river from Hanover. He treated patients in villages and farms that stretched along the whole length of the Connecticut River Valley. The distances were long, and, except for the sometime help of an apprentice or two, he was alone in his practice.

Reasoning that good care demanded both more and better-trained doctors, he wrote to the Board of Trustees of nearby Dartmouth College on August 26, 1796, suggesting that they permit him to establish a medical school under Dartmouth's auspices. Smith generously offered to first pursue further study at his own expense in Edinburgh, Scotland, and also promised to donate laboratory and classroom equipment for the new medical school. He proposed himself as the sole faculty member. Although still struggling to establish the College at the time, the Trustees accepted the offer. They knew a good thing when they saw it.

Smith began lecturing in November 1797 and did virtually all the teaching himself for thirteen years. He soon gained renown for his teaching and his scientific approach to medicine. Before long, student enrollment far outstripped the single room in Dartmouth Hall allocated to the Medical School. Smith, ever the entrepreneur, persuaded the state legislature to provide $3,450 for a three-story building. Completed in 1811, the building stood on the current site of the College's Fairchild Science

Center. In 1813, with Dartmouth Medical School firmly established, Smith moved on to found or help found three more medical schools—at Yale, Bowdoin, and the University of Vermont. In fact, Smith has admiringly been called "the Johnny Appleseed of American medicine."

Thanks to Nathan Smith, Dartmouth was one of the first schools to offer a distinct medical curriculum. While Dartmouth Medical School has undergone many changes—even a refounding in the late 1950s—since its inception more than two hundred years ago, it has remained true to its original purpose: to provide a first-class medical education to a diverse range of students in order to fulfill both the dreams of its students and the needs of the wider community.

Doctors like Smith are woven throughout Dartmouth's history—people gifted in the arts of patient care and teaching, passionate about science, broad and deep in their interests, and committed to a medical school marked by excellence; people like Dr. Dixi Crosby, who founded and staffed "Dr. Dixi's Hospital" on College Street, opposite the medical school; like Dr. Oliver Wendell Holmes, who arrived at Dartmouth in 1838 with his friend Ralph Waldo Emerson and who served for two years as professor of anatomy and physiology; and like Dr. Gilman Frost, the first physician in the United States to perform an x-ray for clinical purposes. Indeed, people like the current faculty of Dartmouth Medical School, who are committed to teaching, mentoring, discovery, and patient care, and who are part of a rich tradition, which they, in turn, enhance. In this book, Constance Putnam introduces us to many of the individuals who helped to chart the institution's course as well as to a number of episodes in its development that have hitherto been largely hidden from sight in the College archives. Readers will appreciate the ways in which Dartmouth Medical School has evolved over the years—as well as the extent to which it has stayed true to Smith's original vision.

Today, Dartmouth-Hitchcock Medical Center is one of the few academic medical centers in the country located in a largely rural area. Dartmouth as a whole is enriched by the presence of Dartmouth Medical School and its clinical partners—Mary Hitchcock Memorial Hospital and the Dartmouth-Hitchcock Clinic. Having grown far beyond Nathan Smith's wildest dreams, Dartmouth Medical School is today the centerpiece of a first-class academic medical center, highly regarded for its research, its teaching, and its practice of medicine.

With its emphasis on quality teaching, critical thinking, research experience, and clinical practice, Dartmouth Medical School can perhaps provide a model for how best to marry the delivery of health care with the teaching of medicine. Nathan Smith demonstrated by his actions a firm belief that medical schools should be attached to academic institutions. Today, the strength of the connections forged between the College and the Medical School testifies to the continuing power of Smith's vision.

Preface and Acknowledgments

CONSTANCE E. PUTNAM

THE BICENTENNIAL CELEBRATION for Dartmouth Medical School (DMS) in 1997 was no ordinary birthday party.* For one thing, the celebrating continued for more than a year, having begun in the autumn of 1996 when the Convocation that marks the beginning of Dartmouth's academic year was dedicated to "200 years of medicine at Dartmouth." This was but one of many slogans put into play in the course of the year, as a stunning array of events unfolded for the enjoyment of numerous audiences. How *does* one do justice to the long and varied history of the "medical school in this College" that was planted and nurtured by Nathan Smith virtually single-handedly two centuries ago but that has changed so much that Smith himself would not recognize it?

One can approach the whole project visually—and that was done. Several exhibits of art and artifacts, mounted in the main corridor of Baker Library and at the Hood Museum of Art and the Dana Biomedical Library, followed in succession. Probably even more people saw the display in the main-entrance rotunda at the Dartmouth-Hitchcock Medical Center during the bicentennial summer or the one that accompanied the major international bicentennial symposium at the Hopkins Center in September 1997.

Ah, yes, the symposium! One can also approach a historical milestone educationally, and that was most assuredly done. The symposium was both the centerpiece and the culmination of the year-long celebration. "Great Issues for Medicine in the Twenty-first Century: Ethical and Social Issues Arising Out of Advances in Biomedical Sciences" was a fitting title. Fifty years earlier, then-president of Dartmouth College John Sloan Dickey had introduced a course for undergraduates called "Great Issues," and in 1960—to cap Dartmouth Medical School's "refounding"—a symposium titled "Great Issues of Conscience in Modern Medicine"

*A summary report of this occasion, with documenting material, can be found in the Dartmouth College Archives.

had carried on that tradition, bringing a star-studded cast to Hanover to challenge and explore pressing matters of medicine in that day. In 1997, the tradition was extended by echoing those earlier titles while looking the future squarely in the face. For what, it made sense to ask, were the concerns for the world of medicine at Dartmouth in 1997—and today and for all our futures—if not the ethical and social issues that continue to arise at a startling rate out of advances in the biomedical sciences? Co-chairing the symposium were Michael S. Brown and Joseph L. Goldstein, co-recipients of the 1985 Nobel Prize in Medicine or Physiology for their work in identifying the process by which receptors on human cells trap and absorb bloodstream particles that contain cholesterol. Their talks—Goldstein on "Burgers, Chips, and Genes" and Brown on "The Making of a Physician-Scientist"—book-ended the formal sessions, though they were flanked by welcoming, opening, and closing remarks from Dartmouth dignitaries: DMS Dean Andrew G. Wallace, Dartmouth President James O. Freedman, and Bicentennial Symposium Planning Committee Chair Heinz Valtin.

It is also possible to approach a celebratory event gustatorially. A summer party open to all residents of the region who are served by the Dartmouth-Hitchcock Medical Center included a day of family fun at the Montshire Museum in Norwich, Vermont, and a gala reception. The opening night of the symposium there was a President's Dinner and at the end of the first full day of the symposium another gala reception. Along the way, with reunion classes in attendance, all present were invited to luncheons and cold buffet breakfasts.

Musically and artistically the bicentennial was also celebrated. A poster was commissioned from noted artist Sabra Field, who produced an original, one-of-a-kind, mixed-media collage of brightly colored paper to be framed and hung at the Medical School. Limited-edition prints and posters made the image collectible by a wider audience. Marilyn "Willy" Black—a local chainsaw woodcarver—was commissioned to produce Nathan Smith in wood. Charles Dodge's commissioned musical work was premièred at the Saturday concert.

Of course, there was more, and the future that was being so much talked about during the symposium is still unfolding all around us. Over-the-shoulder looks at DMS's past (one could hardly celebrate 200 years of anything, without looking back at the road traveled) could in any case not adequately pay tribute to the history of medicine and of doctors at Dartmouth.

And so, a book. Yet it turns out the past is too dense—there are too many heroes and humble participants, too many anecdotes and analyses, too many episodes of interest or import, too many tales and texts, too many documents and discoveries—to hold within the pages of a single book. Hence this volume is itself perhaps best characterized as something of a look-over-the-shoulder that does not (and could not) contain everything of significance to one constituency or another of the family of Dartmouth doctors. Any attempt to write the story of a venerable institution is fraught with difficulties—finding the relevant documents, talking to the right people, unraveling the conflicting stories—but the biggest challenge of all may be deciding what to leave out. Doing even minor surgery on a book manuscript is hard on the surgeon; doing radical surgery (one amputation after another!) was, in this case, downright painful. But if I have done my surgery well, the patient is the better for it. What is left I hope tells enough of the story to satisfy temporary hunger pangs while whetting appetites for further exploration about the resilient and complex contributor to medical education known as Dartmouth Medical School.

And so, as I said, a book. There is precedent. When DMS celebrated its centennial in 1897, Phineas Sanborn Conner—a Dartmouth College graduate (1859) and a distinguished member of the Medical School faculty—not only gave a "historical address" as part of the program, but ten years later published a longer version (on which I rely heavily, as close attention to the notes will show). Then in 1972, shortly after stepping down from his position as Dean of Dartmouth Medical School, Carleton B. Chapman similarly wrote a long essay published in book form, in honor of DMS's "first 175 years." (On that, too, I have frequently relied, as scrutiny of the notes will also reveal.) Three remarks in Chapman's book warrant quoting here.

When, sometime in the early 1990s, Carleton Chapman autographed a copy of that little book for me and offered me "best wishes for your splendid writing project," he was referring to the biography of Nathan Smith that I was endeavoring to complete as co-author with the (then already) late Oliver S. Hayward (*Improve, Perfect, & Perpetuate: Dr. Nathan Smith and Early American Medical Education*, published in 1998 by the University Press of New England). Neither Chapman nor I imagined then that I would be the one to whom he had unwittingly pointed when he wrote, thinking ahead to the medical school's bicentennial, "No doubt some School stalwart, following Phineas Conner's example of 1897, will sum up the record for the two centuries at that time." And though I grew up in the shadow of Dartmouth Medical School and have the right bloodlines for such an effort—my father was a member of the DMS class of 1932—I hardly count as a "School stalwart." Chapman in that same book also said, "It is to be hoped that well before 1997, the bicentennial year, some devoted and energetic soul will have written the definitive history. . . ." Again I must plead nolo contendere: I have been "devoted and energetic," and I have tried to write what would count as "the definitive history" of the school—my readers must be the judges—but I was not even engaged to write the book until the bicentennial was nearly upon us. Thus perhaps I need not be faulted for the fact that I did not finish the book "well before 1997."

With respect to one final remark in Chapman's book, I believe I have done better. Saying that "it is difficult or impossible at present to make much sense, from documentary sources, of the upheaval over molecular biology which rocked the School in the midsixties," Chapman went on: "The future author of the definitive history will have to do what he [*sic*!] can to deal judiciously and at length with that troubled and confused period of the School's life." Certainly I wrote about it "at length"; chapter 10, which covers that contentious period at DMS, is the longest in the book. It may also, by some standards, be the most important chapter, since it appears I am the first to have undertaken to explore the story from so many angles and to lay it out so thoroughly. I have done as much as I could without turning the resulting account into an obsessive monograph on that one topic, which would have overwhelmed the rest of the book. In other words, I have indeed endeavored to be "judicious." Again, my readers must judge my success.

If I have succeeded, it is to a large extent thanks to the willingness of a very large number of people to talk with me quite openly about their experiences and their recollections. I refer to "experiences" *and* "recollections" because it early became evident that recollections were not always accurate—yet the way the experiences are recollected is definitely also part of the story. In order to get as close to the bottom of things as I could, I also decided at the outset that I would not attribute remarks, by name, to those who made them unless those remarks were part of a written record, published or archival—or unless I explicitly asked for and received permission to quote by name. There is good precedent among (medical) historians for doing this; I have in every instance indicated whether the person speaking was a former student or faculty member, or still a member of the faculty, and so on—but I have not identified who said what.

Having decided to follow that policy for the molecular biology chapter, I decided to follow it throughout, when what I was quoting was something said to me in the course of an interview ("interview" includes face-to-face encounters as well as phone conversations, letters, and e-mail correspondence). This may on occasion cause some frustration or annoyance for readers who would like to know "Who said that?"—and who may be a bit surprised, since this book is otherwise so scrupulously documented. But the result, I truly believe, is a fuller and more honest account of several different aspects of Dartmouth Medical School's history in the periods covered that still have living eyewitnesses and participants than would otherwise have been possible. Which brings me to the many people who need to be thanked for making it possible to tell this story fully and honestly.

No book is ever written solely by the author. Acknowledged or not, there are those who support the work that goes into the production of a manuscript in myriad ways. In my case, their number is legion. But I am so indebted to those legions, so conscious of how true the sometimes trite-sounding phrase "I couldn't have done it without . . ." is in this case, that I want to paint a bit of that background for those interested in how a book actually comes to pass.

At the top of the list are the members of the publications subcommittee of the DMS Bicentennial Committee who gave me the opportunity to immerse myself in the history of Dartmouth Medical School. The late S. Marsh Tenney, Dana Cook Grossman, and Heinz Valtin exhibited great patience as it took me well past the end of the bicentennial celebrations to bring this project to a close. My biggest regret is that Marsh, who cared very deeply about having the history of Dartmouth Medical School told, did not live to see the published book. I am grateful for the trust in me that he demonstrated in sharing not only his memories but his unpublished *Memoir*, without which chapter 10 in particular would have been much less rich in detail and nuance. Dana—editor, advisor, fount of knowledge, supplier of information, faithful correspondent, and friend—stayed steadfastly supportive even as I found the schedule slipping yet again. We work together well, and the book is better for her contributions to it. Her willingness to share with me the time and talents of her editorial assistants—first Jonathan Weisberg and then Matthew Wiencke—was a boon; these young men cheerfully tracked down bibliographic details and helped unravel mysteries by scouring the resources of the Dartmouth College Archives for me. Heinz, too, was generous in his enthusiasm for the job I was doing. He and his wife Nancy also opened their home to my husband and me, where we spent a delightful month of house-sitting during one especially intense period of archival work in Rauner Library.

Rauner—still and always Webster Hall to those who, like me, grew up in the area and attended many a concert there—is home today to the Dartmouth College Archives. Countless hours spent there were made pleasant and pleasurable not only by the riches of the archival holdings that yielded innumerable treasures for me but also by the sympathy from the staff that I learned I could count on when some document turned out to be difficult—or even impossible—to find. Nor did any of them ever complain when I asked to have retrieved, again, a box of papers I had already looked through and perhaps just sent back to storage. Nor did any complain when I wrote or e-mailed asking—one more time!—for help. Though many staff members helped me on many occasions (I came to know them all!), the one who stands out above all others is the incomparable Barbara Krieger. Her familiarity with the archives and ability to find items when given only the vaguest description of what they might be called, to say nothing of her constant goodwill and cheerful response to queries, made a huge difference.

The most concentrated periods for me of research and writing were, somewhat improbably, at the Wellcome Institute for the History of Medicine in London (now reincarnated as the Wellcome Trust Centre for the History of Medicine at University College London). Numerous colleagues there cheered me on, buoyed my spirits when the work went slowly, challenged and probed in ways that helped keep me on track. Bill Bynum and the late Roy Porter made suggestions early on and served as mentors without perhaps ever realizing that they were doing so. Three other colleagues who know much about writing institutional histories deserve special mention: Elsbeth Heaman, Keir Waddington, and Lise Wilkinson. Lise has become the best kind of friend and colleague—always supportive, always ready to share what she has learned from her own research and writing experience. Louise Gray shared an office with me and set a good example of hard, steady, and good work.

Others who helped—indeed, who were critical to this project—are the numerous Dartmouth-connected people (current and/or former, faculty and/or students and/or staff) who were willing to be interviewed. Some who were willing never got a chance to do so, because I failed to get back to them; some I talked with only very briefly or so long ago they have probably forgotten the encounters. Some who were of great assistance will not find anything they said directly quoted. Yet all provided details that enhanced the overall picture. Interviews were conducted in person or by mail or e-mail or phone in London and from Oregon to Florida to California to—especially, of course—New Hampshire and many places in between. I learned a lot; I have tried to incorporate much of the best of what I learned into the book. Of particular significance to my work were numerous and extensive communications of various sorts with Thomas Almy and Katharine Swift Almy, R. Clinton Fuller, Howard Green, Allan U. Munck, and most generously Robert

E. Nye, Jr. They know how they helped; I hope that they understand how deeply appreciative I was and am.

Additional individuals who contributed in important ways are Kurt Benirschke, Harry Bird, Barbara Blough, Constance E. Brinkerhoff, John Butterly, Richard Cardozo, Robert Christie, Thomas Colacchio, John Collins, Kenneth W. Cooper, William Culp, Quentin Deming, Merlin K. (Monte) DuVal, Arthur Ecker, James O. Freedman, Robert Gosselin, Paul Guyre, John Hennessy, Shinya Inoué, Samuel Katz, C. Everett Koop, Lisabeth Maloney, Frances McCann, Fletcher McDowell, O. Ross McIntyre, Peter Mogielnicki, Manuel Morales, Edward (Ted) Mortimer, Lafayette Noda, Mayme Noda, Donald Penfield, Stephen K. Plume, Ed Scheu, Molly Scheu, Michael Shoob, Raymond Stephens, Andrew Szent-Györgyi, and Heinz Valtin, James Varnum, Peter von Hippel, William Wickner, and Michael Zubkoff. Also of assistance are several individuals who died prior to my having completed this book: Robert Fairchild, G. Bruce Lemmon, Philip O. Nice, Paul Pagannucci, E. Lucile Smith, Radford Tanzer, and S. Marsh Tenney. My apologies to any whose name I have inadvertantly omitted.

In a special category are those who gave generous financial support toward the publication of this book: Katharine Swift Almy and the late Thomas P. Almy, Ernest J. Moorhead, and Gilbert R. Tanis and the late Frances H. Tanis.

Deans and former deans were of particular importance. I had had the good fortune to come to know the late Carleton Chapman (as indicated above) some time before I was even engaged in this project. I had opportunity for conversations and correspondence with the late Ralph Hunter (whose name was one to conjure with, in my childhood). Conversations with Marsh Tenney happily took place at a point when I was able to benefit directly from his marvelously encyclopedic knowledge of DMS through all phases of its history. Writing this book gave me the excuse and opportunity to meet and talk with Jim Strickler, Bob McCollum, and Andy Wallace; such grip as I (a historian) have on the more nearly contemporary parts of the DMS history is largely thanks to the accumulated decanal insights and wisdom they passed on to me. The only full-time dean since Rolf Syvertsen whom I never met was Gilbert H. Mudge. Conversation with his widow Eleanor Mudge and son John Mudge, who gave me access to a large quantity of papers from Dean Mudge's files, was no substitute for having met him in person, but their generosity made possible a far better understanding of a critical period in DMS history than I could otherwise have had. Similar generosity was exhibited by Janet Bowler Fitzgibbons and her sister Patsy Bowler Leggat, who loaned me a large quantity of papers from the files of their father, John Pollard Bowler; Janet was always ready to answer the variety of questions that emerged as I studied those papers.

Not only Dartmouth people helped. Librarians, local historians, and other keepers of archival records in a number of venues helped. Lucretia McClure and several of her colleagues at Harvard's Countway Library of Medicine answered numerous questions, helping me track down details I would never have found on my own; Toby Appel at Yale's Medical Historical Library did the same. Nancy Richards at George Washington University and Jordan Kurland at the American Association of University Professors (AAUP) offices in Washington, D.C., gave critical assistance. Frank DeMattos, Shirley Parks, and Ron Karr (in Rehoboth, Winchendon, and Lowell, Massachusetts, respectively); Sarah Putnam in Orford, New Hampshire; and Phyllis Lavelle in Bradford, Vermont, each helped answer questions or look for information I had not found and was loath to ignore. Others whose connections with Dartmouth were more tenuous or non-existent but who helped in ways they may not have realized (and may not remember now) include Stanley M. Aronson, Arthur Ebbert, Dan Grossman, Howard Pearson, Andrew Schuman, Marilyn Tobias, and Jeannette Willis. A historian of medicine who is not medically trained is always at risk of failing to understand some medical matter; I am grateful to physicians Christopher Booth, John M. T. Ford, John Henderson, Jerome Nolan, and Henry Vaillant for setting me straight on what no doubt struck them as elementary issues. Carol Bowen, crucially, sent the finished manuscript on its way for me.

If it is true that a picture is worth a thousand words, then on that basis alone I have grounds for gratitude to Penelope Peters, friend and photo researcher extraordinaire. Way beyond her nominal task, she served as a volunteer editor, drawing my attention to places where—as she gently pointed out—what I had written lacked clarity. (She also spared my readers numerous parenthetical asides, but she never got a chance to suggest eliminating this one!) Phyllis Deutsch and Ann Brash at the University Press of New England displayed amazing talent for not making me feel guilty even when I failed to meet deadlines.

Dartmouth Medical School owes a greater debt than it can ever pay—as do I—to my husband, Hugo Adam Bedau. He read every word of the manuscript in its longest form, its several middle-length forms, and its final form; he knows the history of DMS as very few others do. Patient and helpful, willing and able to perform any task I put in front of him to assist me in bringing the project to fruition, he has phoned, written letters, searched through microfiche, looked up bibliographic details, taken notes, read arcane documents—you get the picture. He prodded and he praised. The whole huge project would have taken longer still had he not been standing at the ready, throughout.

Even with so many people to thank, I still cannot lay the blame for errors or failures of interpretation on anyone but myself. I like to think that being "devoted and energetic" counts for something—even though it is certain that not everyone will agree with all my interpretations.

May 2003 *Concord, Massachusetts*

A Technical Note

I have maintained a flexible policy in handling grammatical and orthographic "errors" in quoted material. Many of the manuscripts on which I relied date from a period when spelling, capitalization, and punctuation were by no means so standardized as they are today; I saw little reason always to retain spelling that was likely to distract or—worse—confuse the modern readers. On the other hand, some of the flavor of the eighteenth- and nineteenth-century material would be lost if *all* the nonstandard spelling, grammar, and technical details in the quoted documents were corrected. Thus I decided to follow a very loose rule of thumb, which was to correct without comment the most distracting or confusing "errors" and to leave some of the more charming oddities for flavor. I used "[*sic*]" sparingly, only where it seemed necessary to keep the reader from stumbling or thinking what appeared was a typographical error. My judgment on any or all of these points could be challenged, and I have admittedly tampered with what purists might consider the authenticity of the quoted material; authenticity can be checked via the endnotes, however, and my goal was to make the material accessible and the reading a pleasure rather than a struggle.

PART I

THE FOUNDATION YEARS: INVENTION

CHAPTER ONE

In the Beginning

The scheme, novel and far-reaching, was favorably received . . . and a resolution complimentary to the character and energy of Dr. Smith was passed.
—OLIVER P. HUBBARD[1]

The enterprise was indeed a bold one.
—WILLIAM ALLEN[2]

THE PINES WERE tall and the mud was often deep on the windswept plain that would later become "The Green."[3] But in 1796, with the struggling young college named after the Earl of Dartmouth still less than three decades old, anything like the classic New England college campus of today still lay far in the future.

Nathan Smith's Early Years

Nonetheless, a young and eager (not to say entrepreneurial) doctor named Nathan Smith, practicing in Cornish, New Hampshire, some twenty miles to the south of Hanover and likewise on the Connecticut River, apparently sensed possibility. Call it a vision, call it a dream: Certainly Smith's idea was novel. Something moved him not only to conceive that the fledgling Dartmouth College might be a suitable place to establish a medical school, but also—more startlingly—to believe that he was the man to do it. One of the great unsolved mysteries of early American medical education is and no doubt will continue to be just what it was that gave the thirty-four-year-old Smith the courage of his convictions. He had come to the study of medicine relatively late, and there were many physicians around who had far more experience than he. Why should he have thought he was the one to spearhead an effort to improve medical education in the North Country, and with it, medical care for the people of the rural north?

The nation itself was still young and raw. Up to that time, only three medical schools had been opened, each in an urban setting. Philadelphia was first, in 1765; New York followed in 1767. Then the vigorous and talented John Warren, not yet thirty years old, persuaded Harvard College that he should give anatomy and surgery lectures in Boston in 1782 under the College's aegis; he promptly convinced two medical colleagues (Benjamin Waterhouse and Aaron Dexter) to join his effort and to help assure breadth for the program of lectures he intended to institute. But none of these schools was a plausible precedent for the enterprise Nathan Smith proposed, out in the countryside. (By the time of the first federal census in 1790, the population of Hanover—still only 870 in 1786—had finally passed the 1,000 mark to reach 1,379, of whom 152 were students at the College.[4]) Smith, knowing what Warren had achieved, might have seen it as a model for taking personal initiative. Although no record survives indicating conscious imitation on Smith's part, it is credible that he should have come away from the experience of studying under Warren with the idea that a single individual really could at least start a medical school.

But in the wilderness? For Hanover, at least compared to Boston, New York, and Philadelphia, surely was in the back of beyond. Unless, of course, you lived in an even more remote spot, like Cornish, with its scattered farmhouses. (Even today, the several villages that constitute Cornish together take up only about thirty-five square miles and are connected by winding roads that seem unlikely to lead to each other.) By contrast, Hanover—where the College had recently erected an imposing and handsome new building—must have looked prosperous and important indeed.[5] A town with such an institution surely had an aura of potential that was utterly lacking in Cornish or any of the other Connecticut River Valley settlements with which Smith was by then familiar. Still, notwithstanding the claims of one historian that the "prosperity of the College reflected . . . upon the village," that selfsame college was in severe financial straits. Yet a new meeting house was built in 1795, and a bridge was thrown across the Connecticut River in 1796—so all was not dire.[6] Even so, how and why Nathan Smith should have believed Dartmouth would welcome the idea of a medical school and him as the person to execute the plan must remain a matter for speculation.

Certainly Smith knew his way around, in several senses of that expression. Having moved with his family to Chester, Vermont—only a short paddle up the Williams River from the Connecticut—from Rehoboth, Massachusetts, when he was about ten, Nathan came of age as the eldest of four children left fatherless shortly after the move.[7] He surely would helped out on the farm. He must have learned at least to read and write, probably from his mother, for by the age of thirteen he is said to have been teaching (or assisting) in the local school. That he himself is unlikely to have benefited from much formal schooling is clear from the fact that efforts to open a school in Chester were only just beginning when the Smith family moved there. (Nathan's father, John Smith, was selected shortly after he arrived in Chester to serve on a committee organized to consider where to build a schoolhouse.[8]) On the other hand, from its initial settlement in 1643, the town of Rehoboth had required every resident to attend school (the minister, of course, was the teacher), so young Nathan may very well have received an introduction to the "three R's" there.[9]

The first reasonably reliable record we have of Nathan's youth dates from many years later and is the only first-hand account we have of what turned out to be a signal episode in Nathan Smith's life. The event in question proved so important for the course of Smith's life, and with it for medical education at Dartmouth, that we must be grateful to have it. For if we had more details concerning the first two decades of Smith's life but did not know what happened on this one day, when Nathan was already twenty-two, we would struggle even more to explain subsequent events.

What set this particular day apart was that an itinerant surgeon, Josiah Goodhue, arrived in town to perform an amputation. On this day of days, Nathan Smith found his calling.[10] Goodhue, a physician and surgeon of considerable local repute, was probably a familiar figure; he lived and practiced primarily in the neighboring town of Putney, and the fact that he himself later settled in Chester makes it likely that he was well acquainted there. But an amputation was an event worth witnessing in any case, and so it is probable that a goodly crowd would have gathered for the occasion. More than fifty years later, when Smith died, Goodhue—reflecting on the life and death of his friend and one-time student, Nathan Smith—recalled the occasion as something emblematic of Smith. Goodhue told how Smith had stepped forward when the surgeon called for a volunteer to assist him; he recollected how Smith, apparently overcome with fascination at what he had witnessed and been part of in this small way, asked on the spot whether Goodhue would let him sign on as an apprentice.

Goodhue was understandably hesitant when Smith said he had heretofore only "worked with his hands." The obvious impulsiveness of the young man's request perhaps also gave Goodhue pause. Urging

Smith to get schooling sufficient for acceptance by Harvard College, Goodhue may very well have thought he would hear no more from the youth who had so abruptly concluded that he wished to be a doctor.

Nathan Smith was not one to be easily put off. A few months later, after living with the Reverend Samuel Whiting in nearby Rockingham, Vermont, so that he could conveniently be tutored by that learned man, Smith presented himself to Goodhue once more. The decision Goodhue made at that point to accept Smith as an apprentice turned out to be a good one; the younger man (he was only three years Goodhue's junior) proved an apt and eager pupil. Coupled with how rapidly he had apparently satisfied Whiting's tutorial standards, his quick adaptation to the demands of the doctor's life and the praise Goodhue later heaped on him lead inexorably to the conclusion that Smith was what we would today call "a quick study." Largely unschooled he may initially have been, but he promptly proved himself intelligent, dedicated, and possessed of a marked bent for practical learning based on close observation. Even bearing in mind that the long letter on which we are so dependent for information was written by Goodhue only after he had learned of the death of his close friend and prize pupil, his remarks have the ring of plausibility when measured against what other sources tell us about Smith's subsequent career. Goodhue, at least in recollection, saw in Smith characteristics not common to all "pupils" (as medical preceptees were typically called). "While Smith lived with me the country was new, the roads were bad," he wrote by way of explanation:

> [M]y pupils . . . sometimes objected on account of the road, or inclemency of the weather, but it was not so with him; it was enough to say he might go, and he was gone. Neither the darkness of the night, the mud to his horses knees, or the violence of the storm were any impediments to him. . . . If it should be asked what laid the foundation of Doctor Smith's eminence, the answer is industry. If it should be asked what brought him to the pinnacle of the profession the answer is the most unremitting industry.[11]

Having completed a three-year apprenticeship with Goodhue, Smith struck off on his own, moving to Cornish, New Hampshire, in 1787 to open his own practice. He was then twenty-five. Once again, we are hampered by the paucity of historical records; we do not know how or why Smith chose Cornish. His widowed mother had remarried and moved to Walpole, New Hampshire, not far from Cornish, which may have been a factor. But whatever the reasons, the young doctor chose well. For one thing, the only physician in town was the elderly Dr. Solomon Chase, who had largely ceased seeing patients. For another, Smith soon not only became friends with the extended Chase family but later married into it (on January 16, 1791). The other prominent family in town, the Spaldings, provided him at the same time with his own first apprentice. When Smith moved to Cornish, Lyman Spalding was only a schoolboy of twelve, but he soon manifested a desire to become a doctor. The two became close friends as well as colleagues.

When, after two years of marriage, Smith's childless wife Elizabeth Chase died (on April 24, 1793), the doctor did not have far to look for a new wife. Seventeen months later (on September 16, 1794), he married Elizabeth's younger half-sister Sarah, known as Sally. This would prove a long and fruitful marriage. Sally gave birth to ten children, only one of whom died before the age of twenty; all four sons—like their father—were destined to become doctors (though their medical careers are not part of the story of Dartmouth Medical School).

A Medical Career

After only a couple of years in Cornish, before his first marriage, Smith decided to avail himself of the opportunity for further education provided by the newly opened medical school at Harvard. If any doubts remained about the adequacy of his preparatory education, they were dispelled by his acceptance at Harvard. In 1790, after duly attending the requisite ten-week set of lectures and engaging in some additional private tuition with Benjamin Waterhouse (and no doubt also attending some of John Warren's rather illicit anatomical operations at the Boston Almshouse), Nathan Smith became the fifth graduate of Harvard Medical School.[12] His "inaugural dissertation" at Harvard, "The causes and effects of Spasms in Fevers," was hardly what one would today consider worthy of a doctoral degree, but the published version of this essay and Smith's replies to an anonymous critic are nonetheless worthy of note.[13] In these pages, we have the first concrete evidence of Smith's interest in fevers; thirty-four years after writing his graduation paper, he would publish his most important and most famous work, the *Practical Essay on Typhous Fever*.[14] More important is the evidence provided by Smith's short "dissertation" of what a close observer of disease and of his patients he already was at that early stage. (A century later, a retired member of the Dartmouth medical faculty praised the paper as "the product of an experienced practitioner."[15]) With that, Nathan Smith—the proud owner of an M.B. degree (medical training was at that point still by no means a graduate education, hence the degree was not a doctoral one)—returned to Cornish to take up the reins of his practice once more. By then he was as well trained and systematically educated a physician as custom and educational opportunities in the United States permitted at the time.

The restless desire both to learn more and to share what he knew with other young backwoods boys eager to doctor their neighbors seems to have stayed with Smith. In addition to Lyman Spalding, Jo Gallup—an enterprising young doctor with a practice in Bethel, Vermont—had come to apprentice with him.[16] There may have been others. Frustrated perhaps by the inability to provide systematic instruction for his eager followers, and desirous on his own account to have the advantage of a library beyond what he could accumulate for himself, Nathan Smith somehow conceived the idea that the "literary institution" (as Dartmouth College was sometimes called) just up the road might like to add to its prestige by being able to announce that medical lectures were also available there. In August 1796, Smith sent a letter to President John Wheelock and the "Honble Board of Trustees of Dartmouth College," seeking support for his idea.[17]

Smith's letter is a model of brevity, given the magnitude of what he was proposing, its tone supremely confident. "Gentlemen," he wrote,

> Relying on your Patronage, and being confident, that you will favour any measures, which are likely to promote useful Science, I have ventured to make certain proposals, which, I now present for your consideration.
>
> As we have no medical school in this State where Students in Physic can be regularly instructed in the several Branches of that Science, I propose, if the Honble Board will establish a medical school in this College and will honour me with an appointment in it, that I will go to Edinbourgh in Scotland, and will attend to the Several Branches of Medicine as taught and practiced there & will then return to this College where I will commence public teaching as soon as may be after my return
>
> I am with due Respect your Very Humble Servant
>
> Nathan Smith
>
> Hanover Augt. 25th, 1796[18]

The First Medical Lecture

Smith accompanied his letter with a longer document spelling out in some detail how the medical school at Harvard worked; he clearly intended to use the requirements and administrative arrangements there as a model for his new medical school.[19] He gave no indication that he expected to deviate in any way from that standard, nor did he suggest that the trustees should consider changing anything.

Two points of importance emerge from the form in which Smith made this proposal. One is that he had obviously become convinced of the value of the time he had spent with the clergyman Samuel Whiting, acquiring a basic education. Although he did not want to deprive those who had not had the benefits of a "Public Education" of the opportunity for a medical education, they were to be examined by "the authority of the College on Latin, Erethmatic [*sic*], Mathematics & Natural Philosophy" prior to being examined by the medical professors. A basic education was to be a prerequisite for a medical education. Those who had had prior education would need to be examined *only* "by the Medical Professors on the several Branches of Medicine." Second, Smith's use of the Harvard model underscored that he was not merely trying to organize a course of medical lectures, but that he saw value in having medical education available in association with an established institution of higher learning. The location he had chosen—the small town of Hanover, New Hampshire—was to be neither an excuse for offering second-rate training in medicine nor an impediment to providing anything less than excellent medical instruction.

Smith added a postscript to his covering letter, seemingly anticipating that the trustees might have monetary concerns about his suggested venture. He likewise apparently wanted to demonstrate that, despite the boldness and earnestness of his proposal, he did not intend to importune or force himself upon them: "P.S. I do not consider the Board of Trustees, if they should incourage me in the pursuit of Medical Knowledge as under any obligations to pay any part of my expenses which will accrue in going to Europe, and shall acquiess in their determination respecting a medical Institution at my return."[20] He signed his name once more, as if to make absolutely clear that he really meant what he said. The postscript is, however, at least moderately amusing in retrospect. Smith's cheerful assertion that he would pay his own way is only one among many indications throughout his career that Nathan Smith was hardly a master of finances. The truth is, he did not have the money necessary to carry out his plan for study abroad—a fact of which he was surely well aware. So he may simply, and wisely, have been trying to be politic. (Although he succeeded in borrowing the money he needed, it appears to have taken him twenty years to finish repaying the loan![21])

Smith's declared intention to acquiesce in whatever the trustees decided is the second slightly amusing feature of the postscript. As we shall see, he returned to Hanover after his travels abroad and began holding medical lectures without having received any authorization. What we don't know is whether he advertised what he did as taking place at Dartmouth—but, ex post facto, Dartmouth has been quite happy to insist that the lecture Smith gave in 1797 on (probably) November 22 was the initial lecture at Dartmouth Medical School and thus the founding date of the school. Yet the text of an advertisement that Smith arranged to have published in 1799 (and that he presumably wrote), announcing a new round of medical lectures at Dartmouth, read (in part), "This institution was established in August, 1798."[22] Strictly speaking, that was of course true, since it was not until the August 1798 meeting that the Board of Trustees formally gave approval. Smith himself apparently was not nearly so concerned as subsequent generations have been about the actual date. A few years later, he recounted the early days of the school in a letter: "Respecting the origin of the medical school in this place [Hanover], I gave the first course of Med. Lectures in 1797, begun in Nov."[23] So Smith seems indeed to have done. Here, then, is the thin thread on which the claim of a 1797 founding hangs! Had he been serious about relying on the decision of the Board, one might have thought he would wait for their decision before beginning to lecture.

He did not. One suspects Smith may well have determined already to follow the path he had concluded was a useful one. The fact that the trustees finally did "acquiess" was not the difference between Nathan Smith holding medical lectures and his not doing so, but rather the difference between Nathan Smith holding medical lectures quite on his own and his doing so officially under the auspices of Dartmouth.

The Doctor Goes Abroad

The Dartmouth Board of Trustees took two separate actions in response to Smith's August 1796 letter. The first was to appoint a committee to consider the proposal, overnight; the second was to vote on the committee's report the following day. On such short notice, it is not really surprising that the resolution voted included an agreement that the trustees would "defer further consideration" to their next annual meeting. Even so, the underlying inclination to support the idea in principle seems clear. Behind the restrained words, there is even a hint of excitement at the future prospect:

> Whereas Nathan Smith M.B. has made application to this board to obtain their approbation & encouragement by establishing a professorship of the theory and practice of Medicine for the improvement of the students of this university and others . . . [here the decision to defer was inserted]. In the meantime, though they cannot at present promise any pecuniary compensation, yet from a view of the extensive usefulness of such an institution under proper regulations the board of Trustees do approve of the general object of N. Smith. And from

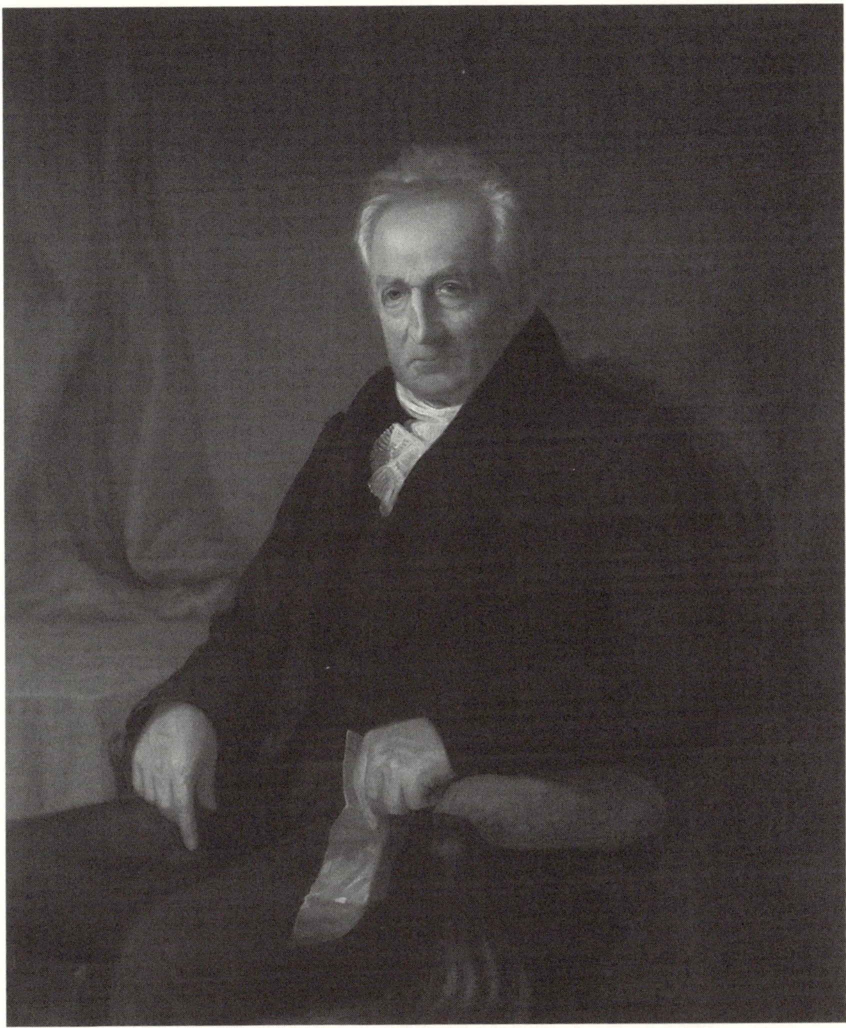

Nathan Smith. Hood Museum of Art, Dartmouth College. Gift of Edmund Randolph Peaslee, Class of 1836.

the opinion which they have of his character and medical knowledge, they could wish that the encouragement for the establishment of such a Professorship may in some future time be inviting. And they feel themselves disposed to afford him all such encouragement and assistance in the laudable pursuit as they shall think and determine their circumstances may admit and his qualifications merit.[24]

Such a response was perhaps as much as Smith could reasonably have hoped for. With no more than this tentatively supportive vote as an official acknowledgment of his undertaking, he set off for Glasgow, Edinburgh, and London just as he had said he would. He also had in hand a letter of introduction to a prominent clergyman in England written by President John Wheelock of Dartmouth. Wheelock's letter gave Smith the encouragement the Board of Trustees seemed reluctant to offer officially, as well as a hint of support (unauthorized by the trustees, incidentally) so strong that it should have buoyed his spirits considerably: "Permit me, Sir, to introduce . . . Dr. Nathan Smith [who] by a resolve of our Corporation, stands now as the only candidate for the Chair of Medical Professor at this University [*sic*]."[25]

Wheelock's letter may not have mattered to Smith; he was probably going to make the trip anyway. Nonetheless, it is an interesting document in light of future developments, for John Wheelock continued to support Smith until they went their separate ways over whether Dartmouth should indeed become a university (as Wheelock and many others were wont to call it) or remain a college (see chapter 2). Hanover was a small and close-knit community; being friends with the president of the College cannot have hurt in the early days of the medical school's existence, and one can easily imagine that Smith himself was much encouraged as he set sail by what looked like good prospects. (There is reason to think the only friend more important to Smith over the course of his Dartmouth career was Mills Olcott, the lawyer who handled all of Smith's affairs even long after his departure from Hanover.[26]) The crisis that would erupt over the College charter and John Wheelock's presidency as well as the impact it had on the shape of the institution came nearly twenty years after these early discussions over the possible establishment of a "Medical Department" at Dartmouth. (We shall return to all that in due course.)

Meanwhile, exactly how to refer to the entity Smith was in the process of trying to establish is difficult to know. It has been referred to in a variety of different ways through its history, especially up to the end of the nineteenth century. The published version of the address Phineas Conner (then a faculty member) gave at the centennial celebration of the school in 1897, for example, included among numerous addenda the following paragraph on the "Name of the School":

> The name of the Medical Department seems to have changed several times. In 1806 the broadside list of students is headed: "Catalogue of the Medical Students and Students of College who attended the Medical Lectures at Dartmouth University" . . . (as far back as Sept. 20, 1781, the Trustees had passed a resolution styling the College a University); that of 1811, "Catalog . . . of the Dartmouth Medical Theatre"; that of 1814, "Catalogue . . . of the Medical Institu-

tion at Dartmouth University"; that of 1817, "Catalogue . . . of the Dartmouth Medical Institution." At some time between this date and 1824 the name "New Hampshire Medical Institution" began to be used and was retained until 1880, though the official title has always been the "Medical Department of Dartmouth College."[27]

As late as 1882, we find on the letterhead on which Phineas Conner recorded students' scores in the surgical examination "Dartmouth Medical. C. P. Frost, M.D., Dean," while Oliver P. Hubbard was turning in grades for the "Chemical Examination Papers 1882" on stationery headed—in Hubbard's hand, to be sure, not printed—"New Hampshire Med. Institution."[28] By the time William Thayer Smith was dean, his letterhead had "Dartmouth Medical School" on it.[29] Why Eugene Orsenigo—a graduate of the class of 1934—should have written, "Dr. William Smith around 1896 gave the school, for once and for all, its official name, calling it the Medical Department of Dartmouth College," is unclear.[30] (To avoid confusion and for consistency's sake, I shall generally use the modern name, Dartmouth Medical School.)

How much effect Smith's visit in Scotland and England actually had on the early shape and later development of the medical school at Dartmouth is impossible to say. We know distressingly little about what he did or learned while he was abroad, despite valiant efforts of more than one researcher to uncover information.[31] Smith himself left very little evidence of what he learned. That may of course not be significant in itself, but if he had come home believing his medical knowledge and skills had been greatly enhanced, it is not unreasonable to think he would have said so, in his lectures. If he did, it does not surface in those student notes that have been most closely studied. On the contrary: William Tully, a student at Dartmouth Medical School in 1808–1809, included a comment in his diary that may be telling, as he summed up "the Doctor's farewell instructions" at the end of the winter course. "First he mentioned the importance of anatomy and physiology," Tully wrote on "Thursday 29th [December]." "He then spoke of the advantages that he had this winter given his class for attaining these branches, and remarked they were *greater than he had in Edinburgh*" (emphasis added).[32] Of course, those valedictory remarks of Smith's to Tully and his cohort of students came more than a decade after Smith had been in Edinburgh, so his memory of what he thought at the time may have faded. On the other hand, we have two further indications that Smith was underwhelmed by the great medical centers he visited in Great Britain. In one of the few letters home that we know about, he wrote to his wife, "I am now in Edinburgh, shall stay here but a few days, shall then go to London." He had already acknowledged, earlier in the letter, that he was "quite homesick," which no doubt affected his mood of the moment; in fact, he stayed well more than "a few days." Still, it appears that his first impressions in Edinburgh inspired no great enthusiasm. He went on: "I have had no material misfortune since I came here; have become acquainted with the Medical Professors here, and am attending their lectures. I have a prospect of accomplishing my purpose."[33] How one wishes he had been more explicit about what that "purpose" was! And how one wishes he had thought Sally might be interested in the content of those lectures. But, alas, he wrote no more letters that have been found.

A letter Smith wrote to John Warren shortly before returning home offers clear evidence that he was unimpressed by most of what he had been exposed to: "I have attended the Medical Lectures and surgical operations in Glasgow, Edinburgh and London and am much disappointed to find that the faculty in this country who have been so much looked up to by our country had so little real merit."[34] That judgment is rather surprising, given the reputation of these medical Meccas. The influence of Edinburgh on the medical school in Philadelphia has been well documented, and it has been said that "much of colonial American medicine" was "in large measure a creature of Edinburgh."[35] Smith's reaction to his time in Edinburgh goes some way toward belying the point, at least as far as the medical school in Hanover was concerned; it also hints again at his confidence in his own knowledge and experience.

Perhaps the chief benefit of the trip was that Nathan Smith became a member of the Medical Society of London, an honor that he referred to so often that we have to infer it pleased him. His membership was thanks to the good services (and recommendation) of John Coakley Lettsom, a towering figure in London's medical world. Smith later contributed two short pieces to the journal published by that society, one of which was his first publication subsequent to the appearance in print of his medical school dissertation.[36] On a professional level, though, the importance of this affiliation is extremely difficult to measure; simply having been able to say that he too had studied in Edinburgh and London may have been a benefit. Certainly not every country doctor (or even every medical professor) in the United States of that day could say as much.

Getting Down to Work

In his original proposal to the Board of Trustees, as we saw, Smith had indicated his readiness to "commence public teaching as soon as may be after my return." He was as good as his word. Arriving home on September 11, 1797, he apparently made the trip between Cornish and Hanover with some frequency almost as soon as he had returned to New Hampshire. What Sally made of this, we do not know. She could hardly have been thrilled; their second son was born while Smith was away, and it is plausible that she would have anticipated some undisturbed family time once he was back. But with help from Rufus Graves, a Hanover merchant, Smith found a place to stay as well as a room in which to hold lectures. And on November 22, 1797, barely two months after he had sailed back into Boston Harbor, Nathan Smith gave his first medical lecture at Dartmouth. He still did not have authorization from the Board of Trustees. Despite having voted to defer further consideration until the August 1797 meeting, the trustees did not take it up then. Smith, after all, was still on the high seas, and the trustees no doubt thought it premature to vote on the merits of letting the young doctor from Cornish begin a medical school until they had evidence that he was still interested in doing so.

Given what we have already seen of Smith's tendency to act precipitately, we should not be surprised that he did not wait another eleven months for the trustees to take formal action. Thus did Dartmouth Medical School come into being—quite unobtrusively, with no fanfare and no formal declaration of its existence. It does not seem to have mattered. At the annual meeting of the trustees in August 1798, everything fell neatly into place—ex post facto. The Board of Trustees took several significant actions in connection with the medical school at that somewhat belated juncture: A committee was appointed to "arrange and report a system to carry into effect a medical establishment at this University"; upon report of the committee, the trustees voted a few days later to "proceed to the choice of a professor of Medicine at this University." Smith was unanimously chosen, the way having been paved by the trustees voting to award him a Master of Arts degree (holding which seems to have been a necessary qualification for being a member of the faculty).[37] All this made eminently good sense, given what Smith had achieved since first approaching the Board of Trustees in 1796. What happened just prior to that vote was less of a foregone conclusion. On the same day, the trustees also voted to award the degree of Bachelor of Medicine (M.B.) to two of the students who had attended the lectures in the autumn of 1797, Joseph ("Jo") Gallup and Levi Sabin, class of 1798. This action in effect ratified the fact that a medical school had existed at Dartmouth College since 1797. Then, in yet another after-the-fact validation of what Smith had done, the Trustees also voted "that the professor of Medicine be authorized to employ such persons to assist him in the duties of his office as he may judge necessary" (provided, of course, that "this board incur no expense in consequence therefore"!) and voted while they were at it to award an M.B. degree to Lyman Spalding—by that time a Harvard medical graduate—who had already been assisting Smith. Unlike the degrees voted to Gallup and Sabin, this was clearly meant as an honorary degree, for Spalding's Harvard M.B. was duly noted.[38]

A "workable system" for establishing a medical school was duly created; it took the form of a set of rules and regulations that once again reflected the Harvard model. Smith was to give "public lectures" on the "three branches" of medicine: Theory and Practice of Physic, Chemistry and Materia Medica, and Anatomy and Surgery. The Board's stipulations were set out in detail:

1.— Lectures shall begin on the first day of October annually and continue ten weeks, during which time the professor shall deliver lectures on the three branches each day Saturdays and Sundays excepted as shall be agreed by him and the president and other executive officers.

2.— In the lectures on the Theory and Practice of Physic shall be explained the nature of diseases and method of cure.

3.— The lectures on Chemistry and Materia Medica shall be accompanied with actual experiments tending to explain & demonstrate the principles of chemistry and an exhibition of the principal Medicines used in curing diseases and also an explanation of their Medicinal qualities & effects on the human body.

4.— In the lectures on Anatomy and Surgery shall be demonstrated the parts of the human body by dissecting a recent subject if such subject can be legally obtained, otherwise by exhibiting anatomical preparations and which shall be attended by the performance of the principal capital operations in Surgery.

5.— The Medical professor or professors shall be entitled to the use of the library and apparatus equally as the other professors and to all honorary privileges attached to a Collegiate profession.

6.— Medical students under the private instruction of a Medical professor and all students while attending lectures shall be entitled to the use of books from the College library under such regulations as the President shall direct they having given sufficient bonds to the Treasures for the payment of all fees fines & forfeitures.

7.— Medical Students shall be subject to the same rules of Morality and decorum as Bachelors in Arts residing at College.

8.— No graduate at any College shall be admitted to an examination for the degree of Bachelor in Medicine unless he shall have studied Medicine with some respectable practising physician or Surgeon two full years and attended two complete courses of public Medical lectures at some University.

9.— No person not having received the degree of Bachelor of Arts at some University shall be admitted to an examination for the degree of Bachelor of Medicine unless he shall have studied Medicine three full years with some respectable practising physician or surgeon, attended two complete courses of public Medical lectures at some University and shall appear upon a preparatory examination before the President & Professors to be able to parse the English and Latin languages to construe Virgil and Tully's orations, to possess a good knowledge of common arithmetic, Geometry, Geography, and Natural and Moral Philosophy.

10.— All examinations for a degree in Medicine shall be holden publicly before the executive authority of College by the Medical professor or professors, at which time each candidate shall read and defend a dissertation on some medical subject which shall have been previously submitted to the inspection & approbation of the Medical professor or professors & President.

11.— Every person receiving a degree in Medicine shall cause his dissertation to be printed and sixteen copies thereof to be delivered to the President for the use of the College and Trustees.

12.— The fee for attending a complete course of Medical lectures to any person not a member of some class in College shall be fifty dollars, this is, for Anatomy and Surgery twenty-three dollars, for Chemistry and Materia Medica seventeen dollars, and for the theory and practice of physic ten dollars.

13.— The fee to be paid by the members of the two Senior classes in College who shall attend those lectures shall be twenty dollars for a complete course, that is, for Anatomy & Surgery eight dollars, for Chemistry and Materia Medica seven dollars and for the Theory and practice of physic five dollars.

14.— Any person having attended two complete courses of public Medical lectures in any University shall be admitted *gratis* to any lectures.[39]

The fact that these rules and regulations were not wholly original is of little importance. Why should Smith not have taken advantage of whatever curricular experience he had gained? What mattered was that the Board decided to go ahead with the project at all. Here was the chance Nathan Smith wanted: to offer formal medical education to the boys of northern New England in a way that would make them college men, members of an educated elite. The aim was to raise medicine from the "low state" to which he and his mentor Josiah Goodhue believed it had fallen.[40]

And so it came to pass. Dartmouth Medical School was officially established, and the College had its very own professor of medicine. Formerly merely a small-town doctor, Professor Nathan Smith, M.B., A.M., Corresponding Member of the Medical Society of London, was officially ready to continue what he had begun in November 1797.[41]

CHAPTER TWO

Pressing Forward

Here, then, was a man who for Dartmouth men in particular may well serve as their ideal of a doctor. . . . possessed of originality of thought, of energy, of resourcefulness, . . . an accurate and keen observer . . . ; he had the sound judgment of a great teacher. —HARVEY CUSHING[1]

Nathan Smith—Physician and Educator

WHAT SORT OF a man was this medical pioneer, Nathan Smith? Answering this question provides insight into the kind of place Dartmouth Medical School was in its early days. Expressions of doubt about Smith's extraordinary capabilities are in very short supply. Instead, one story after another appears in letters from Smith's students, sent home or to friends, all testifying to his stellar qualities. In a fragment of an undated letter, Samuel Elder—a student of Smith's in the autumn of 1811—told his unknown addressee that he "went to Dartmouth College and there pursued the study of medicine under Dr Smith in whose praise as a man of genius and science too much cannot be said."[2] A. T. Lowe, who received his Dartmouth medical degree in 1816, reflected many years later on what it was like to be one of Nathan Smith's students. He wrote, in part: "The very high reputation universally accorded to Dr. Smith at that period, not only in New Hampshire but throughout New England—perhaps a reputation never before so generally awarded to any member of the profession in this part of our Country—had inspired me with a respect;—almost with awe—for one so distinguished."[3] Yet observations of this sort are too general to tell us much and must be treated with caution precisely because the praise is so lavish. More helpful are stories like the one that A. B. Crosby recounted for his colleagues in the New Hampshire Medical Society in an address he gave in 1870, particularly when coupled with commentary like Crosby's own in this instance. "I have recently learned an incident that still further illustrates Dr. Smith's sagacity," he began, and went on at some length to tell how Smith had responded to the account of a sailor whose dislocated hip was cured in a most extraordinary way:

On one occasion [a friend who was a sea captain] told Dr. Smith that on his previous voyage one of the sailors dislocated his hip. There being no surgeon on board, the captain tried but in vain to reduce [reset] it. The man was accordingly placed in a hammock with the dislocation unreduced. During a great storm the sufferer was thrown from the hammock to the floor, striking violently on the knee of the affected side. On examination, it was found that in the fall the hip had some how been set. This interested Dr. Smith wonderfully, and he questioned the narrator again and again as to the exact position of the thing, the knee and the leg, at the time of the fall.

From this apparently insignificant circumstance, Dr. Smith eventually educed and reduced to successful practice the method of reducing dislocations by the manœuvre, a system as useful as it is simple, and as scientific as the principle of flexion and leverage on which it depends. *Had this incident been related to a stupid man, he would have seen nothing in it, or to a sceptic, and he would have discredited the whole account, but to a man of genius it furnished a clue by which another of Nature's labyrinths was traced out* [emphasis added]. This system is by far the best ever devised, simplifying and rendering easy the work of the surgeon, while reducing human suffering to its minimum.[4]

On the basis of many stories like this, latter-day disciples and enthusiasts still speak with admiration for Smith. A former DMS dean, inspired to reflect approvingly on Smith as the 200th anniversary of the institution's founding approached, had this to say: "Nathan Smith must have been a most formidable and capable man—intelligent, venturesome, committed, but restless. How else could one account for his peripatetic manner and success?"[5] Another such admirer has said that Nathan Smith, in his own way, definitely took a scientific approach to clinical work; he early developed the capacity to recognize what was unknown, to appreciate what was not working, and to question dogma.[6]

A good example of just this feature of the way Nathan Smith worked can be found in his "Dissertation on scirrhous and Cancerous affections," unfortunately neither polished nor published.[7] Nonetheless, there is much of value in it, showing as it does not only those Smith character traits so often cited, but also his effort systematically to analyze the cases he encountered. He began by expressing dissatisfaction with the then-current definitions of "scirrhous and cancerous affections":

The usual description of cancer as given by authors who have written on the subject as it relates to outward appearances is correct in a majority of cases but there is considerable variety in the symptoms of that malady especially in its early stages, so much so that even those who have seen considerable practice are not always able to determine the true nature of the disease on its first appearance, but such definitions give no clue to the pathology of the complaint.

After proffering a definition of his own (rather convoluted and not of particular interest here), Smith explained how he intended to proceed in his paper—giving as he did so a perfect example of inductive reasoning: "Before I attempt a pathological theory of cancer I shall give the history of several cases which have fallen under my care and observation, and from facts noted in those cases shall endeavor to draw certain conclusions relative to the nature of the disease and the proper method of opposing it."

Neither the details of the case histories Smith spelled out nor his conclusions matter so much as the care he evinced in the task he had undertaken. After giving the history of the first case, for instance, he concluded as follows:

In performing the operation I cut round the sore in the edge of the sound scalp and dissected it off down to the pericranium which appeared healthy, but did not at that time remove the enlarged gland. The wound appeared well for several days but then it began to put on a cancerous appearance round its edges. I again removed the diseased parts by cutting the scalp at a greater distance from the sore and dissecting it off with the pericranium down to the skull. At the same time I removed the tumor on her neck but all to no good purpose. Both wounds soon became truly cancerous and she died of the disease in June following the first operation.

Medical historians as well as admiring Dartmouth doctors have also heaped praise on Smith. Smith had, we are told, an "active and constructive mind"; he was "New England's grand old man of medicine," and the "dean of medical professors in New England."[8] He was "undoubtedly the region's most influential medical man outside Boston,"[9] and he has been referred to as "the formidable Harvard graduate" (this latter is somewhat misleading, given the brief period Smith spent at Harvard).[10]

In addition to being peripatetic—another reason for calling him "New England's grand old man of medicine"—Smith was also willing to give advice and even prescribe through the mails. He also kept in touch with former students, answering questions and sharing his own experiences. In one such letter to Lyman Spalding, for instance, Smith was responding to an enquiry about goiter. He stated with confidence that it is rare except in the inland parts of the country, and that it is more common in the children of parents who have moved inland from the seacoast than in the children of parents born and raised in the interior; his effort to connect parentage with what we now know is basically an uninherited deficiency problem was not a very accurate piece of epidemiology, though it does present him as an astute observer of his patients. (He also told Spalding he thought goiter was becoming less common, as may well have been the case.[11])

In an undated letter from Smith to a John Powers (probably the Dr. John D. Powers who was a contemporary of Smith's and practiced in Woodstock, Vermont), Smith went into considerable detail about how one of Powers's patients should be treated. The letter is a striking example of the care Smith took in responding to a colleague's request for advice. He could count on Powers (like most physicians of the day) to prepare his own drugs and roll his own pills.

Dear Sir
Respecting Mrs. Thomas's case I would advise to give her the Tincture of Blood Root and Laudanum. Make a strong Tincture of the Blood Root & give 40 drops with 15 drops of common Laudanum morning—Also
Make a decoction of the Root of common milk weed called silkgrass—& let her take from half a gill to a gill four or five times each day if that quantity should offend her stomach or should prove cathartic you may diminish the dose & if it should have no sensible effect increase the dose— —
If the above remedies should prove ineffectual you may try the following, that is

R_x Squills ½ drachm[12]
Digitalis 1 scruple
Opium 1 scruple
Tartar Emetic ½ grain
Simple Syrup QS [Quantum sufficiat]
Mix & make 20 pills
Dose one pill night & morning

While taking the above pill let her
Take the following, that is,
R_x Island Marse 1 oz.
Liquorice Stick ½ oz.
Put into a pint & half of cold water and simmer over a gentle fire to a pint
Take this in divided doses in the course of 24 hours & continue to take in this quantity daily
N.B. I am inclined to think that it would be well to take a small bleeding from the arm say about eight ounces, & if the effect should be to diminish the cough & hoarseness I would repeat it again in about a week & continue to repeat it according to the effect—
I would bleed the first time before you begin the medics I have ordered
I am with sentiments of esteem your Obedient Servant

Nathan Smith[13]

Smith was clever, inventive, thoughtful, reflective, and resourceful as well as willing to share what he knew. No wonder he was called a "man

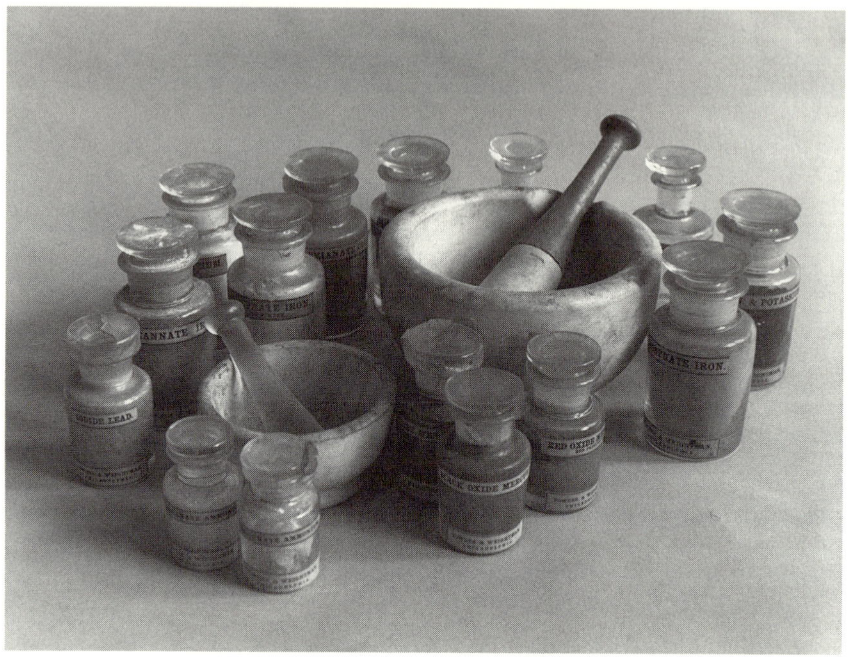

Jars of medicinal chemicals and mortar and pestle. Stoughton Museum, Dartmouth College. Courtesy of Joseph Mehling, Dartmouth College.

of genius" and enjoyed "a very high reputation." Yet despite the tales of his having managed to teach the medical school curriculum single-handedly for more than a decade—tales that have taken on a near-mythological status (see, for example, the discussion of his having held not a "chair" but a whole "settee" of professorships, in chapter 3)—Nathan Smith apparently did not really want to manage on his own. When the trustees voted to add a professor of medicine to the faculty, it will be recalled, they also voted "that the professor of Medicine be authorized to employ such persons to assist him in the duties of his office as he may judge necessary." Since even with the addition of Smith the entire Dartmouth faculty would still comprise only five men, it is highly unlikely that this vote was the result of calculations by the trustees that it would be a good idea to have more than one person engaged in teaching the medical curriculum.

Teaching Chemistry

We can with some confidence suppose that the trustees were aware—even without Smith drawing their attention to it—that he had already, in the first year of not-yet-actually-approved lectures, asked for and received assistance from Lyman Spalding. Smith's asking Spalding to assist him that first autumn is remarkable, considering that the younger man was only twenty-two. Lyman must have proved himself an apt and congenial preceptee; Smith otherwise presumably would not have created this additional opportunity for close collaboration. Indeed, Smith's confidence in Spalding was considerable. The young man—when only twenty-one—had served as Smith's *locum tenens* while the latter was in Europe.[14]

Even more to the point was Spalding's preparatory education, considerably more substantial than Smith's. As a friend of the family, Smith would have been well aware of this. Lyman was a graduate of Charlestown Academy (in New Hampshire), where he had studied Latin; at Harvard, he had been tutored in French. That in turn meant he could read the work of French chemists like Antoine Lavoisier (1743–1794) and Claude Berthollet (1748–1822), who were just then bursting onto the intellectual landscape and slowly changing chemistry into a less-primitive science than it had been. While at Dartmouth, Spalding prepared a kind of student handbook for chemistry terms based on the work of the French scientists, which he distributed in later years to colleagues much as scholars today hand out reprints of their articles.[15] The chemistry mentor at Harvard for both Smith and Spalding had been Aaron Dexter, a key figure in the teaching of chemistry in America; he had early introduced "French chemistry" to the New World. Spalding's little book was, in turn, fundamental to the dissemination of the new chemistry throughout the country.[16]

In Smith's hands, the chemistry being taught was—and would remain—elementary in the extreme, despite his exposure in Edinburgh to Joseph Black and perhaps also Thomas Charles Hope (who became conjoint professor with Black, probably about the time Smith was in Scotland).[17] William Tully, while a student at Dartmouth, in a moment of uncharacteristically generous praise once went so far as to say of Smith's "Introduction to Chemistry" lecture in 1808 that "What he laid down was done with great precision, and his divisions were lucid and satisfactory."[18] On the other hand, another student two years later left a record that exposes just how modest Smith's grasp of chemistry was. Andrew Mack dutifully wrote down Smith's two-dozen-word definition of chemistry from the opening lecture of that course in the autumn of 1810: "Chemistry," Smith pronounced, "is that science which treats of the action of one body upon another," action that was "explained in relation to mechanical action or power."[19]

Such an exquisitely unsophisticated understanding of chemistry did not separate Smith from most others of his era, however. Certainly when he hired the Hanover merchant Rufus Graves to assist him in chemistry (after apparently struggling along on his own for several terms when he could no longer persuade Lyman Spalding to stay, or even come to Hanover for a brief stint, to help), the instruction in this basic science can hardly be said to have improved. It is quite unclear what made Smith think Graves was qualified for the task, notwithstanding a latter-day claim that the faculty was "strengthened by the appointment of Rufus Graves," as if making chemistry "for the first time, a separate branch" was by itself a measurement of "improvement."[20] Successful entrepreneur and businessman though he may have been, Rufus Graves was no Lyman Spalding; Smith may simply have been desperate to share what was for him a difficult task. Looking back years later, another student—Isaac Patterson—said of Graves's efforts that he "gave a few lectures on this subject, but not having any apparatus for experiments, it did not amount to much."[21] Lack of equipment was a constant problem for early chemistry teachers in the New World, not least because there were too few glassmakers, which meant that retorts and other laboratory glassware had to be imported or done without. On the other hand, the student Ezekiel Dodge Cushing wrote home in 1809 complaining about having been up "performing chemical experiments till 3 o'clock in the morning two thirds of the time since the lectures have begun." *Some* equipment must have been available.[22]

The significance of all this for the history of the medical school lies not in the quality of the teaching of chemistry, whether it was done by Smith or by one of those he hired to do the job. Chemistry was a science in its infancy, and few if any had the remotest inkling of how critical an understanding of chemistry would later become for the study of medicine. Rather, what is striking here is that Nathan Smith—despite being clearly uneasy about his own abilities in chemistry—from the outset wanted to make sure it was part of the curriculum. Whether he was initially simply aping Harvard, where he had, after all, had the opportunity to study some chemistry under the eccentric Aaron Dexter, or whether here as in so many other areas he had an instinctive sense of what mattered and what would turn out to be important, we cannot know. But when the trustees requested that their professor of medicine teach the science course in the College as well, he did not refuse. They offered no remuneration for this work, any more than they did for his medical lectures, but in this regard, the trustees were simply following the usual practices of the day. The standard procedure in medical schools well into the nineteenth century was for students to pay lecture fees directly to the professors (admission tickets were issued to each student upon payment of the fee)—which then, collectively, generally constituted the entire compensation for the professors in question. A bit extra might come from actual graduation fees, though at Dartmouth the Board had been careful to specify that these fees were to be shared: "one half part of the fees for confering [*sic*] the degree of Bachelor of Medicine *pro meritis* be a perquisite to the President and the other half be a perquisite to the Professor of Medicine."[23] So the College was to benefit financially—without having to incur any direct costs—as a result of having added a member to the faculty.

We know something about the extent of the assistance Spalding rendered thanks to a letter he wrote to a friend: "I have resided at Dartmouth College for a few weeks. . . . While at Hanover, I prepared all the Chemical Suspensions . . . for Dr Smiths Lectures in the fall of 97. . . . The fall course I had the soul [*sic*] management of as well as profit—I expect to continue in this branch."[24] If this was literally true, it means Smith himself managed to avoid teaching chemistry as long as Spalding was around; it is difficult to imagine that he would otherwise have waived his right to the fees (the "profit") from that course. Yet when he had no one else to help, he taught chemistry himself.

There are other reasons for spelling out the story of these early efforts to include chemistry in the curriculum. First, though the arrangements seem to have been handled quite informally, Smith's (or Spalding's) teaching of chemistry in the College meant a precedent of sorts was being established from the outset for making dual appointments between the College and the Medical School.[25] Second, it could be argued that with the inclusion of this collegiate science course, the medical school curriculum embraced both clinical and basic science work from the start, at least in principle.

Student Attitudes

Clinical courses were at the heart of what Smith taught at Dartmouth, and they were no doubt what he did best. We have records of these courses in two forms. A handful of surviving letters from students, usually to their parents, includes tales of going on house calls with Smith—a physically rigorous opportunity for "making rounds" that was available often even before the lecture term began. William Tully, though he did not participate, recorded one such example. Smith was to operate on an aneurysm, but the patient was sixteen or more miles away, and Tully disdainfully observed that it wasn't worth the effort: "Many of the medical students, in this instance, were unwise enough to be at much pains and expence to hire horses and to post off, break-fastless, to the patient's house, not to return, probably, till midnight, a dollar or two expended, a day's study lost, them selves fatigued, and six-cents worth gained." *He* was occupied with his books, he insisted, and did not expect to gain anything while at Hanover "from seeing practice." Such benefits as would accrue to him would be "derived solely from the Anatomical Museum, the lectures, and the library."[26]

Others were considerably more enthusiastic.[27] Furthermore, such outings would come as no surprise to students who had already spent time as apprentices (as most would have), for "riding with the doctor" was a standard part of that form of training. En route to the patient's house, we learn both from these student letters and from some of Smith's own letters, the students would have a chance to listen to Smith lecture, or at least talk about the case they were going to see or similar cases he had previously encountered.

Beyond such letters, numerous student notebooks have survived, some of which contain remarkably full records of what Smith (and other faculty members, later) said in their lectures. These notebooks are by no means unique to Smith's students or to students of medicine. First the lack and then the expense of textbooks meant that most students had none; the result was that lecturers spoke slowly enough to allow those listening to make thorough notes if they were so inclined. Some actually seem to have written the lectures down verbatim (others, admittedly, took very sketchy notes indeed). As has been pointed out, since "the ancillary requirements for the medical degree, such as a knowledge of Latin, Natural Philosophy and so forth, were tested at graduation time, if at all, rather than as a condition of admission to the course . . . [there is] great variance in literary standard among the extant notebooks of the period."[28] The more diligent students transcribed their notes in the evenings. Some borrowed notes from fellow students to copy. Others, like Calvin Gorham, wrote notes that show quite a low literary standard and surely were not copied at all.[29] Still other notes are so handsomely written that we have to conclude they must have been copied later; they are very complete, neat, and expensively bound in leather. Those who did copy their own or someone else's notes must have devoted an exorbitant amount of time to the process—though remembering that there were few texts to be studied, we can appreciate why the time might have been thought to be well spent.

Perhaps the most striking feature of Smith's lectures, as evidenced in student notebooks, is the way he shaped and changed his lectures depending on the cases he was treating at the time. He used actual cases as illustrations in his lectures, frequently commenting about the status of patients under his care. According to one student, "he usually commenced [his lectures] with some anecdote that happened in his practice and proceeded in a conversational style—his talk was full of practical instruction."[30] As a result, the lectures were often quite lively; students must have gained from them, almost as much as they did from riding out with Smith, a sense of direct involvement in the world of medicine.[31]

Another extremely important characteristic of Smith's lectures was his repeated emphasis on using observation to determine results of remedies. To claim that Smith's approach was an early example of what is now called "outcomes research" would be going too far, but his characteristic crisp dismissal of the work of physicians who relied on "theory" instead of close observation of how patients actually fared is found in many of the lecture notes. A splendid example appears in an anonymous set of notes from 1811–1812. Following what he wrote down on November 2, 1811, on the "Lecture introductory to the Theory and Practice of Physic by Nathan Smith," the unknown student recorded in careful detail the following opening paragraph of "Lecture No. II. Nov. 4th, 1811. P. Smith":

> The Nosologies of Medical Writers have been numerous, but most of them vague and established on principles which have no foundation in nature. Hippocrates indeed wrote usefully while describing diseases, and the various effects which remedies have on the system. The Galenic system . . . was inadequate and unsupported by facts. Boerhaave's explanation of this Doctrine on mechanical Principals [*sic*] was Still farther from the truth, and wholly unfounded in nature. Dr Cullen's spasmodic Theory and his arrangement is no more than a list of Diseases, his numerous divisions are unwarrantable in any known operations of the living principle. . . . I shall attempt in the course of our investigations to make such practical divisions of the diseases which affect the differ[ent] general systems of the living principle as shall according to my observation, lead to a successful application of remedies.[32]

This passage is doubly significant. In addition to demonstrating Smith's inclination to rely always on commonsense observation and "nature" rather than on abstruse theory (though he was not alone in this, his view was unusual), it clearly illustrates his boldness and self-confidence. By this time Smith had been teaching for more than a decade, so he certainly should have been familiar with the work of his forebears; his willingness to criticize them, however, is noteworthy. Smith's approach gave medical education at Dartmouth a rather different emphasis from what it had in the hands of many other teachers of medicine at the time. It was both more practical and more closely focused on clinical realities.

Anatomy in the Curriculum

Lyman Spalding was not the only former student Nathan Smith called upon to assist him. Leaving aside the estimable Rufus Graves, a student of Smith's if at all only by virtue of being in the chemistry course taught largely by Spalding, the other prime example was Cyrus Perkins. But by far the most dramatic appointment Nathan Smith made was Alexander Ramsay—in 1808—to teach anatomy. The flamboyant Scotsman, considered by many the outstanding anatomist of the day, created a considerable stir in Hanover, quite out of proportion to the brief time he spent there.[33] Yet the fact that he was sought out and persuaded to come at all is another indication of the seriousness of Nathan Smith's intentions and his dreams for Dartmouth Medical School.

Unlike chemistry, anatomy was understood by everyone to be central to the medical curriculum; it was also one of the branches of medicine in which Smith was most skilled. This makes all the more striking his wanting to bring to Dartmouth someone who could be expected to upstage him on the very platform where he played so brilliantly. We learn both that Smith was undaunted by the social and personnel challenges presented by the irascible and egocentric Ramsay, and that Smith's own ego was unlikely to hamper opportunities to advance the program he envisioned for the school. The clearest statement of Smith's view is in a letter he wrote to Lyman Spalding: "Dr Ramsay is in my opinion the best anatomist in the United States. I have seen his anatomical preparations & have heard him lecture." The praise seems genuine.

Another reason Smith may have been eager to bring Ramsay on board was that he was, himself, so busy. In an earlier letter to Spalding, he had asked his young protégé—by that time with a practice of his own, in Portsmouth, New Hampshire—to place an ad in the Portsmouth paper announcing Ramsay's course on "Anatomy & Physiology." The ad copy, which Smith provided to Spalding, included the information that Smith himself would be teaching a chemistry course ("as usual") prior to Ramsay's course, then "a compleat course of practical surgery, founded on the principles of Anatomy & Physiology" (this was obviously to follow Ramsay's course), and finally "Lectures on the practice of Physic."[34] By having Ramsay teach anatomy and physiology, Smith not only got a break but was free to sit in on those lectures and demonstrations himself, if he wished. Indeed, he also made clear to Spalding in the later letter that he was counting on acquiring more "preparations" (done by Ramsay) for his own "Anatomical Museum" of specimens as a side benefit of the visitor's work. However much he already knew and had taught, Smith wanted the best for his students—and was not too proud to step aside when he found someone he thought could do an even better job than he.

When Ramsay left after a single term, Smith's motivation for asking the trustees to establish a separate chair in anatomy and then hiring his former student Cyrus Perkins for the position presumably had more to do with how overworked Smith was than with any expectation that Perkins could improve on Ramsay. For all his competency, no one has ever suggested that Perkins was in Ramsay's class as an anatomist. But Smith must have known exactly what he was getting in this colleague. Perkins's entire medical education had been under Smith's direction, after all, and Smith probably knew many details of the eight years of experience in private practice that Perkins had to his credit by the time he was appointed to the Dartmouth faculty.[35] Furthermore, it is clear the heavy workload was finally beginning to trouble Smith. His appeal to the trustees was quite explicit on the matter, and their records quote him as follows:

> Your memorialist presents that finding the Labors required of him as a teacher of medical science too great and more than he can perform with convenience to himself and advantage to the public, he prays that some other person may be associated with him in that department and that such associate be appointed Professor of Anatomy, and that he himself be excused from teaching in that branch.[36]

No doubt Perkins offered some genuine relief, and he and Smith seem to have gotten along reasonably well (they even formed a practice partnership together that lasted until Smith left for Yale).[37] And as we will see in chapter 3, Perkins's appointment as the first additional member of the medical school faculty officially recognized by the trustees (as opposed to the interim hires made by Smith on his own) marked an important step forward for the still-young school.

End of an Era

The Smith era effectively ended when Nathan Smith tendered his resignation in 1813 to accept a call to Yale. (Reuben Dimond Mussey, the first truly important figure on the faculty after Smith, began his long career at Dartmouth the following year.) With Smith gone, Nathan Noyes—another of the earliest Dartmouth Medical School graduates, one of three who earned an M.B. degree in 1799—helped Perkins by serving as a lecturer in the theory and practice of medicine for a year.[38] Earlier, on at least one occasion, Noyes had also come to Smith's rescue by lecturing on chemistry while Smith was out of town; Tully said he "had been for some years a Tutor of the College and Assistant Lecturer to Smith." As for the help Noyes rendered in chemistry, Tully said nothing of the content of the lectures, but focused instead on the fact that Noyes, "having had an earlier education" than Smith, had "more and better words at command than the good doctor; and from not being called to converse so much with the ignorant people of country places, his style was much less colloquial."[39]

But Perkins, having preceded Mussey on the faculty, was the senior member of the team once Smith left. Whatever his merits as a teacher—one student found some aspects of his lectures "tedious," but also said he had "never seen surgical instruments handled with more skill and adroitness"[40]—today Perkins is more especially remembered for having been on the losing side, a disaffected faculty member, in what has come to be called the "Dartmouth College case."[41] The fight over whether the College charter could be altered unilaterally by the state legislature in a manner that would turn the College into a public university was a matter of considerable political importance. Furthermore, the lasting significance of the case (argued before the Supreme Court, famously, by Daniel Webster on March 10, 1815) goes far beyond the confines of Dartmouth and Hanover to the issue of how sacrosanct the founding principles of eleemosynary institutions are. It did not directly concern Nathan Smith's enterprise, which was still seen as a "department" within the College rather than as a separate "school." Only if it were the latter could it have been plausibly argued that the College really was a "university" already.[42] Even so, not least because of Perkins himself, the fight did have a dramatic effect on the medical school.

The complexities of the case, both in its institutional politics and its larger legal ramifications, are beyond the scope of this study.[43] What really mattered was that John Wheelock and his partisans on the Board of Trustees seemed eager to let the state legislature have a role in altering the original design of the institution. For a short time, despite the institution's small size, it split into two. Both "College" and "University" held classes; students answered to the same class-ending bells, and passed each other on The Green, and they even held separate commencements.[44] Though the medical school itself avoided division, there was considerable tension in the air. Perkins was deeply committed to the University; Reuben Mussey was equally devoted to the College. How fully Wheelock appreciated the differences between the two men is not clear. In laying out his side of his fight with the trustees, he wrote that Perkins was a man with "correct and enlightened views," and went on to observe—somewhat lamely—that "Professor Mussey has lately been associated with him, as successor of Doct. Smith." He ended that particular passage by insisting that if the medical school was to survive, it would have to "sever the chain, that holds it to the College, or produce a reform in the Board, which manages its concerns."[45] Mussey's behavior shows that he thought otherwise.

The uncertainties over the institution's status almost certainly played a role in Smith's decision, once he had joined the Yale faculty, not to return to Dartmouth again after he had come up from New Haven to teach one course of lectures in 1816. His position was awkward. Personally sympathetic to Wheelock, he was also indebted to the *College* Board of Trustees—which had appointed him but had ousted Wheelock.[46] And then there were two boards—one for the College, one for the University—and two presidents: William Allen was named president of Dartmouth University (after John Wheelock's death, who had briefly been reinstated as president by "his"—University—Board), and Francis Brown became president of Dartmouth College. Confusion reigned. For Smith, who knew all parties but had already left Dartmouth once, choosing sides between these presidents or between Perkins and Mussey—both former students of his—cannot have been a comfortable prospect. President Brown made it clear he would have liked Smith to continue teaching for the College.[47] Yet the legislature was in the process of trying to strike down the authority of the College trustees, and until the matter was settled, it could have been argued that it was technically illegal to teach for the College. Cyrus Perkins was willing to wear his heart on his sleeve and to declare unequivocally for the University side; Smith was more cautious, apparently supporting the College but somewhat disingenuously implying he could not afford the risk of doing so publicly. And so he resigned, writing to Brown, "I beg leave through you to request the Honorable Board of Trust for Dartmouth College to consider my office as vacant."[48] He may have simply decided Yale offered a better opportunity. That the situation at Dartmouth nonetheless concerned him is clear from a letter he had written to Mills Olcott the week before he resigned:

> Since I left Hanover the affairs of Dartmouth College & University as well as the church difficulties have pressed considerably on my mind as I feared that there might be some thundering about the place of holding their respective com-

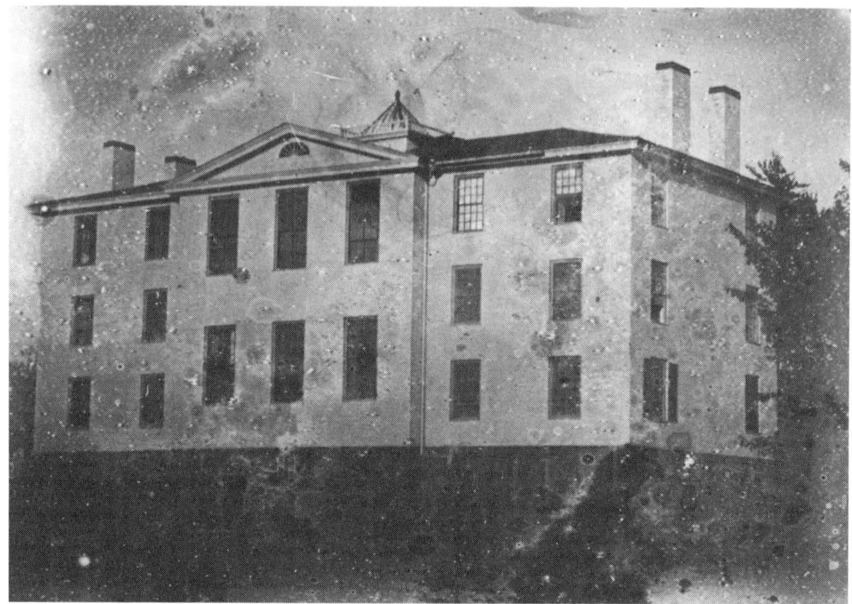

Nathan Smith's Medical House, built in 1811, the first purpose-built medical building in the nation and probably the oldest photo of the building. Photo made from a daguerrotype at Dartmouth dating probably from the 1850s. Courtesy of Dartmouth College Library.

mencements, at length a lucky thought came into my mind which I hope might obviate all difficulty on that head. The thought is that as the colleges of late have but one exercise each there will be ample time in the campus of one day for both parties to show their prettiest on the stage if the time is equally divided between them. Therefore let them agree to do so and let the two presidents toss up for the first going in . . . I think by a little alteration to the business you may bring the thing about in this way.[49]

Earlier yet he had expressed anxiety about whether the situation might get out of hand: "If there should be a prospect of a pitched battle between the College & the University I hope it will take place before my arrival as I have not forgotten the sage advice of Fallstaff [*sic*] that it is best to come in at the beginning of a feast & the latter end of a fray." How worried he really was can be questioned, given the lighthearted and somewhat sarcastic remark in the same letter that "Good Old Dartmouth has become very famous of late & excites more attention than any College or University in the country."[50]

Smith's Legacy

The most tangible feature of Smith's legacy at Dartmouth Medical School that remained after he left was his "New Medical House," completed in 1811, the first structure in the United States built expressly for and devoted solely to medical education.[51] The story of how this fine edifice came to be built is a complicated one that illustrates both Smith's determination and his lobbying skills—for he succeeded (against considerable odds) in persuading the New Hampshire state legislature to contribute funds for the building. The money Smith got from the State proved not to be enough—not surprising, since the legislature had not allotted the sum he had requested. Smith at one stage also insisted, wisely, on more expensive construction than was originally planned. He dug into his own pockets to cover the costs.[52] The building would prove its worth, staying in use as the centerpiece of Dartmouth Medical School until it was razed—amidst vigorous cries of protestation from many quarters—in 1963. At that point, it was the oldest structure in the United States that had been built explicitly for medical education and was still in regular use for its original purpose.[53]

The students and the impressive record of the way Dartmouth Medical School's influence spread is a less-tangible but even more-important aspect of Nathan Smith's legacy. One of the clearest manifestations is the number of his students who became medical educators themselves. A prime example is Jo Gallup, one of that first pair of young men to be granted a medical degree from Dartmouth. Smith would surely not have been sympathetic with some features of the way Gallup—who was something of a lightning rod for controversy[54]—practiced medicine.[55] But there is no doubt how the citizens of Woodstock, Vermont, felt about him. Gallup not only settled there to practice; he ran a cottage hospital and his own school of medicine. "The majority of the people of Woodstock favored Dr. Gallup who had been a resident of the town for thirty-four years. . . . Dr. Gallup had a high reputation as physician, author, and educator, that extended throughout the state."[56]

Another Dartmouth medical graduate who taught in Woodstock for a while was Gilman Kimball; he was "Lecturer in Surgery" there, "a position he held for several years. . . . He also taught at the Berkshire Medical Institution during the years he was teaching at Woodstock. He was a man well known in the profession, the author of several books on medicine and the editor of a medical journal." Kimball practiced for some years in Lowell, Massachusetts.[57] And among the founders (in 1818) of the medical college in Castleton, Vermont, was Theodore

Woodward, who also had been a student at Dartmouth Medical School.[58] Lyman Spalding, about whom we have already heard so much, was the first president of the College of Physicians and Surgeons of the Western District of New York in tiny Fairfield, New York (to give the full name to what was generally referred to simply as "Fairfield"), and several Dartmouth graduates taught there at one time or another.[59] More modestly, Moses Swett—a student of Smith's at Dartmouth in 1809—served as an anatomy demonstrator for Alexander Ramsay that year and later performed the same service for Smith himself at Bowdoin.[60]

Also among Smith's protégés were the two who faced off against each other in the University–College fight—Cyrus Perkins and Reuben Dimond Mussey. Once the legal case was settled and it was clear that the College had won, Perkins left for New York. By that time, Smith had acquiesced (for the nonce) in Yale's request that he teach exclusively at Yale. Thus Dartmouth Medical School was briefly left with no one but Mussey. It could have done much worse; Mussey not only stayed—in the process becoming an extremely important transitional figure between the Smith era and all that was to follow—but served the institution well for many years. With Smith and Perkins both gone, it was suddenly possible for the trustees to appoint a new generation of faculty to join the reliable Mussey. When they did so, as we shall see in the next chapter, the first overtones of a more systematized approach to course offerings and less parochial teaching appointments became audible in the distance.

PART II

NINETEENTH-CENTURY PROGRESS

CHAPTER THREE

Creating Shadows of Their Own

This is the hour after the hour of arrival. —JOYCE HORNER[1]

The Medical School Comes of Age

AND SO THE deed was done. Thanks to Daniel Webster, Dartmouth College was saved from becoming a university—in name if not in fact. To this day, the great orator's ringing peroration before the United States Supreme Court, "It is, sir, . . . a small college, and yet there are those that love it," remains the single most famous line ever uttered about the institution of which Dartmouth Medical School is a part.[2] Superficially, it might seem that adherents of the medical school should have supported the idea of a "Dartmouth University," for the existence of professional schools beyond the undergraduate level is generally precisely what turns a college into a university.[3] But Nathan Smith and Reuben Mussey had taken the part of the College, the College side had won, and Cyrus Perkins (supporter of the University cause) had left Hanover for New York. For better, for worse, Dartmouth remained a college, and Nathan Smith's medical school was about to enter a new phase of life.

The crisis in institutional organization and governance may have helped, in a perverse sort of way, for it was in the aftermath of the jibes exchanged between colleagues unsure which way to turn that Dartmouth Medical School began to mature into a forward-looking institution. With Perkins's departure, the school lost the person whose appointment in 1810 to head a separate department of anatomy and surgery was the first step in the move toward specialization that continues today. Once the air cleared, the medical faculty consisted only of Reuben Dimond Mussey and the chemistry lecturer James Freeman Dana. The trustees were in a position to rethink the medical education being offered in

Hanover. As the third decade of the century opened, with Nathan Smith fully engaged elsewhere, it was clear that the Smith era was truly over. Dartmouth was no longer on his agenda.

Mussey was the bridge between old and new. His ties to Smith—his erstwhile mentor, instructor, and then academic colleague—were never so strained as relations between Perkins and Smith became. Thus what was essentially a new generation was free to put its own stamp on Dartmouth Medical School without repudiating the past. The trustees took the dramatic step of formally identifying four separate and reasonably well-defined chairs for faculty in the "Medical Department." The trustees' minutes for the meeting of August 22, 1820, record the decision:

> Resolved that the Faculty of the Medical department consist of
> 1st The President of the College
> 2 A Prof. of Surgery, Obstetricks, and medical Jurisprudence
> 3 A Prof. of Theory & Practice of Physic, Materia Medica & Botany
> 4 A Prof. of Chemistry, Mineralogy & the application of Science to the Arts
> 5 A Prof. of Anatomy and Physiology.[4]

No longer would one or two men have to carry the entire load; the intention was clearly to cease relying solely on a single individual of outstanding capabilities. (Further evidence of the effort to improve the curriculum was the faculty vote that students would not be allowed to take a course of lectures from only one of the professors, unless they had already had two full courses of lectures at Dartmouth.[5]) Mussey had been hired in 1814 with almost as broad an agenda as Smith himself initially had. (His original appointment was as Professor of the Theory and Practice of Medicine, Materia Medica and Therapeutics, and Obstetrics.) He would now be able to choose which of the disciplines he wanted to teach from among the array of subjects to be included in the curriculum. He still took on a lot, replacing Theory and Practice with Surgery, keeping Obstetrics, and adding Medical Jurisprudence. But at least he had more colleagues.

Harvard-trained James Dana was promoted to Professor of Chemistry (responsible also for mineralogy and "the application of Science to the Arts"). Daniel Oliver—like Dana, a Harvard man, with the added benefit of a medical degree from Pennsylvania—was to teach Theory of Physic, and Materia Medica and Botany. Another important addition to the faculty was Usher Parsons, who had a Harvard M.D. Having served with considerable distinction as a surgeon in the War of 1812, he seems also to have taught some surgery along with Mussey, even though his official appointment was as Professor of Anatomy and Physiology.[6] Thus the division of labor appears to have been somewhat arbitrary. It was Oliver, not Parsons, who later published a physiology text. Further, Oliver had served as a lecturer in chemistry for a year (1815–1816) before Dana was appointed to that post; he could presumably have been made professor of chemistry instead of Dana in 1820.

Arbitrarily assigned or not, the significance of these several appointments lies less in who taught what than in the dramatic growth they marked in the staff of the medical school. Never before had there been such a degree of quasi-specialization in the traditional subject matter. No lingering sense could remain that Dartmouth Medical School was one man's school, handed on to that man's successors. Of the solid new faculty quartet, only one—Mussey—had had either direct association with Nathan Smith or a Dartmouth degree. He had both. The others, Harvard graduates all, no doubt brought a rather different perspective to the task of teaching at Dartmouth.

Parsons, who had a young Dartmouth man (Jesse Smith) to assist him as Lecturer in Anatomy for his first year, nonetheless stayed only two years. But Dana stayed six as professor, following his four as lecturer. He somehow inspired the trustees to give additional prominence and support to the teaching of chemistry. In their October 1820 meeting, they voted to give him, as Professor of Chemistry, $300 over and above student fees, "provided he shall remain in Hanover & give Lectures . . . to the Students, on the subject of the application of Chemistry to the arts."[7] In a way, of course, this simply echoed what seems to have happened when Nathan Smith and Lyman Spalding were asked to open their chemistry lectures to undergraduates.[8] But no extra remuneration was ever afforded Smith and Spalding for this additional duty, and the vote of the trustees to give Dana added compensation for what appears to be simply part of the job is somewhat surprising. On the other hand, it may be that this was meant to recognize it as a joint appointment with the College. In 1826, however, Dana left Dartmouth for the College of Physicians and Surgeons in New York (Fairfield); it has been suggested that at least part of the reason was that Dartmouth "'lacked the atmosphere favorable to investigation and scientific leadership.'"[9]

Oliver, like Mussey, stayed until 1838, thus adding continuity and stability to the growing institution. When Parsons resigned, Mussey was appointed Professor of Anatomy in addition to the other positions he already held. Physiology seems to have fallen from the curriculum again, at least as a separate course, until Oliver picked up that responsibility in 1831.[10] In any case, "physiology" at the time was largely anatomy, there not having been enough experimental work done to turn physiology into a genuine discipline in its own right. The years Mussey and Oliver gave to the institution in the end far outstripped Smith's term of service, signaling in another way a new phase in the school's history.

Among the most significant features of Oliver's tenure on the faculty was that he was the first in what would eventually be a long line of those who officially taught in both the College and the Medical School. In 1823, "recognizing the fact that the medical faculty served both medical and College students, the Trustees set up the first joint faculty appointment," as one historian has pointed out. Daniel Oliver, Professor of the Theory and Practice of Medicine, later Professor of Physiology, and sometime Professor of Medical Jurisprudence, also became Professor of Intellectual and Moral Philosophy in the College.[11] This may be among the reasons that Oliver was called "the finest scholar connected with the College" by a contemporary, though that of course tells us nothing about his teaching abilities.[12] He was also the first member of the medical faculty not to engage in medical practice, which some may have thought marked him as a true scholar.[13] In 1840, he published the first edition of his textbook, *First Lines of Physiology: Designed for the use of students of medicine*, in Philadelphia; a second edition followed the next year. An impressively early attempt at a physiology textbook, this was well enough received that a Boston publisher brought out a third edition ("with corrections and additions") in 1844.[14] Oliver's presidential address delivered before the New Hampshire Medical Society in 1833, published, "by request of the Society," was on a subject dear to Oliver's heart: temperance.[15]

An even more important figure in the school's history, in part because he was associated with the institution so long, was Reuben Dimond Mussey. His connection with Dartmouth spanned nearly four decades. Having received his A.B. from the College in 1803 (he was a classmate of George Cheyne Shattuck, another of Smith's protégés—the two of them were at Smith's side together when the older man died[16]), he did not proceed to the study of medicine quite so promptly or directly as some of his friends. He originally thought he would become a minister.

Once set on the path of medicine, however, he became an earnest and steady practitioner of both the art and the science of medicine as well as a much-admired medical teacher. Having added further study in Philadelphia to his tutelage at Dartmouth under Nathan Smith (where his M.B. degree was granted in 1806 and converted to an M.D. in 1812) and a practice in Essex, Massachusetts, Mussey earned an M.D. from the University of Pennsylvania in 1809. This combination armed him with absolutely the best medical education available in the United States. He then settled in Salem, Massachusetts; he and Daniel Oliver were at one point surgical partners.

Mussey, "an independent-minded researcher" who "successfully challenged several prevailing medical notions," made his mark as an exper-

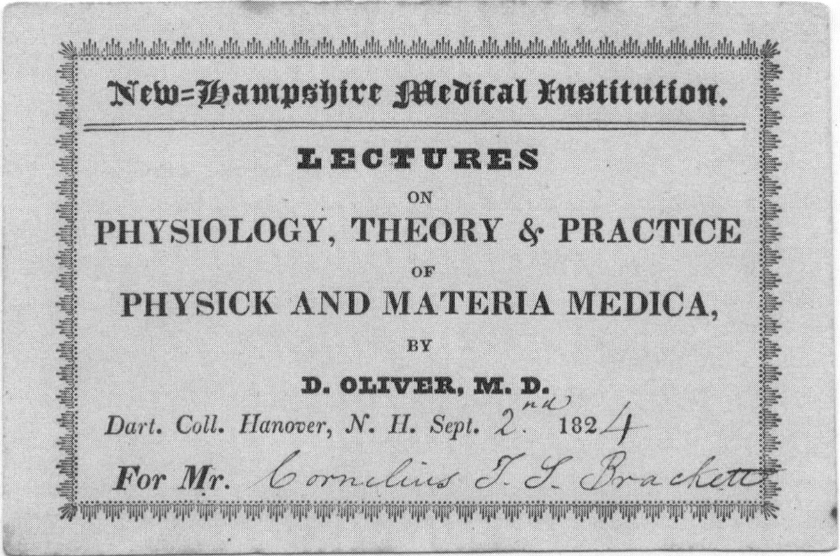
New-Hampshire Medical Institution.

LECTURES
ON
PHYSIOLOGY, THEORY & PRACTICE
OF
PHYSICK AND MATERIA MEDICA,
BY
D. OLIVER, M. D.

Dart. Coll. Hanover, N. H. Sept. 2nd. 1824

For Mr. Cornelius J. H. Brackett

Lecture ticket for Cornelius J. H. Brackett to attend lectures on Physiology, Theory and Practice of Physic and Materia Medica. Gift of D. Oliver M.D., 1924. Courtesy of Dartmouth College Library.

imental scientist most dramatically "by soaking himself in tubs of water containing different chemicals and administering appropriate tests before and after each immersion," proving to his satisfaction that human skin was absorbent. This was in direct contradiction of claims of the great Benjamin Rush (who theorized that substances could not be absorbed through the skin).[17] His account of these experiments is a marvel of careful description, but his results lead one to suspect that he almost certainly failed to guard adequately against contamination. To his credit, though Mussey was convinced he had demonstrated that soaking in bath water infused with rose madder (the root of *Rubia tinctoria*)—for example—did indeed alter the color of urine, he was nonetheless cautious in making his claims. Saying there was much work still to be done, he insisted that it "would be an extremely limited view of the subject, should we suppose that Nature prepared the cutaneous absorbents for the purpose merely of taking in an infusion of madder."[18]

Nor was this Mussey's only piece of scholarly work. He wrote a substantial article called "Fracture of the Neck of the Thigh-Bone" (after he had left Dartmouth and was professor of surgery in the Miami Medical College at Cincinnati, Ohio), in which he reported on a series of cases and then compared and contrasted the views of various distinguished members of the profession. An earlier letter to the editor of the *Boston Medical and Surgical Journal* also related cases from Mussey's practice—five successful bi-lateral lithotomy operations, and two very different but equally successful operations for osteo-sarcoma. One was of the lower jaw; the other, of the os humeri and the scapula, required removal of "the arm and the entire shoulder-blade, with the acromial half of the collar-bone."[19] All this in a period when many medical faculty were not bothering to publish at all. Among Mussey's important operations was a successful ligation of the carotid artery, worth boasting about in a newspaper advertisement for the school.[20] One later commentator on the history of Dartmouth Medical School went so far as to say that Mussey was "almost . . . as active and well known as was his predecessor [Smith], and very much of an investigator covering several fields outside his specialty."[21]

Mussey was a true generalist. "He was a vegetarian, a prohibitionist, an anti-tobacco protagonist, and an accomplished musician, playing the first double bass viol to come to New Hampshire and being one of the founders of the Handel Society of Dartmouth."[22] He was a lean and earnest-looking man—seeming indeed not very robust, just as one might expect of someone who had concluded he did not have the physical stamina required to become a minister. Portraits show him hollow-cheeked and unsmiling. His publications on temperance, tobacco, and the "friends and . . . foes" of health indicate that the serious and stern demeanor was likely a matter of settled character and not just for show.[23] Furthermore, it was Mussey's newspaper account of the case of Laura Bridgman—deaf and blind from the age of two—that led Samuel Gridley Howe to take her on as a kind of reform project. Together, Bridgman and Howe helped make history at the Perkins School for the Blind in Boston.

It may have been Mussey who suggested the innovation in medical school procedures that resulted in the New Hampshire Medical Society sending delegates to attend and participate actively in examining medical degree candidates, beginning in 1820.[24] Certainly on other occasions it is clear that Mussey was materially involved in every aspect of the Medical School's operation. Prior to the first formal appointment of a medical school dean late in the century, it was the secretary of the medical faculty who effectively played that role.[25] Mussey was the first of nine who held the joint position of secretary and treasurer; he was the incumbent for six years (1814–1820).

In 1835, when it became evident that Daniel Oliver was thinking about resigning, the trustees asked Mussey to undertake a national search for a professor of chemistry and to make visits to such candidates as necessary in order to find some "suitable person" to be appointed professor of natural philosophy and mathematics as well as professor of chemistry. It was a tall order, but the man eventually given the job—Oliver Payson Hubbard—turned out to be another major figure on the Dartmouth landscape, as we shall see in the next chapter.

Two years later (in 1837) Mussey, too, decided to resign. He wrote a letter of resignation that was a model of rectitude fully characteristic of the man. The minutes of the trustees from their Commencement day meeting in July 1838 read thus:

The following Communication was received from Professor Mussey.

Dartmouth College July 25, 1838

Dear Sir Permit me, through you, to tender to the Hon. Board of Trustees, my resignation of the Professorship I hold in this institution. I need not state the motives which have led to this decision as the most important of them are already known to you, but in retiring from this field of Labour in which I have been occupied for twenty four years I cannot help expressing the wish that Dartmouth College may flourish till literary institutions can no longer bless Mankind
Very sincerely & Respectfully
Pres.[t] Lord Yrs R. D. Mussey[26]

The contrast with the trustees' account of votes surrounding Nathan Smith's two resignations is striking. Smith's initial departure was recorded with words of stiff formality, in the midst of the College versus University turmoil: "Whereas Doctor Nathan Smith has expressed to this board his desire to resign his office as Professor in this College; and as he has neglected to perform the duties of a Professor for fifteen months past, Voted his resignation be accepted; and that he be no longer considered professor in this College."[27] When he resigned again, after having taught one final term in 1816, the record of it was even more brisk: "Voted That the resignation of Doct[r] Nathan Smith of his Office of Professor of Surgery and of the theory and practice of Physic in this College be accepted."[28] Mussey's resignation was handled more graciously and with more attention to the kind of administrative detail characteristic of a more mature institution.

Although Mussey did not explain in his letter why he chose to resign—the recipients of the letter were aware of the reasons, he said—we know that he, like Smith, went from Dartmouth to another medical school. (He had already, while at Dartmouth, also spent time lecturing both at the Medical School of Maine, in Brunswick, and at Fairfield.) Upon leaving Dartmouth, Mussey went first to the Medical College of Cincinnati, where he taught for fourteen years; subsequent to that, he once again followed in his mentor's steps by helping to found yet another medical school, this time the Miami (Ohio) Medical College, which he served for five years.[29] Like father, like son: Mussey became a physician in spite of himself. Like teacher, like student: Mussey became a medical educator with broad influence. In 1870, four years after Mussey's death, one of his successors on the Dartmouth medical faculty called him "a gentleman whose reputation as a physician and surgeon has been hardly second to that of any man in America." Even allowing for some degree of sentimental hyperbole (Mussey's death was still relatively recent, and the occasion for the remark was the anniversary of his death), it is an impressive testimony. The speaker went on: "I need only write the name of Reuben D. Mussey to recall to the friends of medicine in New Hampshire the memory of an eminent Christian, a learned physician, a world-renowned surgeon, the best labors of whose most creditable life were devoted to the good of our state, college and commonwealth."[30]

A Parade of Talent

After Reuben Dimond Mussey, another fifty men would serve on the faculty of the medical institution in Hanover during the nineteenth century—and this number does not include those like Benjamin Hale who taught chemistry to medical students but whose appointment was in the College, nor does it count the two dozen men who served as all-important "demonstrators" in anatomy (their names appear in the catalogues for the years they were so employed, but they were not considered faculty members).[31] The period of years that individuals spent as members of the faculty is quite varied. Some stayed only a year: Hiram McNutt was an assistant lecturer in obstetrics in 1869–1870; Arthur Herbert Kimball was an instructor in anatomy and physiology in 1875–1876; Arthur Mead Edwards lectured in chemistry in 1871 only; and James Henry Pooley was a lecturer in surgery in 1877–1878. Others, professors all, stayed decades; partly as a consequence, their names are much more familiar to faithful followers of Dartmouth's fortunes: Dixi Crosby, Edmund Randolph Peaslee, Lyman Bartlett How, Carlton Pennington Frost, Edwin Julius Bartlett, William Thayer Smith, Gilman DuBuois Frost, John Martin Gile, Oliver Payson Hubbard.

Less well known but deserving the prize for the most extraordinary names are Charles Beylard Guérard de Nancrède (who joined the faculty in 1887 as a lecturer in surgery), Tilghman Minnour Balliet (who taught therapeutics beginning in 1893), and his 1890s colleague Solomon Solis Cohen (a lecturer in therapeutics for two one-year stints). The faculty was an eclectic lot, and stories of interest could no doubt be told about each of its members. Unfortunately, the paucity of archival materials in some instances and of space here makes it necessary to include only fragments of the careers of a few.

The number of subjects taught—by the faculty as a whole and by some of its individual members—also ranged widely. Several faculty members, especially in the later years of the century, took charge of only one relatively narrow area—like "Medical Jurisprudence" (sometimes called "Legal Medicine")—as Joel Parker did in the period from 1845 to 1857. (Narrowness of curricular responsibility aside, during these years, we are told, Parker was one of only two DMS faculty making significant contributions to professional literature.[32]) Others, in the tradition of Smith and Mussey, taught whatever needed to be taught and shifted fields readily and apparently almost at will. Edward Elisha Phelps, for example, over a period of thirty-five years beginning in 1841, taught Materia Medica, Medical Jurisprudence, Medical Botany, Therapeutics, Theory and Practice of medicine, and both Pathological Anatomy and General Anatomy. (More will be said about who taught what in chapter 4.)

Of those who stayed only briefly, the most famous was Oliver Wendell Holmes, the man chosen to pick up some of the slack created when Mussey and Oliver resigned. Holmes had made clear in a letter to Mussey on July 12, 1838, that he would accept the job were it offered to him,[33] which may have helped Mussey reach the decision to resign. At their meeting in July 1838, the trustees "Voted by Ballot and chose Oliver Wendell Holmes Professor of Anatomy" at the same time they were choosing Dixi Crosby as "Professor of Surgery & Obstetricks" and Elisha Bartlett as "Professor of Physiology, Medical Jurisprudence & materia medica."[34] But also at that meeting, immediately after accepting Mussey's resignation, the trustees requested Mussey to continue to lecture the next term (as they did Oliver, as well, when they accepted *his* resignation). Thus it appears that although Holmes was appointed to succeed Mussey, he did not do so immediately. When he wrote to his brother-in-law, Usher Parsons (who had earlier held the anatomy chair himself), in August 1838, Holmes not only said that he thought the Dartmouth job "a very agreeable appointment" but mentioned that he wouldn't have to lecture until the following August.[35] Holmes's handwritten text of his "1st Introductory Lecture" is headed simply "Aug. 1839" (the second is similarly dated: "Aug. 1840").[36] A lecture ticket admitting "Charles D. Cleav[e]land" to Holmes's lectures is dated August 8, 1839, making that seem the likely beginning of Oliver Wendell Holmes's brief tenure as a member of the Dartmouth Medical School faculty.[37] We know the terms ran from August to November and that

Holmes's resignation was accepted by the trustees at their January 1841 meeting. Thus it appears that, although Holmes may have been technically a member of the faculty from 1838 to 1841 (having been appointed in 1838), by prior agreement he actually taught only twice, in the autumn terms of 1839 and 1840.[38]

The two terms Holmes taught at Dartmouth were in any case long enough, as indicated, to give the institution its claim on this particular celebrated New England figure. Nor does anyone at Dartmouth seem to mind Holmes's disparaging remarks about the school's location in the boondocks. After a visit to Hanover in May 1839, Holmes wrote to Dixi Crosby exclaiming over the wonder of having gotten home safely. "[C]ontrary to my expectations," he wrote, "I arrived in Boston in one whole piece. I thought I should have been a living museum of comminuted fractures before I had ploughed through twenty miles of what you call *The Road* by a singular misnomer, in New Hampshire."[39] Indeed, a historian of the school claimed that Dartmouth has always "taken pride in" Holmes's association with the institution, despite the fact that his "reputation as a professional teacher and writer was in later years so overshadowed by that of the Poet and the Autocrat."[40] And although Holmes's reputation is indeed today primarily as a writer, it is true that he "earned his living throughout most of his life as a professor of anatomy"—and that Dartmouth gave him his first academic appointment. (Official College records indicate Holmes was professor of both anatomy and physiology; how separate the two disciplines really were is open to question. Holmes thought of himself more as an anatomist than as a physiologist.) Townspeople attended his lectures "in search . . . of the fun which cropped out so often in [them]."[41]

The most frequently quoted remark connecting Oliver Wendell Holmes to Dartmouth appears, however, to be based on an error. Writer after writer (and speaker after speaker) has claimed that Holmes quipped about Nathan Smith that he had held not a *chair* in the newly fledged medical school at Dartmouth, but a *whole settee*.[42] The truth seems to be that Holmes made the remark about Albrecht von Haller, the great Swiss professor at Göttingen whom he had especial reason to admire.[43] Von Haller not only held three professorships (in anatomy, botany, and medicine) and carried out investigations in physiology, but—like Holmes—was an accomplished and published poet as well.[44] Of course it may be that at some point Holmes quoted himself, so to speak, and applied the remark to someone else—for instance, Nathan Smith, who of all those peripatetic, multi-talented, and multi-disciplined medical professors of early American medical education probably most deserved the implied accolade.[45] Still, for all the brevity of his tenure at Dartmouth, Holmes has a firm place in the long and distinguished line of holders of the chair in anatomy at the school. Nor did he shake Dartmouth dust off his feet altogether when he left at the end of the term in late 1840; eighteen years later he returned to give the commencement address.

The Crosby Contribution

Dartmouth has been blessed by connection with several families that contributed more than one member to the faculty. The earliest and undoubtedly the most remarkable example of such a family is the one to which Dixi Crosby (1800–1873) belonged. He was another of those appointed along with Holmes at the time of Mussey's and Oliver's resignations; indeed, parts of Mussey's many-legged chair were divided between Holmes (anatomy) and Crosby (surgery and surgical anatomy). Crosby and his descendants were to play important roles in Dartmouth and Hanover medicine.

The Crosby story actually begins not with Dixi, but with his father Asa Crosby (1765–1836), also a physician. Asa spent only his final days in Hanover, but his second son Alpheus (1810–1874)—an "infant prodigy"—at the age of nine and a half passed all the entrance examinations for Dartmouth College. He entered college at the age of thirteen, in 1827, after his older brother Dixi had graduated from the medical school. (Alpheus, fulfilling his prodigious promise, became a professor of Greek and Latin in the College; he was granted emeritus status at the age of thirty-nine.)

This aside on the father and the younger brother merely sets the stage; it shows that the contribution made by the two Crosby family members most frequently mentioned—Dixi and his son Alpheus Benning Crosby (1832–1877) called "Dr. Ben"—was not the only place where Crosbys and Dartmouth crossed paths. A third son of Asa, Thomas Russell Crosby (1816–1872), studied medicine with both his father and his older brother Dixi and also became a physician. He, too, taught at Dartmouth, though in the College's department of natural history rather than in the Medical School. Thomas was another of those young men (like Reuben Mussey) who studied medicine only because they did not think they were fully capable of being ministers; his health was considered not good enough. Although one historian called this a "mysterious conclusion," to think that "the life of a physician would make fewer demands upon one in poor health than that of a minister," in fact the decision was more common than mysterious, as has been well documented.[46] (Another example tangentially relevant to our story is Nathan Smith's youngest son, John Derby Smith, who—having been ordained a Congregational minister—likewise took up the study of medicine when he had to stop preaching because of throat trouble.[47])

Having earned his medical degree from Dartmouth in 1824, Dixi began his faculty career when he accepted the offer of a position as professor of surgery and obstetrics fourteen years later, in 1838.[48] He would remain on the faculty until 1870. (He had a further Dartmouth connection, having been one of James Dana's preceptees.) Such was Dixi Crosby's talent that even someone seeking to praise him cautiously (saying that he was a "top notch man [but] perhaps not as great as his predecessors in medicine in ability") acknowledged nonetheless that he was "a man of fame well deserved."[49] He was bold, innovative, and successful as a surgeon; he came to be considered "head of the medical profession of the state"; was, as a lecturer, "clear, dignified and incisive"; and during the thirty-five years he lived in Hanover, "no personality in the community was better liked and more esteemed than Dr. Dixi."[50]

Nor was Hanover alone the beneficiary of his ministrations. He practiced across much of northern New England, as well, in direct continuation of the pattern set by Nathan Smith. Even more significant was Crosby's successful establishment of a hospital in Hanover sometime before 1850; it closed when he retired in 1870.[51] In 1824, an ad for the Medical School masquerading as a news item, which appeared in the *Boston Telegraph*, had boasted of the fact that an "Infirmary, on a limited scale, has been commenced at Hanover, by the Medical Professors.—Boarding places have been engaged for patients who may need surgical operations, and for a small number laboring under chronic diseases."[52] But Crosby's hospital was less ad hoc, no mere "infirmary" with "boarding places." Performing operations for his students in the Medical House, he would then transport the recuperating patients across the road to his hospital for further care.[53] Not until late in the century would anyone take steps again toward organizing such an institution, an indication of how far ahead Crosby was in his thinking. It was he, also, who "introduced ether anesthesia to Hanover" after going to Boston to learn how to use it shortly after the initial demonstration at the Massachusetts General Hospital on October 16, 1846.[54] A portrait from near the end of Crosby's life shows him full-bearded and with heavy eyebrows, an imposing figure who looks the part of a medical pioneer and community leader.

By the time "Dr. Ben" arrived on the scene, the Crosby medical tradition was well established. Ben is said to have accompanied his father

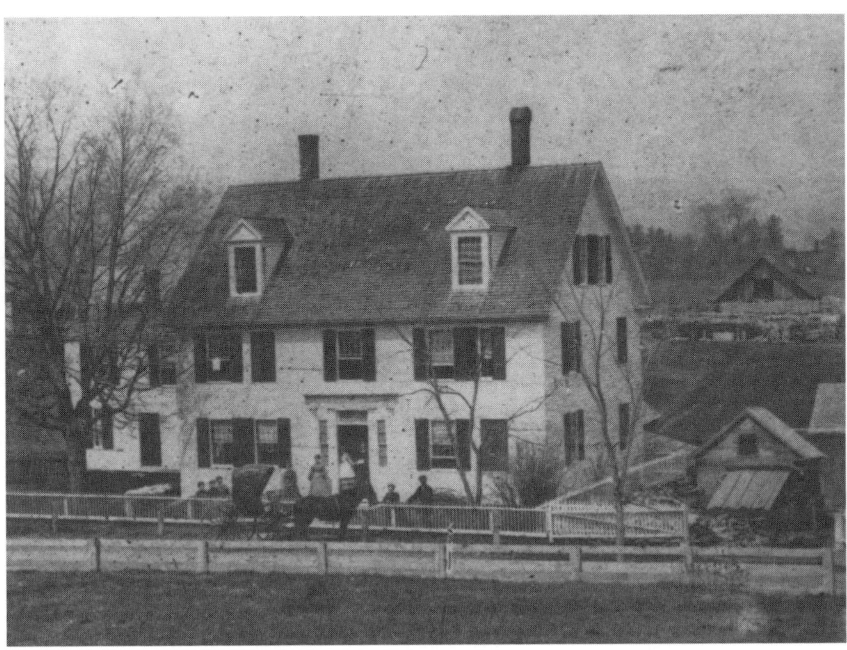

Dixi Crosby's Hospital, North College Street. Courtesy of Dartmouth College Library.

on house calls—even to have assisted in minor operations—already as a boy. He received his medical degree from Dartmouth in 1856, served briefly in the Civil War, and then returned to Hanover where he was made an assistant professor of surgery in 1862. The way the notice of his appointment is worded in the trustees' minutes is startling today, in that no effort is made to disguise the nepotism: "Resolved that the consent of the Faculty be given to the request of Prof. Dixi Crosby that his son, Dr. Alpheus B. Crosby, be appointed Assistant Professor of Surgery," which resolution was unanimously adopted: "Voted, that, Alpheus B. Crosby be and hereby is appointed assistant Professor of surgery."[55] He was soon promoted to associate professor, and in 1869 to professor of surgery, thus taking over that portion of his father's responsibilities.[56] A year later, Dixi retired. A mark of the esteem in which his colleagues held him is that he was designated "Professor of Surgery Emeritus." When he died three years later (in 1873), an obituary noted anecdotes illustrating Crosby's intrepid approach to surgery, from early in his career, and credited him with several surgical firsts; he was also said to have had "a nature so fearless, and so fertile in expedients."[57]

His son Ben, who succeeded him, died just four years later, at the age of forty-five—perhaps in part because he did not know how to say "no." (In 1870, he was identified in print as professor of surgery at the University of Vermont, the University of Michigan, and the Long Island College Hospital as well as at Dartmouth.[58]) Yet the Crosby medical line did not die out with Dr. Ben. Neither of his sons—the second Dixi Crosby (1869–1900) and William Pierce Crosby (1874–1914)—lived even as long as he had, but the younger Dixi was an 1891 graduate of Dartmouth Medical School and William, class of 1898, practiced for a while in Hanover.[59]

The stories of Mussey and of the Crosbys (father and son) are easy to tell, because they seem so straightforwardly positive. The same cannot be said of every member of the faculty, as the following two cases—very different from each other—illustrate.

The Removal of Benjamin Hale

Benjamin Hale had been appointed professor of chemistry in the College in 1827; he also taught mineralogy.[60] At the July 1835 meeting of the trustees it was resolved that the professorship in chemistry, mineralogy, and the application of science to the arts that had been established in 1820 "is hearby repealed." The medical faculty was authorized to hire a "suitable person" to lecture to the *medical* students on chemistry and mineralogy. Ira Young, professor of mathematics and natural philosophy, was to be requested to lecture on those subjects to members of the upper classes in the College; custody of the mineralogy cabinet was handed over to him as well. Thus Hale's job was eliminated out from under him.[61]

Such clarification as there is for why Hale was removed from office comes not from the Trustees Records, but from a series of privately published documents. Hale's own *Valedictory Letter to the Trustees of Dartmouth College* (October 27, 1835) ran to more than twenty pages and was full of indignant outrage. Then came *Professor Hale and Dartmouth College*, signed simply "Alumnus," an essay of similar length written in support of the trustees' position. A third, longer essay (more than thirty pages) carried the title *Remarks on a Pamphlet Entitled "Professor Hale and Dartmouth College."* Signed "Investigator," it was intended to demolish, point by point, everything in the pamphlet it was attacking; the claim was that the trustees had abused their power irresponsibly. Suffice it to say that the College did not handle matters smoothly, even if it had reasonable grounds for wanting to be free of Hale.[62]

That the Hale affair was distressing to more than one individual is clear from the fact that A. B. Crosby, in an address before the New Hampshire Medical Society, could not resist resurrecting the episode years later. Though he dispensed with details of how matters had worked out, he shared his understanding of the reason for the vote to abolish the chair in strong terms:

> I cannot forbear to recall for an instant the name of Professor Hale, who, after serving the college in the chair of Chemistry for a few years, lost his connection with the institution in a manner by no means creditable to the trustees. Professor Hale was an Episcopalian, and was wont to hold the service of the church of England at his own house, for the benefit of whoever might choose to come. This course was obnoxious to the college fathers, who were at the time strongly sectarian. The board determined on his removal, but as it was found that it could not be legally accomplished under the college charter, the Alexandrian method of treating this heretical [Gordian] knot was adopted. A vote was passed abolishing the Professorship of Chemistry.

In a final jibe at Dartmouth, Crosby added that "Subsequently, as President of Geneva College, Dr. Hale passed a most useful life." He quickly softened the blow, going on to insist that "Whatever may have been the derelictions of Dartmouth in the past, I am proud to say that her spirit is liberal and catholic now."[63] Whether the grounds for Hale's removal were in fact religious or financial or something altogether different, Dartmouth's treatment of him does, in retrospect, seem both crude and conniving.

The Oliver Hubbard Affair

Another more complicated story that shows all was not always well in the halls of medical academe at Dartmouth concerns Oliver Payson Hubbard (1809–1900) in the early years of his long career. Few can match Hubbard in both longevity and variety of roles played at Dartmouth. Not only was he a long-time member of the Medical School faculty who also taught undergraduates, but he was for six years (1839–1845) both treasurer and secretary of the medical faculty; holding the latter position, it will be recalled, was tantamount to being dean.[64] In addition, Hubbard was for fourteen years (1851–1865) the College librarian, and it was he who conferred the medical degrees at the October 30, 1863, commencement, in his role as "President pro tem of Dartmouth College."[65] (Hubbard's "Lecture Introductory to the Eighty-Third Course of Lectures"—not the only time he performed this duty—seems to be one of the few such Medical School inaugural addresses to have been preserved in print.[66])

Hubbard, with an A.B. earned at Yale in 1828, began his Dartmouth run quietly enough in 1836 as an associate professor of chemistry and pharmacy in the medical school (promoted to full professor in 1838) and professor of chemistry, mineralogy, and geology in the College (or, depending on the source one consults, as "Professor of the Physical Sciences"—a title that appeared for the first time with his appointment).[67] Thus he had already been teaching at Dartmouth for a year when he earned his M.D., in 1837, at the Medical College in Charleston, South Carolina. In 1838 his title at Dartmouth became "Hall Professor of Mineralogy & Geology and Professor of Chemistry," in recognition of a major donation from Frederick Hall of the class of 1803 (and, at the time, president of Mt. Hope College).[68] He did not retire until 1883, when he was granted emeritus status; he lived another seventeen years, dying only as the new century began in 1900.

This brief chronology hides a major controversy, a tale of faculty politics over a complaint that dragged on for years and resulted in one of the longest committee reports in the records of the trustees. The difficulty began at the trustees' January 1841 meeting. There is an explicit statement that Hubbard was to be "Professor of Chemistry and Pharmacy" in the "Medical department" (in addition to his teaching in the "Academical department," that is, in the College); it was acknowledged that "the effects of his labours would be advanced by a change of his relation to the Medical department of the College." But then there is a notice that his salary was to be paid retroactively from April 18, 1836, despite the fact that he did not actually begin until August of that year—because he had arrived in April (ready to teach) "in pursuance of a previous understanding that his duties were then to commence." A hint that he must also have asked for more money is a further note indicating an inability to raise his salary, but promising that it would be increased (to $1,000 per annum) at such time as the Board was able "to advance the salaries of the other Professors to that sum."[69] One interpretation goes like this: You do have a grievance (because you came ready to teach, in good faith, prior to when it turned out you were actually needed, and so you legitimately expect to be paid for that), and, yes, it would be only reasonable to raise your salary—but we can't now and in any case won't until we can raise the salary for the other professors as well.

That would seem to have been the end of the matter—unless what happened five years later is part of the same misunderstanding, by then escalated. In January 1846, the trustees' records show that Professor Hubbard was to be told he was expected to "refund the graduating fees from the Medical Students, which he has received, and that the treasurer of the College be notified of this vote."[70] Hubbard appears not to have been pleased, according to a note in the minutes of the July 1846 meeting.[71] The next day it was voted to refer Hubbard's "bill" (as it was then being called) to the Prudential Committee for settlement.[72]

Not until a special adjourned meeting in January of 1848 do we finally get some fuller sense of what the issue was. "The Committee on Prof. Hubbard's Memorial made its Report, which was accepted, as follows"—nearly five full pages, detailing the complaint and all considerations.[73] Hubbard believed he was entitled to a share of the fees paid for medical lectures over and above his salary, and he believed he was entitled to the graduation fees paid by medical students. He based his case on what he insisted was an explicit condition he had imposed in accepting his election to the professorship. In the committee's view, the matter was far more important than a mere financial disagreement with a particular professor. Rather, it had to do with the very fundamental issue of the relationship between the College and the Medical Department, including which of them was to have responsibility for paying which faculty members. To the extent that the trustees were right—and they appear to have been, citing as precedent "the difficulties experienced under the former organization of the Medical Department, when the Professor of Chemistry was connected with the College only as a professor in that department"—their conclusion seems reasonable: "It did not occur to [the Board] that by electing [Hubbard] to fill the Professorship, they were laying themselves under obligations to alter their original design in a point so important and fundamental as diverting a portion of the proceeds of the Medical Lectures from the College Treasury." As a consequence, "With every feeling of respect and kindness toward Professor Hubbard and a desire to do every thing that can be done, consistently, to render his situation satisfactory, the Committee see no good reason for diverting any portion of the income of the Medical Lectures from the College Treasury."

The report ended, and the trustees' records moved on to the next item on the agenda; there is no evidence of further unpleasantness or disagreement on the matter. In other words, though Hubbard appears to have considered himself quite wronged—for several years—once the matter was thoughtfully and carefully worked through (with Hubbard having won only a very partial victory), there seem to have been no hard feelings on either side. A year and a half later, a special vote of the board turned up $150 for use in the department of chemistry, mineralogy, and geology—that is, Hubbard's department.[74] Though Hubbard must have been disappointed with the committee report on his "Memorial," either out of institutional loyalty or out of a sense that his complaint had been treated with the seriousness it deserved, he continued to go about his business as a faculty member for many years. As mentioned earlier, he was elected librarian in 1851,[75] and when he resigned that post in 1865, thanks were voted him "for his long and faithful services as Librarian of the College."[76] But the successful management of this little-known challenge to the authority of the Board, in a matter that was indeed "fundamental and important," tells us much about the maturing of the institution.

More Faculty

The total cast of characters on the nineteenth-century medical school faculty—fifty strong—is too large to permit doing them justice here. Yet three father–son tandems beyond the Crosby duo must at least be mentioned. Carlton Pennington Frost has already been named as one who served for many years as both secretary and treasurer (and de facto dean) of the medical faculty. A few years later, his son Gilman DuBois Frost would hold the same position. Gilman—whose membership in Phi Beta Kappa is some measure of his abilities—initially taught German and Latin right after college, but he eventually followed in his father's footsteps by becoming a lecturer in anatomy at the Medical School (C. P. Frost was first appointed in 1868; G. D. Frost in 1893), much as Ben Crosby succeeded Dixi Crosby in the surgery chair. Though nepotism is again certainly evident, the sons were extremely able. Dartmouth benefited greatly from having them pick up where their fathers left off. A third such pair crosses the border at century's end to influence events at Dartmouth well into the twentieth century. John Martin Gile—another of those who would over the years of a long career at Dartmouth teach half a dozen different subjects—joined the faculty in 1896. Among the responsibilities he relinquished when he retired in 1925 was the position of instructor in physical diagnosis. (He was also the Medical School dean for fifteen years.) His son J. F. Gile, an instructor in anatomy from 1922, became instructor in physical diagnosis on his father's retirement; he would in addition be one of founders of the Hitchcock Clinic in 1927. Finally, in the twentieth century, there would be the appointment first of Colin Campbell Stewart II in 1904 and then of Colin Campbell Stewart III in 1931. An entire book could be written on these father–son pairs.

One faculty member who is less often mentioned, but who nevertheless had an enormous impact on the Medical School and its future, is Edward Elisha Phelps. A member of the faculty for more than thirty years (1841–1875), he too had a record of having taught a wide range of subjects. His longest-lasting contribution to Dartmouth Medical School came about not as a result of his teaching, but his practice, of medicine. A wealthy New York lawyer, E. W. Stoughton, Esq., with no Dartmouth connection except for having been one of Phelps's patients, offered a gift of $10,000 to the Medical College "to establish a Museum of Pathological Anatomy" in 1871. He was explicit that his generosity had been inspired by affection for Phelps and gratitude for his professional services. Stoughton had, he wrote to Phelps, "an earnest wish to benefit an Institution with which you and your distinguished associates have been long and usefully connected, and which through your and their efforts has done much service in the training of youth for the practice of your noble profession." That gift made it possible to establish a genuine "Museum of Pathological Anatomy," which came to be known as "The Stoughton Museum."[77]

Students and Student Life

Our knowledge of what student life at Dartmouth Medical School was like in the nineteenth century is limited; records are spotty, but a few stories must be told. Certainly some students were virtually destitute. One example of a severely impoverished student is Eleazar Burbank, a nongraduate of the class of 1816. Young Burbank is said to have walked to Hanover from Scarborough, Maine—well over a hundred miles—to study under Smith, and later to have walked home because he could not afford to pay fares for the journey. It has also been speculated that his failure to graduate had to do not with any inability to write the required thesis, but with a lack of funds to pay the cost of a degree.[78]

In 1825, an event transpired that involved a number of students whose actions might have been motivated in part by poverty. Exactly how many students took part in this particular episode we do not know, but nearly two dozen took the trouble formally to make a declaration of innocence. "To the Medical Faculty of Dartmouth College," one of these notes began: "Having been suspected of being concerned in the clandestine removal of the books belonging to the Dartmouth Medical Society from the Library room during the present term, I hereby declare upon the honor of a gentleman & the faith of a Christian, that I have not had any agency either directly or indirectly in the transaction, and that I had no knowledge of it, or of its authors before it was committed." This one was signed "14 Dec 1825. Lewis Colby." Another nineteen notes—some identical (except for the signature), others in a very slightly modified version—can be found today in the College archives.[79] What the actual motivation was, or what became of the books, we do not know. Perhaps it was theft (or attempted theft); books were expensive and far more difficult to obtain than they are today. (Some two decades earlier, Nathan Smith had complained to his recently departed student George Cheyne Shattuck about having suffered "a prodigious loss of books." Whether students borrowed and failed to return or did, in some instances, actually steal the books is not clear—but there is no reason to think Dartmouth students of the early nineteenth century were generally less responsible in such matters than students elsewhere, or since.[80])

One student who received his medical degree in 1824 (the year prior to the assault on the library holdings)—Charles Knowlton—had an especially unusual career and made a singularly important contribution to the lives of numerous young people quite apart from his career as a practicing physician. Though Charles was married, he could not afford to have his wife join him in Hanover (she stayed with her parents); he was "shy and retiring" and probably not very well (he was "continually troubled with digestive problems and headaches").[81] Knowlton's ("abject") poverty was enough to persuade him to join the ranks of those who engaged in grave robbing to earn cash. As a result of one such episode, he spent two months in jail in Worcester County, Massachusetts. Found not guilty on the charge of grave robbing, he was nonetheless convicted of having conducted an illegal dissection.

Grave robbing and even illegal dissection would not by themselves be enough to distinguish young Knowlton's career from that of many of his contemporaries (see chapter 4). Rather, it was his publishing efforts—not the routine medical articles written in his later days, but his second book—that make him stand out among not only Dartmouth men but nineteenth-century physicians more generally. In 1832, a small volume called somewhat mysteriously *The Fruits of Philosophy* was published in New York; the author, identified simply as "A Physician," was in fact Charles Knowlton. The title notwithstanding, the book was in effect the first common-sense birth-control manual written deliberately for ordinary young couples who might want to delay or limit the size of their families. As such, it caused a fair amount of uproar particularly among a certain class of pious, self-appointed protectors of public morals.

When Knowlton acknowledged that he was the author, he suffered the consequences—having to put up with three separate trials (one resulted in a fine, a second in three months in jail). Even so, some 10,000 copies of his book were sold in less than a decade. In 1834, the book appeared in England. There, too, it continued to sell; it became the precipitating cause in the arrest and subsequent prosecution of Charles Bradlaugh and Annie Besant in 1876. Their "crime" was not merely that they were freethinkers and ardent enthusiasts for birth control, but that they had published Knowlton's book after its earlier publisher had pleaded guilty to publishing an obscene book (a plea that obviated any need for prosecutors to examine the book's contents). Bradlaugh and Besant were committed—among other things—to true freedom of the press. Once it was known that the trial had to do with publishing an "indecent, lewd, filthy, bawdy, and obscene book," sales skyrocketed. Knowlton, by that time long dead, would no doubt have been puzzled, or at least bemused. He was—perhaps unwittingly and unintentionally—a pioneer in a field that remains as relevant as it is controversial (for some) today.[82]

William Tully had a very different experience at Dartmouth. A priggish and comfortably well-off young man from Connecticut, Tully went to Dartmouth after having done his undergraduate work at Yale. The diary he kept in 1808–1809 is an often-cited record of what life was like for medical students in Hanover at the beginning of the nineteenth century. Like many a Yale loyalist in subsequent years, he found both Hanover and Dartmouth definitely infra dig. At Dewey's Tavern, where he first sought a room, he complained of "a sour landlord, and a very dirty bar room full of persons of all descriptions." The Bush Hotel, to which he then repaired, was not much better: "we entered a spacious, ill contrived, unfinished, and uncleanly house." Desperate, he and his companion stayed anyway. But when they woke up the next morning, he reported, "I reflected, with considerable dissatisfaction, on my reception, and subsequent entertainment, in Hanover. . . . When I got up, I found the house quite as slovenly as it appeared last night."[83]

A student writing to a friend more than three decades later painted a picture in a brief letter that has parallels to Tully's remarks in tone as well as content: "The next day about midnight I came into this place," Leonard Spaulding wrote to James Farrar in 1842. "I was somewhat disappointed . . . —it is not as handsome a place as I had expected to find." Here he sounds like Tully, except that he continued: "But it is good enough and I shall find no fault with it." He was less concerned with dirt and lack of civility than with the lack of piety. "There are not so many pious people in the place as I imagined, and there are a great many profane persons and sabbath breakers. There is a good deal of riding round on the sabbath among a part of the people. A very few, compared with the population, attend the church."[84]

The most striking dissimilarity between Spaulding and Tully was their relative enthusiasm for their medical studies. Tully devoted considerable space in his diary to criticizing the lecture style of Smith and the visiting anatomist Alexander Ramsay (though in the end he admitted he had come to admire both).[85] Young Spaulding, in contrast, seemed pleased with the academic offerings despite the fact that he clearly found the course rather too challenging:

> I have to work hard. We have from five to six Lectures a day, each one an hour long. I am [as] well pleased in attending Lectures as I could reasonably expect. It is difficult to retain even the smallest portion of what I hear. The Lectures commence at 8 o'clock in the morning and continue till 12 with an intermission of one or two minutes between the lectures. . . . The fifth Lecture comes at 4 o clock P.M., and Tuesdays we have 2 in the afternoon, commencing at 3 o'clock making 6 in one day. I take notes and copy them off after the Lectures. So, nearly my whole time is occupied in hearing Lectures and copying notes. I find I must do every thing I intend to do at the proper time. If I neglect copying notes to day I shall have no time tomorrow.[86]

Spaulding did not stay at Dartmouth; he returned instead to his native Massachusetts and earned an M.D. the following year (1843) from the Berkshire Medical College.[87]

A letter from another nongraduate of a few years later gives us even more detail about the life of a student at Dartmouth Medical School in the 1840s. Charles Boyden, like Leonard Spaulding a Massachusetts boy, entered Dartmouth in the fall of 1848. He had something of a Dartmouth pedigree: Joseph Boyden—also from Beverly, Massachusetts (and presumably his brother)—appears in Dartmouth records as a nongraduate of the medical school class of 1833; more to the point, Charles's "Pa" was Wyatt Clark Boyden, an 1819 Phi Beta Kappa graduate of the College and an 1826 medical school graduate. We do not know why Joseph left without his degree, but Charles's failure to stay seems to have been because he could not resist the lure of the gold fields in the West.[88]

Charles's letter is a long one, giving us insights into his own habits and attitudes toward scholarship as well as into some aspects of how the school was run. "My Dear Parents," he began, on November 9, 1848:

> I have been much to blame for my negligence of writing you; I am very sorry for it, and will endeavour to do better in future. The Lectures closed on Monday. The Graduating Class, consisting of ten members, were examined on Tuesday and the forenoon of Wednesday, and received their Diplomas in the afternoon

in the Chapel, after the delivery of an Address from Dr. [Joseph H.] Smith of Dover, who is one of the Delegates from the N. H. Medical Society. . . . The Course of Lectures was throughout of high character as to the talents and ambitious endeavours in teaching, of the Professors. The Students were generally inclined to study and to improve their opportunities. The Graduates of Colleges were not generally superior to those who had not graduated. The best scholar in my opinion, was not a Graduate. I presume that I have attended at least two thirds of the Lectures. I have taken Notes, which are generally full.

—Of Prof.	Parker's lectures	— 2 pages		
Of "	Crosby's	"	—27 pages	
Of "	Phelp's [*sic*]	"	—18	"
" "	Hubbard's	"	— 8	"
" "	Roby's	"	— 5	"
" "	Peaslee's	"	— 7	"
In All——			67	"
Notes of Sermons—			3	"

I have also read the four Gospels in Greek, with the help of a translation. I am far from boasting of my application. I confess, am sorry for it & hope to do better—My Studies & other actions generally have been more the fruit of impulses than a true abiding principle, lighted by a steady aim for a grand result. I think however that I have learned enough to make a good Quack.[89]

William Child, a member of the medical school class of 1857, wrote a steady stream of letters to his wife while he was serving in the Civil War as an assistant surgeon in the Union Army. Detailed though his communications were, they tell little of medical interest beyond repeated observations about how dire the situation was for many of those wounded in battle, according to the author of an article based on those letters. Five days after the Battle of Antietam, for instance, Child wrote home: "Day before yesterday dressed the wounds of 64 different men—some having two or three [wounds] each. . . . The days after the battle are a thousand times worse than the day of the battle, and the physical pain is not the greatest pain suffered. . . . The dead appear sickening, but they suffer no pain. But the poor wounded, mutilated soldiers that yet have life and sensation make a most horrid picture."[90]

Learning no more than we do from these letters about Child's medical experiences (or competence), we gain little in the way of insight into how he did or did not benefit as a result of having attended and grad-

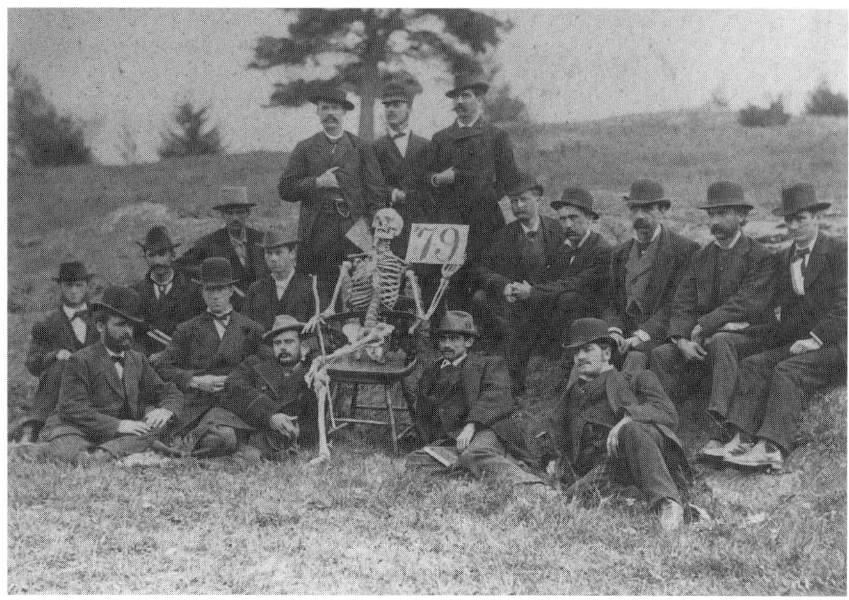

Class of 1879, posed with their "teaching assistant." Courtesy of Dartmouth Medical School.

uated from Dartmouth Medical School—though we know he was promoted to major and became his unit's chief surgeon. The story of William Child is nonetheless important, because he was the kind of young man Nathan Smith had in mind when he founded the Medical School. Born and raised in Bath, New Hampshire, some forty miles north of Hanover, Child was a prototypical local boy who took advantage of the fact that northern New England provided an opportunity for an academic medical education.

John Goodrich Henry, who graduated from Dartmouth Medical School in 1881, also left a cache of letters. His missives, written to his fiancée, are—in sharp contrast to Child's communiqués—full of rich detail about his medical work. Furthermore, Henry's story gives evidence both that those who needed medical assistance looked to Dartmouth and that a kind of old-boy network was definitely in place by the 1880s. Once again, we see how the medical school at Dartmouth played a role in bringing medical care to the people of northern New England.

In 1881, H. B. Flanders, the doctor serving the small village of West Fairlee, Vermont (about twenty miles north of Hanover, a few miles back in the hills), wrote to Frost at Dartmouth Medical School. No longer in good health, Flanders was looking for a doctor to help him out and possibly take over his practice. The timing turned out to be good. Frost sent the letter to John Henry, who had some eight months earlier graduated at the head of his medical school class, urging him to consider this chance to get into private practice.[91] Henry had already accepted a staff position in a privately run asylum in Winchendon, Massachusetts, but—having become engaged to Lola Manzer of that town—was apparently eager to earn more money than he could there. Dr. Flanders had an established practice, into which Henry was able to step—and needed to, since Flanders really was not at all well (he died a few weeks after Henry arrived). Life in the hill country was hard, and many of the people in the area worked at the Ely Mines. Such employment is bound to result in injuries; the new young doctor had plenty to keep him occupied. "I have been so busy this week that I hardly know which end my head is on," Henry wrote (August 15, 1881), and then "My work is getting the best of me" (September 18, 1881), and "I don't know how much longer I shall manage to exist if this run of work continues at the present rate" (November 6, 1881). Yet he did not seem to mind. He often reported proudly how many patients he had seen in a single day (and sometimes how much money he had taken in), with obvious satisfaction.

On the other hand, Henry was touchingly candid about how much his contacts with Frost (and others) in Hanover meant to him—when he could find time for them. Early on (August 21, 1881) he wrote enthusiastically, "Prof. Frost from Hanover was here last week and called to see me. You bet I was glad to see him." Three months later, he wrote somewhat plaintively, "I wanted awfully to go down to Hanover last week but could not leave my typhoid patients"—but he was also able to find grounds for pleasure in the situation as well: "Goodness heavens, here I am only one year out from College, tied up with so much practice that I cannot leave even for a single day" (November 20, 1881).

The most striking feature in the letters is not the range of cases that Dr. Henry found himself caring for, but his self-confidence and apparent competence. One measure is his willingness—one might even say eagerness—to take on the local "Dr. [Timothy G.] Simpson, our worthy competition" (August 21, 1881), whose care Henry repeatedly indicated was sub-par if not downright suspect.[92] Yet Henry was not averse to getting a second opinion on his own cases: "Had Dr. [Harry Bruce] Allen from White River Junction in consultation on one of my cases day before yesterday," he wrote on one occasion (October 6, 1881).[93]

Of course he could not save all his patients. "I have crawled out of one bad place. A week ago I had 3 or 4 cases which promised to die, and all are now on the high road to recovery but one, and she promised well till yesterday, when she had a hemorrhage from her bowels (a case of typhoid fever) and now will die." He was not oblivious to the sadness of the situation: "She is a splendid woman," he went on, "and has a large family of children, two of whom are now sick with the fever. There have been eight cases in that house this fall" (November 6, 1881). Hard-working, intelligent, competent, eager—John Goodrich Henry was a credit to Dartmouth Medical School. After returning to practice in Winchendon and marrying Lola Manzer, he established the first hospital there.[94]

This race through the nineteenth century gives only the barest sense of some of the leading figures on the Dartmouth Medical School faculty and what student life was like. As with most institutions, the main body of DMS developed tentacles so numerous and so intertwined that it is not possible here to trace each to its end. Some observers have suggested that there were "really no important events taking place in the medical department" in the middle part of the nineteenth century.[95] Those present at the time would have been unlikely to concur.

CHAPTER FOUR

Curricular Change

History is full of instances in which erroneous assumptions, so firmly held that their truth is never called in question, blind men to a truth which would otherwise be obvious. —SIR FREDERICK W. ANDREWES[1]

Expanding the Curriculum

As THE MIDDLE of the nineteenth century approached, there were at least some who believed the medical school at Dartmouth was making a valuable contribution to medical science and medical education in New Hampshire. Thomas Chadbourne, an 1813 graduate (he earned a second M.D. thirty years later, from Castleton Medical College in Vermont), was an established member of the state's medical community; he practiced in Concord for half a century.[2] In an undated communication, "Part of Delegates Report on the Examinations of 1845" (which he had written "to the New Hampshire medical Society"), Chadbourne's enthusiasm for Dartmouth Medical School is obvious:

In conclusion, your Delegates would again urge upon the consideration of the Society the claims of this school of medicine, not because "it is one of the oldest Institutions in the country," for it might be in decripid [*sic*] old age,—not because the Professors "are zealous in the discharge of their duties" and are "*endeavoring* to elevate the standard of medical science and striving to place the Institution on a firm basis," but because they *have* done all this. Neither would we appeal to the *patriotism* of the profession to sustain this school because "it is our *own*, & the only one in the State,"—It may be all this & yet unworthy [of] our patronage. But we would respectfully invite our brethren before sending their pupils elsewhere to examine & candidly compare the privileges enjoyed here with those of other kindred Institutions. We would refer them to the Library, now numbering over one thousand volumes of well selected Books, mostly modern, with a valuable collection of coloured plates and engravings illustrating the various departments of medical science. Then the *Museum* of *Materia Medica* and *Medical Botany* in which may be seen samples of all the medicines now used in actual Practice, together with beautifully coloured engravings of all the medical Plants described in the United States Dispensatory. . . . Next the *Anatomical Museum* containing more than 300 preparations . . . the whole well arranged and classified.[3]

What is not immediately clear is whether this glowing report reflected any real changes in the school's curriculum or its quality. More than three decades earlier, in 1812, the New Hampshire legislature had been faced with a petition from Nathan Smith for additional state funds to "defray the expenses of finishing the building" (known as the "Medical House"). Although the report of the duly appointed committee included a reminder that "Dr. Smith has legally conveyed one acre . . . of land, and assigned . . . anatomical and chemical apparatus to the state" and that the building itself as well as the land and all that apparatus was to be "exclusively the property of the state, on the death or removal of Dr. Smith, from the medical school." Although the committee report was favorable, the extra funds were nonetheless denied. Levi Jackson, writing for the legislative committee, concluded his assessment as follows:

At present, the medical institution at Hanover affords to students of medicine all the means of a correct and useful education. The number of students for the last three or four years, we believe to have been greater than at any medical school in the United States, that at Philadelphia excepted.[4] The reputation of the school is deservedly high. Its connection with Dartmouth College increases the usefulness and celebrity of that literary institution. On the whole, we do not hesitate to declare that this medical school is worthy [of] the patronage of the legislature.[5]

Written by a nonphysician, this report was of course not so detailed as Chadbourne's, but the overall impression given is certainly still of a judgment of quality. So what, if anything, was different?

Spot checks through the century will have to suffice to give us some sense of what was considered important or essential as both the School and medicine itself changed. We have already seen how chemistry, in particular, presented a challenge for Nathan Smith and his early colleagues. Even when James Freeman Dana and subsequent science instructors like Benjamin Hale and Oliver P. Hubbard joined the faculty, the focus of their teaching was geology—which basically meant mineralogy—though Hubbard's title in 1837 was "Professor of Chemistry." His counterpart in the College, Professor Ira Young, kept the telescope in his own back garden until Smith's former student and old friend George Cheyne Shattuck gave the College money enough to construct a proper observatory.[6] In 1836 Hubbard also wrote a letter of complaint about facilities at Dartmouth to his father-in-law, Benjamin Silliman, the outstanding chemistry professor at Yale who was to become the most influential chemist of his generation. The laboratory, Hubbard opined, was "almost a *nonentity*." He did, however, have high praise for the library collections (which included a complete run of Silliman's own *American Journal of Science and Arts*).[7]

Dartmouth did not suffer alone, however. Colleges and medical schools generally struggled over how, or whether, to teach chemistry, hampered as they were by poor equipment as well as a good deal of poor teaching. Theories about phlogiston—a substance supposedly emitted during combustion—had chemists everywhere squabbling among themselves. Still, by 1838 a few colleges did at least have lab assistants as well as professors of chemistry, and by the 1850s America was gradually becoming less dependent on imported glassware. Yet as late as 1869, when Charles Eliot became president of Harvard, one of the first reforms he considered it necessary to implement was enlargement of the chemistry laboratory. Some indication of how novel chemistry was as a medical school subject can be seen from the fact that even under Eliot, it was not until 1890 that the Harvard faculty introduced a new course in "medical chemistry" for first-year students who had satisfactorily passed an examination in undergraduate chemistry studies. And as Harvard historians have noted, Eliot was actually "remarkably uncertain about the role of his own subject, chemistry, in medical teaching."[8] (This was despite his arguing forcefully that medical education badly needed attention; he made reform of the medical school's administration and curriculum one of his first goals.[9]) So strongly did Eliot feel about the issue that he raised it already in his inaugural address. Science teaching, he pronounced, should be done with "objects and instruments in hand—not from books merely, not through the memory chiefly, but by the seeing eye and the informing fingers."[10] One can imagine that Eliot would have very much liked the therapeutics textbook (more a reference book, actually) published by Robert Thaxter Edes in 1887, shortly before his brief stint on the Dartmouth Medical School faculty in 1891–1892. In the preface, Edes wrote that he had "constantly endeavored to utilize and . . . harmonize the data of experimental physiology and chemistry with those of thoroughly digested experience."[11]

Among the reasons for difficulties in chemistry at Dartmouth were the purely administrative complications that arose from having faculty with dual appointments, as we saw in the controversies over Benjamin Hale's status on the faculty and over Oliver Hubbard's claim to fee money over and above his salary. When Hubbard resigned the chemistry chair, we find in the trustees' records the same language used as when Mussey was made a committee of one in 1835 to find a "suitable person" to teach chemistry. Once again, in 1867, the trustees reported the need to look for "a suitable person to give instruction in Chemistry."[12] Two years later, the ongoing concern was noted again in the trustees' records.[13]

Some hint of the nature of the concern over how much and what to teach under the heading of "science" appears in a letter from E. W. Dimond, a chemistry instructor in the College, to the then-president of the College, Asa Dodge Smith, early in 1869. "If Prof. Hitchcock is here only six weeks there will be three weeks this term and the five weeks in the summer term during which the Seniors will have no studies in Science."[14] If medicine was in "a low state" in the days of Josiah Goodhue and Nathan Smith, inspiring Smith to found the school in the first place, medical science seems to have continued in that condition for decades. In fact, the author of one history of the School simply says briskly that the "content of the Chemistry that was taught is . . . problematic." Those were kind words, a generous assessment.[15]

In 1878 a step forward in the teaching of science was taken when it was decided to hire a second person to teach chemistry; Edwin J. Bartlett was elected to assist Hubbard.[16] How promptly that appointment resulted in raising the standard in chemistry courses is open to debate. Consider Bartlett's own reflections (forty-five years after he was hired) on the state of affairs at the time:

> "Chemistry is no use anyway", said the student. And he was right as it was taught, as it had to be taught. A few lectures and no laboratory work, or the minimum of elementary fumbling was all the student got. If he could pass the ABC's of chemistry and glibly supply a few formulas of no more value in themselves than the spelling of c-a-t, he never wanted to hear of it again. And yet he was going forth to aid the most complicated chemical machine in the world to do its work aright. The time was not ripe. The older practitioner knew no valuable chemistry; it had not been brought into practical form for the student.[17]

Five years later, in 1883, the trustees took still further action in their continuing effort to improve the teaching of chemistry: "Dr. Frost appeared in behalf of the Faculty of the Medical College to ask if opportunity can be given to the Medical Students for Laboratory work and instruction in Culver Hall, whereupon Voted. That the Board is disposed to grant any facilities to the Medical Students whi[ch] are practicable without prejudice to the present occupants of the buildings."[18]

Such arrangements were in fact satisfactorily made—though it took time. In 1892, a communication from Bartlett (by then promoted to full professor) was received concerning the need for more "accommodations" (space) in the "chemical laboratory."[19] Occasional notes like this in the trustees' records constitute evidence of a growing understanding that science (chemistry in particular) was crucial to medical and "academical" study alike.[20] And for all the difficulties that chemistry presented, no one seems ever to have considered dropping it from the curriculum. In 1893 a professorship in biology was added along with professorships in history, social science, and bibliography, and an instructorship in "Physical Training." Obviously this was a time of general expansion of the curriculum in the College.[21]

What looks like the first real shift in emphasis in the science curriculum came with the formal introduction of "medical botany" as a discipline in its own right. From the outset, "Materia Medica" had been taught; it was one of the several "branches" the trustees approved as part of the curriculum in Smith's day. A science course of sorts, it was more in pharmacy than pharmacology. Although the trustees had resolved in 1820 that one of the members of the "Faculty of the Medical department" should be "A Prof. of Theory & Practice of Physic, Materia Medica & Botany," and Daniel Oliver was appointed to fill that position, a later list of what he taught does not include "Botany," medical or otherwise.[22] (How "medical botany" differed from "materia medica" would in any case have been as much as anything a function of the particular interests of the instructor in question.) It appears that the medical school was already forty years old before a course actually called "Medical Botany" was first offered (in 1838), by Stephen West Williams, and it did not last long.

Three years later, Edward Elisha Phelps replaced Williams as lecturer in medical jurisprudence and medical botany, but medical botany seems to have been dropped after 1849; thereafter it does not appear as an area of responsibility for anyone in the list of faculty. One factor may have been that Phelps was teaching such a large array of subjects; he was listed as *professor* of materia medica and later of therapeutics as well. After many years as professor of the theory and practice of medical as well as of pathological anatomy, in 1871 he added general pathology to his professorial offerings. Small wonder that he was no longer teaching medical botany, which by that time had in any case gone largely out of fashion. As early as the end of the first third of the century, botanic medicines had come to be largely the province of the followers of Samuel Thomson, the first "to capitalize on the growing suspicion of the medical profession," and other "irregular" practitioners.[23] The growing popularity of a certain amount of therapeutic nihilism led to a decline in enthusiasm for intervention in the form of any kind of medicines and drugs—except in minuscule quantities.[24]

Obstetrics and the diseases of women and children became a course in its own right—the topics were presented together—for the first time in 1838.[25] John Delamater, twelve years after receiving his medical degree from Berkshire Medical College, had joined the Dartmouth faculty in 1836 as professor of the theory and practice of medicine; two years later he became professor of materia medica, obstetrics and the diseases of women and children. The latter responsibilities were picked up in 1840 by the estimable Dixi Crosby, who taught these subjects (along with others) until 1870—except that the diseases of women as a separate course was turned over to Edmund Randolph Peaslee in 1868, who had been teaching anatomy and physiology. Peaslee, incidentally, had published a path-breaking text, *Human Histology*, in 1857, among the earliest in this field.[26] His most important work, *Ovarian Tumors*—first published in 1872—was used as a standard text for many years.[27]

In 1881, the trustees voted "That the following professorships be established in the New Hampshire Medical College [yet another name for Dartmouth Medical School] but without giving their occupants a vote in the medical faculty: viz. A professorship of mental diseases, a professorship of Laryngology, and a professorship of ophthalmology." Elected, respectively, were the three men who had already been lecturers in these fields at Dartmouth: Jesse Parker Bancroft, Louis Elsberg, and William Wallace Seely.[28] There was at least talk about introducing hygiene as a course also as early as 1881.[29]

That there were misgivings about this move emerges in a letter from one of the well-established faculty members—Professor Lyman B. How—to Frost: "If Elsberg and Seely and Bartlett and Bancroft all give special courses, I don't see how we can get in a course on Hygiene this year. And I am not in favor of trying unless we can get some first-rate man like Billings."[30] The trustees finally established a chair of hygiene in 1895; Granville P. Conn was "unanimously elected Professor."[31] Then, when Conn retired in 1909, Howard Nelson Kingsford added hygiene to his teaching assignments, which already included histology as well as bacteriology and pathology. The curriculum was becoming crowded, though not until several years into the twentieth century were *clinical* surgery or *clinical* medicine listed among the disciplines being taught. The former seems to have been offered first by William Thayer Smith.[32] John Martin Gile took over clinical surgery in 1910; that same year, Gilman DuBois Frost became the first professor of clinical medicine.[33]

Anatomy and the Need for Cadavers

A constant—and constantly troubling—part of the curriculum from the beginning was anatomy. No one doubted its value, nor were qualified instructors in short supply. All concerned agreed that an anatomy course was a critical part of what any medical school should offer. The problem, beginning already in Smith's day, was how to get enough bodies (or "subjects," as cadavers were somewhat euphemistically called) for students to do the work they needed to do. (One of the reasons Smith left Dartmouth for Yale was his hope that in New Haven he would have less difficulty finding and acquiring cadavers, as well as less direct personal responsibility for doing so.) And the need for "subjects" was the major theme that, all during the nineteenth century, ran through the curriculum melody—no matter how many variations on it were played. Dartmouth was no different from other medical schools in this regard. At all medical institutions, "body-snatching" was an issue. The problem was only very partially and unsatisfactorily solved by changes in the laws governing the acquisition of bodies, despite A. B. Crosby's claim in 1870 that "[m]odern legislators, wiser than their fathers, have rendered it easy for the medical student to legitimately pursue the study of practical anatomy without wounding the sensibilities of the living and without desecrating the graves of the dead."[34] But as has also been pointed out, "[e]nactment of laws is one phase of the problem, their enforcement is quite a different matter. The vast majority of illegal disinterments were not discovered. . . . Arrests and indictments were few, and convictions yet fewer."[35]

By comparison to other towns and cities that were home to medical schools, however, Hanover was relatively quiet when it came to body-snatching and the digging up of bodies. A few minor fracases over such "resurrectionist" activity—alleged or actual—have taken place over the years in and around Hanover, clearly perpetrated by Dartmouth students.[36] And at least one future faculty member, Dixi Crosby, apparently arrived in Hanover to begin his life as a student with a body in tow. Gilman D. Frost, in the "Introductory Lecture" that it was his turn to give in 1895, told the story as follows:

> The difficulties in the way of obtaining an adequate supply of material for dissection in those early days are illustrated by the experiences of one of Dr Mussey's pupils, Dr Dixi Crosby, who graduated here in 1824. After the custom of those days when he left [the town of] Sandwich in this State, he came to Hanover for the study of medicine, he brought with him a body for dissection, doubtless obtained in a questionable manner. His townspeople hearing of this fact became much enraged & made many threats of future vengeance. Crosby, however, did his dissecting undisturbed, and when he settled later, chose Sandwich to begin in, & within a short time built up *an excellent* practice.[37]

So at least in some instances, outraged citizens could be mollified. The faculty was undeniably grateful to Crosby for his ability to acquire cadavers. At an 1848 faculty meeting it was voted (without comment) "to purchase of Dr. Crosby three subjects which he had procured last spring, for use during the present course of lectures & the next annual course, for the sum of $90."[38] Such affairs were often handled completely matter-of-factly.

At the tail end of the nineteenth century, the problem still existed. Winding up his centennial oration, Phineas Conner—who after one year as a lecturer in surgery had been professor of surgery for twenty years—railed against the status quo:

> If Dartmouth is to give proper fundamental training, she must have and continue to have the right of legitimately securing ample anatomical material. If she does not get it and cannot get it, her decay is as certain as fate. If she is worth saving, let her have what she needs. . . . Let the State, let the town, let the Judiciary decide which it prefers, educated physicians in whose hands may rest the life or death of the best beloved, or sentimental regard for the welfare of the animal, and half civilized worship of the decaying body. Give Dartmouth the needed means and facilities for teaching and she will be a training school of the highest order, fitting her men to later learn the practical work of the profession in the midst of the diseases and injuries of the great cities.[39]

Between the purchase of Crosby's cadavers and the time of Conner's address there were many similar pleas and expressions of concern. Two of the letters from How to Frost that have survived make especially vivid just how awkward and difficult it could still be in the early 1880s to obtain bodies, despite the legislative act whose passage had led Crosby to enthuse that the problem was solved. From Manchester, New Hampshire, where he lived and practiced when he was not lecturing in Hanover, How wrote:

> I cannot get anything here in the city—not at present at any rate.
>
> The alms house of this county is way over to Wilton—ten miles out in the woods from anywhere. I have been trying to get a chance to go over there . . . but it has been so all fired cold and business has been so unusually driving I have not yet found an opportunity. However, this past week I have got on a new scent and shall follow it up. I understand blockade running is renewed in New York and Montreal now and that you are being better supplied than you was [*sic*]. Arrivals are reported here also.[40]

Another letter a little more than a year later carried a more optimistic report:

> I have been over to Wilton—a whole days journey. Started at 8 A.M. by [train] via Nashua [changing trains in Nashua to get from Manchester to Wilton]; then rode from Wilton village with Dr. Geo. Hatch, 80, five miles to the County Farm way up on the side of Temple mountain. . . . It is terribly healthy up there and almost everybody dies of old age—of the dried up form at that. There were three unclaimed bodies there last year that would have been useful—two fair

ones and one suicide a first rate one. The Suptdt is a very sensible fellow and will do anything in his power.[41]

The problem would persist for at least another fifty years.

Curricular Reform

Professor How's correspondence leaves us with another useful bit of insight into curricular concerns during the latter part of the nineteenth century. In an unusually detailed letter to Frost early in 1878, the extent of How's interest in reshaping the curriculum becomes clear. While others may have been equally engaged by the subject, their proposals (if written) for just how the proper division and balance in the curriculum was to be achieved have not survived. How's letter helps show how complicated a matter it was to work out the schedule at a time when there was no established or agreed-upon precedent.

I think my chair should be divided and a course and a half of lectures allowed for the two departments [Anatomy and Physiology]. . . . I told you last Fall I was ready for a division of my chair, but I have never seen how it could be done and suitable time secured with the existing order of giving the various courses. But all is changed now and your idea of including Obstetrics and Gynaecology in one 3/4 chair opens the way in part for the carrying out of an improved schedule. We thus gain 1/4 for a chair of Physiology and the other 1/4 can be obtained by cutting down Chemistry to a 3/4 chair. We shall then, I think, have as many lectures on *Chemistry* as are given in country schools and we shall have a course and a half on Anatomy and Physiol.—the same as is given at Burlington [University of Vermont] and Bowdoin [Medical School of Maine]. . . . Making these changes, a schedule of lectures could be made on something like the following plan to which I can think of no considerable objection.

Whole course divided into eighths.

1/8	2/8	3/8	4/8	5/8	6/8	7/8	8/8
Surgery				Practice			
Anatomy				Ordronaux[42]	Chemistry		
Obstet. & Gynaecol.			Physiology		Therapeutics		

Physiology will thus begin before Anatomy is completed. I think this would be no disadvantage for so short a time; the lectures could be so arranged as to *dove*tail into each other. Chemistry could be written where Physiology is above, but it would be very inconvenient for us all to get along in the laboratory together. As to the desirability of the above changes my mind is fully made up. But can we bring them about this year?[43]

The similarities to and differences from other fully laid-out schedules of lectures—like the one that follows next, from three decades earlier—are instructive, though we do not know precisely all the shifts and changes that were made in the intervening thirty years. The term beginning in August 1846 was to run sixteen weeks (the year before it had been only fourteen weeks) and the schedule was to be as follows:

Voted . . . the first 8 weeks be as follows:

	8 A.M.	9 A.M.	10 A.M.	11 A.M.	4 P.M.
Monday	Surgery	Theory & Practice	Chemistry	Anatomy	Theory & Practice
Tuesday	Surgery	Theory & Practice	Anatomy	———	Mat. Medica
Wednesday	Mat. Med.	" "	Chemistry	———	Theory & Practice
Thursday	Surgery	" "	Chemistry	Anatomy	Theory & Practice
Friday	Surgery	" "	Chemistry	Anatomy	———
Saturday	Mat. Med.	" "	———	———	———

The Schedule for the last 8 weeks of the term is arranged as follows:

	9 A.M.	10 A.M.	11 A.M.	3 P.M.	4 P.M.
Monday	Crosby	Hubbard	Peaslee	Crosby	———
Tuesday	Crosby	"	"	"	Phelps
Wednesday	Phelps	"	"	"	———
Thursday	Crosby	"	"	"	———
Friday	Crosby	"	"	"	Phelps
Saturday	Phelps	Crosby	———	———	———

Lectures on Medical Jurisprudence were to be "superadded to those contained in the Schedule," and given in the last part of October.[44]

Since at least the early 1840s, there had been a summer term. A notice in the *Boston Medical & Surgical Journal* announced that the Dartmouth Medical School faculty was to offer a three-month summer session, "a systematic course of instruction."[45] The use of the summer term for visiting professors was a way to bring more and different lecturers to Dartmouth than the school could otherwise possibly have afforded. The result (for many years) was a split faculty, with only some in residence. Scheduling the nonresident faculty was typically an awkward and time-consuming business. In 1881, Louis Elsberg wrote to Frost, in part, as follows: "In answer to your kind letter of yesterday I want to say that I look forward to being with you to lecture, with very much pleasure. Can you arrange to have the lectures either very early in July or else in September? I have an idea of running over to London to attend the

International Med. Congress but will not go if *going & lecturing in Hanover* are incompatible."[46]

Other pieces of correspondence in the archives indicate that ad hoc scheduling of this sort was not an isolated occurrence, that numerous members of the faculty were nonresident instructors, and that there was often uncertainty about just what lectures would be given in a term. On February 21, 1890, David Webster wrote thus to Frost: "Your favor informing me of my election to the Professorship of Ophthalmology in Dartmouth Medical College has been received. Please convey my thanks. . . . I would prefer to begin my lectures on the 16th of July, so as to get through with them early and have the month of August to spend in vacation." Eighteen months later, on August 16, 1891, Charles Loomis Dana also wrote, proposing a new arrangement for *his* lectures, saying to Frost:

> I am anxious to do all I can in my professional chair but I can not at present afford to devote two weeks to lecturing. As it happened my week last year cost me a good deal. It is quite natural you should not care to try new hands; but I should certainly not recommend [John Winters Brannan] if I did not think it would be advantageous to the school. . . . The only scheme I can propose now would be this: I will begin lecturing Sept. 7th & lecture for a week; to be followed for a week by Dr. Brannan.[47]

These individually made arrangements were critical, we are told. It "would not have been possible to secure lecturers of the highest ability had it not been for the attractions of a Hanover summer and of a session which at its longest continued from the middle of July to Thanksgiving, thus allowing those who must return to metropolitan engagements to give their lectures in the first half."[48]

A complex exchange between Frost and Alfred Mitchell at the Medical School of Maine over exactly what should be offered, and when, gives insight into efforts in the 1880s to develop standards for the medical curriculum that would then be followed by each of the three medical schools in northern New England. What courses should constitute a complete program and who would give the lectures were only part of the issue. Lengthening the course of study—the advisability of increasing it to twenty weeks—was also on the agenda as one way to raise standards. A memo and letter from Frost to his colleagues on the faculty explained what had emerged from the meeting:

> The object of this meeting was to consider a proposition to lengthen our terms of instruction to twenty (20) weeks. The result of conference was that we submit to the Faculties of the several Colleges the following propositions.—
> Prop. 1 After the Session of 1885 the Requirements for Graduation shall be
> (1) Three years Study of Medicine

(2) 21 years of age
(3) Two Courses of Lectures of twenty weeks each
(4) Fifteen months between beginning of first course & end of last
(5) A Preliminary (entrance) examination
(6) The final Examination to be written.
Prop. 2 After 1885
(1) Three years Study of Medicine
(2) Two Courses of Lectures of *16* weeks each
(3) Fifteen months between beginning of 1st & End of Last Course—
(4) 21 years of age
(5) Preliminary (Entrance) Ex- [*sic*]
Prop. 3 After 1885
(1) Three years of Study of Medicine
(2) Two Courses of Lectures of 16 weeks each
(3) Fifteen months between beginning of 1st & End of Last Course—
(4) 21 years of age . . .
Respectfully Submitted, C.P. Frost
When ought to be added our present requirement of *dissection* of what parts of the cadaver.

In the accompanying letter, Frost clarified several points and gave his position.

Gentlemen,

. . . We stated to the gentlemen the difficulties which seem to me to be almost or quite insuperable in our case to lengthening our term to 20 weeks. The tendencies of the Schools are to have a vacation in July & Aug. . . . So we can hardly begin earlier than we now do. . . . With our present corps of teachers we cannot begin later or continue much later without very serious inconvenience. Bowdoin can very easily begin so as to get 20 weeks before the College Com. in June. Burlington does not wish to lengthen the term but possibly will if Bowd. & Dart. do so. They feel happy now & swear they will have 300 students next term. They have just issued an edition of 70.000 Announcements at a cost of $3000 & intend to send one to Every doctor in the U.S. of America & contiguous Nations. . . .

While I greatly favor the 20 weeks term on general principles I cannot vote for it in our case—& can only vote for the 2^d^ Proposition with the Dissection classes added & No 6 of 1st Prop.

Respy, C. P. Frost

At the bottom, the votes of the faculty members were recorded. The most complete response came from Phineas Sanborn Conner: "Yes to the full five [in fact there were six] parts of Prop. 1. With the added dissecting classes—and an additional one providing for the appointment of a Supervisory Committee to watch Burl^ton^ which has all the vices of N.Y. without its virtues. Add on the extra 4 weeks anywhere in the course of the year and fight Burlington with its own weapons." This final remark showed that cooperative efforts were likely to go only so far; there was genuine competition among the New England medical schools and some concern about Dartmouth holding its own.[49]

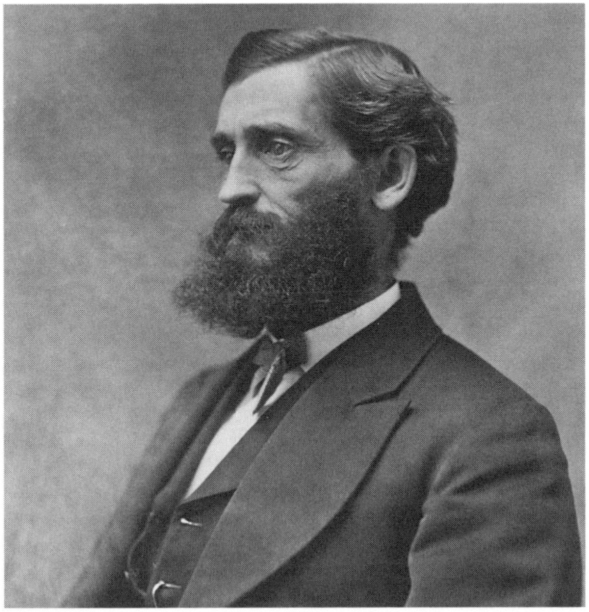

Carlton P. Frost, DMS class of 1852. Courtesy of Dartmouth Medical School.

Course Content

Unfortunately, the evidence we have about the actual content of courses is fragmentary. Course catalogs as we know them today did not exist for most of the nineteenth century.[50] More typical were brochures like the one from 1825 that listed the faculty, mentioned the four lectures daily "in the various branches of medical science," and then in six pages of prose gave a general description of what the school had to offer. The extant pamphlets show gradual growth in the size of the faculty and consequently in what could be offered to students. The 1840 "Annual Circular," for example, boasted—in addition to the president, three faculty members, and two New Hampshire Medical Society delegates (also listed in the 1825 brochure)—two lecturers, one demonstrator for anatomy, one curator of the museum, and one librarian. That year the faculty was for the most part in residence; a note was appended indicating that "All the Faculty, with the exception of Dr. [Stephen West] Williams, will lecture during the whole term."

The 1841 flyer, like the one from 1840, also announced that "Private Medical Instruction" was available without clarifying just what that meant. An addition to the usual material was a page on which the names of graduates and their thesis titles were listed. In 1844, what appears to be a new feature was the list of the thirty-eight operations students had had the opportunity to see performed before the class (or elsewhere, for those able to attend); reasonably full course descriptions were included as well, as they were also in 1846. The announcement bulletins for 1874, 1875, and 1876 contained lists of prizes and of textbooks being used—but no course descriptions.[51] Finally, by 1895, the "Circular of Information, Dartmouth Medical College" included a schedule of classes as well as such details as the fact that an innovative recitation term of twenty-three weeks was to be followed by the lecture term of twenty weeks, which in turn was to be followed by an exam. (The way the recitation class altered the curriculum is discussed in chapter 5.) The very fact that such brochures continued to be published on a fairly regular basis is one indication that an effort was being made to regularize degree requirements; this was made easier by the relative stability of the faculty over several decades.

Despite these brochures, it remains difficult to determine exactly what was being taught. Even a close study of all the extant student notebooks would not give anything like a complete picture, because which notebooks from which courses happen to have survived is quite chancy. Jesse Little, for example, took notes on Reuben Mussey's "Obstetricks Lecture 1st" on November 14, 1826, but fewer than fifty pages of notes altogether appear in this part of his notebook. (Turning the book around and reading from back to front, we find more than a hundred pages that begin with notes on "Theory & Practice," taken from Daniel Oliver's course in 1824.) Lewis Emmons's "Medical Notebook 1827–1830" is in two volumes, one of 100 pages and the other twice as long (with some blank pages) and in a neat hand; more could clearly be learned from his notes.[52] There is, however, no way of knowing why students broke off in their note taking where they did—whether the lectures ended or the students ran out of paper, lost interest, or quit attending lectures. And the quality of the notes varies a great deal.

Professors' lecture notes could in principle provide information on course content. Few seem to have been left. One example, from much later in the century, is the bound and typed set of notes for twenty-eight lectures on gynecology, by Paul Fortunatus Mundé, who taught that subject for twenty years (1880–1901), first as lecturer and then as professor, following Edward Swift Dunster's two-year stint as professor of gynecology. Mundé later also became professor of obstetrics in 1888, once again following his colleague Dunster. A note headed "1885" and inserted in the volume of notes lists the lecture titles in a rather different order, indicating that he at least varied the sequence of topics somewhat from year to year. A few corrections inserted in hand and some underlining for emphasis give these notes an immediacy that is utterly lacking when all we know is the name of the course or what discipline a given professor was supposed to teach.[53] Another distinguished member of the DMS faculty in gynecology, who may very well have used his own books as course textbooks (at Dartmouth and elsewhere—he taught at several institutions), was John Osborn Polak; his *Manual of Obstetrics, Students' Manual of Gynæcology* and his *Pelvic Inflammation in Women* each went through several editions.[54]

A very different kind of insight into what students were doing, seeing, and learning comes from the letter written by Charles Boyden, a portion of which was quoted earlier.

> There have been about twenty operations during the course, including 10 excisions of the tonsil, 9 amputations above the knee, 2 for Cataract, 1 for fistula lachrymalis, 1 for Necrosis, 2 for Hydrocele, besides others upon tumours & wounds. Dr. Peaslee's private term for the study of Anatomy & Physiology commences not quite three weeks hence, on the 30th of Nov. & ends about the 10th of Feb. Dr. Crosby probably, and Dr. Hubbard will not commence until spring. During this Vacation, I have access to the Library and liberty to examine the articles in Dr. Hill's Apothecary store. Dr. Hill remembers Pa as a Classmate in his first course of Lectures.[55]
>
> Hanover will be comparitively [*sic*] quiet soon, as most of the students will be absent keeping school.[56] . . .
>
> I have $10. In about a month, I shall want more . . . to pay my tuition fee $15; and to pay my present board & incidentals. It will cost me this winter probably some more than two dollars a week for board, rent, wood & oil. . . .
>
> I see no advantage in removing from this place for [a] good while to come. Now I am in Hanover, I wish to understand the place & and Professors pretty well.

We are further indebted to Boyden for not wanting to waste the rest of the sheet of paper, for he then proceeded to give summaries quite unlike the notes most students actually took in class. The result is that, instead of the precise words of the professor, we get a student reaction to what was being taught. Boyden went on, thus:

> Dr. Crosby's Introductory.—He had an experience of nearly a quarter of a century. Upon this he should found his lectures; not giving the theories of others, but his own observations.
>
> To understand simple truth, few words are necessary. His style would be practical or axiomic. We had done well in chooseing our profession. There is always much practice to be done. Surgery at the present time is advanced more than ever before—and as illustrious Professors & Masters adorn the sciences as ever did at any period. We have ample encouragement to proceed.
>
> How shall we obtain practice?—the diploma is of no assistance, knowledge is the power. The Master of one book or one system is the man. Good habits

are necessary. We should determine to stand or fall on right principles. No matter what book we study or where we go to practice—get knowledge, it is wanted and we shall be found out.

Pfo. Parker's Introductory.—Medical Jurisprudence may be subdivided into *Medical Jurisprudence*, a department of law and *Legal medicine*, a department of medicine. We trace this branch of study to Germany.

Its Professorships have been established within the present century.

A physician should have some knowledge of the nature of legal evidence, otherwise he will not understand many questions that may be put him and be exposed to other difficulties in the delivery, which may subject him to mortification. If he should thereby lose his temper he would be likely to be a loser, as the Lawyer is at home & fighting with his own weapons. &c.

Prof. Peaslee's Introductory.—A humerous [*sic*] exordium was pointed with the motto—"Be shure you are right, then go ahead." "Ne quid Nimis" or the not medicating too much is a point in which the Profession has much improved within the last fifty years. Medicines never heal, but they do assist Nature—the vis naturae Medicatrix which preserves the equilibrium & restores it, either alone or with the aid of medicine.

When the recuperative energy is unimpaired, use no medicine (of any power at least) in slight illnesses and the mildest forms of self limited diseases. Medicine is essential in severe cases. Be not exclusive in practice, but like the Bee, cull the good wherever found.

And then, abruptly, he was at the end of the page. Urging his parents "Please to write soon," he signed off.[57]

Doctors in the Making

The number of students to whom this ever-changing curriculum was being taught fluctuated wildly during the nineteenth century, in the latter years reaching more than 100 with some frequency.[58] Of course more is not necessarily better. One thing we do know, quality and qualifications apart, is that representatives of minority groups were few and far between among the students. (The complete absence of women is notable but hardly unusual for the times.) There was a curious remark in a letter the student Parsons Whidden wrote in 1828 to the effect that the "The Girls don't attend the Chimical Lectures as they have hereto fore."[59] Far from being an indication that female students had been admitted at that point, however, this is just another instance of the fuzzy line that was drawn between "public lectures" on the one hand and academic lectures open only to students who could produce admission tickets for which they had duly paid. We learned earlier that townspeople flocked to Oliver Wendell Holmes's lectures. Prior to that, too, we know that Alexander Ramsay gave lectures that were genuinely open to the public. He was not only to teach anatomy but to offer a course on "natural theology" as well.[60] William Tully had worried that "[t]he ladies," who were invited to attend Ramsay's "hints, on Medical Education," might "Tumble to pieces."[61] Later in the century a custom was established of having a different member of the faculty each year give a formal "Introductory Lecture."[62] The general public—including women—attended. The faculty minutes from August 3, 1880, begin thus: "The Lecture Introductory to the Eighty-Fourth annual Course of Lectures was delivered in the Medical Lecture Room, by Prof. L. B. How . . . in the presence of a goodly number of Gentlemen of the College and their wives together with ladies & gentlemen from the village citizens & Strangers with a large number of Medical Students."[63]

In 1852, Dartmouth missed a dramatic opportunity to set a historical precedent when it refused the "request of Miss Emily Blackwell of Cincinnati to be admitted to the present course of lectures." At their August meeting, the resident faculty (comprising Crosby, Phelps, and Peaslee) "Voted that in the opinion of this Faculty we should not be justified by the medical profession of New England in complying with her request."[64] Blackwell, whose sister Elizabeth had recently graduated from Geneva Medical School in New York (making her the first woman in the United States "to receive a diploma from a regular medical school") was not to be deterred. She found a warmer welcome in her home state of Ohio, at Western Reserve Medical College, from which she graduated in 1854.[65] Women applicants just were not taken very seriously at Dartmouth. In the trustees' records twenty years later, there is a note that the "question of admitting females to the privileges of the College [never mind the medical school] was referred to a committee"—which was to consist of the president and three others. Whether the committee ever reported back is not clear. No move was made in favor of admitting women for many, many decades.[66]

As for minority students, the record is also very thin. A few did make the cut. In at least one case Dartmouth did, to its credit, take a bolder stand than a fellow institution had. Samuel McGill, a young black man from Liberia, had been sponsored by a group of liberal religious leaders who supported his study of medicine at Washington College (one of Baltimore's several medical schools) in the mid-1830s. Predictably, McGill was not welcomed—though one might not have expected the student body to object so vigorously as to go on strike. McGill's chief benefactor, one Moses Sheppard, stood by his protégé, and "after much negotiation, secured entrance for [him] to Dartmouth College. . . . In due course Samuel McGill was graduated with an MD and honors from Dartmouth College."[67] Discussions of only a few other "Negro" or "colored" students appear in the faculty minutes: Dempsey Rollo Fletcher in 1846, Isaac H. Snowden and Alexander Lang in 1851, and Daniel Laing in 1854.[68] Fletcher graduated from the medical school in 1847 and Laing in 1854; Snowden is listed as a nongraduate of the class of 1851. Dartmouth clearly was not a vigorous pioneer in making medical (or general academic) education available to members of minority groups, despite having been founded for the purpose of assisting Native Americans.

The students who did graduate with medical degrees from Dartmouth, however, were for the most part ones of whom the school could be proud. A dozen or so of the early graduates from the school's history were among those who helped found the Maine Medical Society in 1820. James Goodwin, one of those founders of the Society, told a tale about himself that makes him sound like exactly the kind of bold and self-confident surgeon of which Nathan Smith was the premier model:

> Other doctors had been called in consultation, and all of these refused to have anything to do with murdering the patient as they harshly called my suggestion that amputation ought be done and at once. So I got the patient's consent . . . [and] set to work as rapidly as I could. . . . Everything went well that day at least. We had a very anxious time during convalescence, but it finally came out all right, and the patient grew up to be over seventy years or more before she died.[69]

Examinations

But how much were the students really learning? An accurate assessment is not easy to make. We have already seen the rather discouraging account of chemistry that Edwin Bartlett gave retrospectively, and Charles Boyden's summary of introductory remarks made by various professors at the beginning of the term—while interesting—provides too little information to make a judgment. Only occasionally do we have a record of what questions were being posed to the students. Some idea of what students were expected to have learned can be deduced from the examination questions, of which scattered examples are still extant. (See Appendix B on page 294 for the 1888 version.) Most are cryptic, however; since students were examined orally, it is not surprising that the professors simply made notes to themselves about the topic on which they planned to grill the students. Thus, for instance, on a scrap of paper dated June 1886, we find six items listed—including "Peculiarities of the RT Auricle" and "Ligaments of the knee joint." A sheet headed "Examination in Therapeutics, 1880" is a bit more discursive, with nine items of the following sort: "Tonics—Define. Give difference between tonic action of Iron and Quinia"; "Opium—Dangers from its use with the very young—How use safely?"; and "Vomiting: Measures & Means for its arrest."[70] But if we look at some of the records of student performance in the final exams, we can at least see what their examiners (professors and delegates from the state medical societies) thought of them.

In a notebook "Kept by Dixi Crosby" (as noted on its frontispiece), the "Results of Examinations of Candidates for the Degree of MD" at the end of each term, commencing with the year 1841, are listed. (This particular record runs to 1860; where results from 1842 and 1843 should be, the pages are blank.) The examinations for 1856 have some special interest, because among the candidates was none other than the future faculty leader, Carlton P. Frost. (A local boy, he had prepared at Thetford Academy, in nearby Thetford, Vermont.). Frost was not the weakest student—but neither was he the strongest, if the recorded examination results can be taken as a fair measure.

Among those on deck for the "Medical Examinations Nov. 11. 1856," C. W. Hunt of Gilford, New Hampshire (No. 8 on the exam list), had some manifest difficulties:

> Anat. & Physiology—Well
> Chem and Pharmacy—Poor
> Mat.. Med & Therapeutics—Fair
> Theo. & Prac & Pathol^{y}—well
> Surgery & Obstetrics.—[blank]

Delegates NH. Med. Soc^{y}
W. H. H. Mason Fair
Hosea Pearce well

In contrast, the next young man to face the examiners—Paul Merrill of Augusta, Maine (No. 9)—shone in every area:

> Anat. & Physiology—Very well
> Chem and Pharmacy—*Excellent*
> Mat.. Med & Therapeutics—Excellent
> Theo. & Prac & Pathol^{y}—very well
> Surgery & Obstetrics.—[blank]

Delegates NH. Med. Soc^{y}
W. H. H. Mason Excellent
Hosea Pearce Excellent

Comments on the performance of other students examined that day include "Fairly," "Tolerably," "Good," "Pretty well," "Very fair," and "Quite well." Despite the curious mixture of adverbs and adjectives that

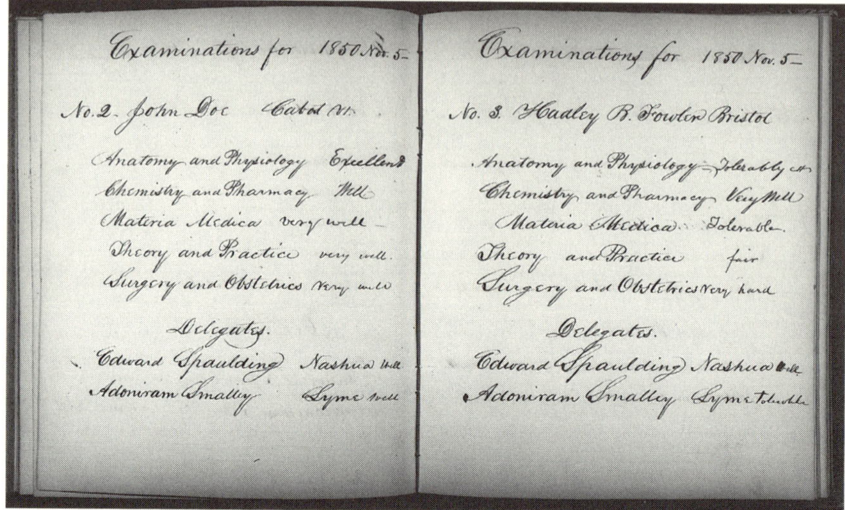

Examinations for 1850 Nov. 5—

No. 2. John Doe Cabot Vt.

Anatomy and Physiology Excellent
Chemistry and Pharmacy Well
Materia Medica very well —
Theory and Practice very well.
Surgery and Obstetrics Very well

Delegates.
Edward Spaulding Nashua well
Adoniram Smalley Lyme well

Examinations for 1850 Nov. 5—

No. 3. Hadley B. Fowler Bristol

Anatomy and Physiology Tolerably well
Chemistry and Pharmacy Very Well
Materia Medica Tolerable.
Theory and Practice fair
Surgery and Obstetrics Very hard

Delegates.
Edward Spaulding Nashua well
Adoniram Smalley Lyme Tolerable

Examination document showing grades, 1850. Courtesy of Stuart Bratesman, Dartmouth College.

bespeaks a lack of agreement on the vocabulary of the rating system, all this seems reasonably straightforward—except for the occasional blank space after one or another subject. A dramatic example of this appears in 1858, when George William Gove of Whitefield, New Hampshire, was passed with high marks in three subjects—"Chemy & Pharmacy *Very Well*; Mat. Med & Therap. Exceedingly well; Theo. & Prac & Path°ly Very well indeed"—but without any comment at all for either "Anaty & Physiology" or "Surgery & Obstet."[71]

In 1876, at least one student was rejected outright after the examinations on 30 October. Asahel Wellington Hamlin of Bowdoin, Maine, had an average grade of 3.44 on a scale of 1 to 7 (the system had been altered by then), with only a 1.5 in anatomy and physiology. And the next day, George Edward Leit [*sic*—his surname was actually "Leete"] was "Advised not to appear before the Delegates but to wait till the June examination & try again."[72]

As the century moved on, instead of the faculty gathering as a panel, students were tested separately in the various disciplines, with each professor responsible for his own subject. In 1881, Lyman B. How wrote to Frost, who was trying to collect the student grades from the scattered faculty, to report scores for seven students on the examination that covered both anatomy and physiology. Two of the students had earned marks of 3.43 and 3.0 respectively (very low scores), which moved How to unburden himself more generally on what he thought their status should be:

> Hathaway and Morse I vote against; no recommendation to mercy in their case. Not one of them was as good as he ought to have been considering the advantages afforded. There is a vast unexplored territory in Heath's Anatomy and Dalton's Physiology yet before nearly all of them and when Gray or Quain and Carpenter are mentioned imagination stands aghast and the new comet is nowhere. I hope they will never wander into those devius [*sic*] mazes and never more get out.

He signed off in Latin, as he frequently did: "I remain, De profundis cordis, Tuus L.B.H."[73] The other instructors apparently had rather different views, for both James Newton Hathaway and Charles Alfred Morse graduated in the class of 1882.[74] By September of that year, How was being even more blunt about his dissatisfaction with some students. He recorded grades for twenty-three successful candidates in the anatomy and physiology examination, but he also had a list of eighteen unsuccessful candidates. That list of names is headed simply "Strangulati pro bono publico."[75]

Edwin J. Bartlett saw the whole examination ritual (at least as he reflected on it later) as somewhat more benign than How's sarcastic dismissal of those who failed might lead one to imagine it:

> Later the methods of the concourse prevailed and each doctor had his prey—each lion a Christian so to speak—who rotated at the tap of the bell. The touch of the examiner in Chemistry was light [here he was speaking of himself]. . . . Physiology seldom offered obstacles. But you may be sure that the instruction in Practice, Surgery and Obstetrics was well explored, as was to be expected of busy practitioners who wanted to know the latest doctrines. The occasion was intimate and in retrospect agreeable, though at the time it suggested too much the intimacy of the surgeon or the dentist. But the best students were as well-prepared and ready then as now, and it was a pleasure to hear the learning flow forth.[76]

Plus ça change . . .

The medical school's 1827 catalog—such as it was—included in the prose section an explanation of the relationship that had existed since 1821 between the "Medical Institution at Hanover" and the "New-Hampshire Medical Society"; the Society's delegates had a duty to make a report each year "respecting the condition of the medical school." The delegates, we are told, having been present during the examinations, were impressed by the fact that the student performances were "with very few exceptions . . . highly satisfactory." (One cannot help but wonder, if that was the case, why medical degrees were conferred on only eight of the twenty-eight examined!) "It was thought," the report continued, "that more attention had been paid to preparatory studies in this class, than in many classes which had gone before them." Clearly, there was interest and concern about standards. Satisfaction with the current state of affairs was registered with the observation that a "large proportion of [the students] appeared to be gentleman of education and refinement, and bid fair to do honour to the institution and the profession at large."[77] Overall, through the decades, complaints about students seem relatively rare (though there was the occasional student who was denied his degree).

A student's academic performance was at times of less concern than his "moral character." In 1810, in what appear to be the first changes to the founding articles of 1798, the initial stipulation was that "each person previous to his becoming a [student] member of the Medical Institution be required to give satisfactory evidence to the Executive Officers of College that he sustains a good moral character." In addition: "That it be required of Medical students during their residence in the vicinity of the College that they conduct themselves respectfully towards all the Executive officers of College and if any of them should be found guilty of immoral or ungentlemanlike conduct the executive may expel them from the Institution."[78] Two years later, it was decided that only those students who were not college graduates needed to provide evidence of their good character (those who had survived college being presumed already to have demonstrated that they were gentlemen—if not saints—and scholars of good morals). This was now the second rather than the first rule: "Those who have not received a Collegiate education shall, previous to examination give satisfactory evidence to the President and Professors that they possess a knowledge of the Latin Language and of natural & experimental Philosophy; and also that they sustain a fair moral character."[79] Then, in 1820, reference to moral character was omitted; though attendance at chapel was urged, it was explicitly not required.[80] By the time the "Statutes of the Medical Institution of Dartmouth College" appeared for the first time in printed form in 1842, the requirement that the student "give satisfactory evidence to the Faculty" of sustaining a "good moral character" (along with a knowledge of Latin) was back, although this time it was required for "Medical Graduation" rather than for matriculation.[81]

Thus it is not surprising to find suspicion of the *lack* of proper character being investigated with utmost seriousness. The 1845 faculty records contain the following:

> In consequence of a report strongly implicating the moral character of one of the candidates for the degree of M.D. examined yesterday (No. 15) [Charles Harvey Rowell] having reached the Faculty, the individual alluded to was summoned before the Faculty & the Delegates, and required to answer to the charges which had been brought . . . an alleged attempt at swindling a fellow student by passing a $10 fraudulent bill. The charge however could be substantiated only by probabilities; and in the absence of *positive proof* of intention to defraud, it was
>
> Voted that all proceedings against the accused candidate be discontinued for the present; & that he be allowed to receive his Diploma this P.M. with the others of the graduating Class . . . provided he will previously produce a certificate of good moral character . . . as the accused of his own accord had volunteered to do.

This condition was complied with, and Rowell received his Dartmouth medical degree in the class of 1846.[82]

The students were, by and large, diligent and committed. The sacrifices required to spend time attending medical lectures, and the difficulties presented by the subject matter itself, were sufficient to guarantee earnest and serious behavior most of the time. Once again, we gain insight from Edwin Bartlett's reflections:

> The order of a medical school was self-regulated and peculiar. The jovial medic, cramped and constrained during a long morning spent on the hard seats of the amphitheater, had a way of easing joints and nerves before and after lectures by singing, stamping and the most boisterous horse-play, sometimes passing a man up from the lowest tier of seats to the top with shrieks and howls of artless glee; but the minute the lecturer entered the room all noise stopped as though the sportive crew had been changed to stone, and no body of men could have been more quietly attentive. One jocund act perhaps encroached a bit, but it had salutary qualities of discipline. When a student arriving late had the hardihood to descend to his seat in attempted stealth, feet all over the room beat time to his soft steps, and when he placed his anatomy upon his chair a deafening crash marked the instant of contact. The effect was ludicrous in the extreme and few men made a second attempt. Other disturbance was unknown, and the hour was always the lecturer's opportunity, though his audience was quick enough in recognizing whether he was giving value for their time.[83]

The matter of "giving value for time" was increasingly a concern of the faculty. As the nineteenth century drew to a close, evidence mounted that the faculty and the administration alike considered the responsibility of offering high-quality medical education a serious matter. We turn next to some of the new issues of institutional relations and faculty governance that emerged as the school grew.

CHAPTER FIVE

Shaping the Institution

Vita brevis; ars longa; occasio celeris; experimentum periculosum; judicium difficile.

[Life is short; art long; opportunity fugitive; experience delusive; judgment difficult.]
—HIPPOCRATES[1]

Creating a Strong Faculty

ONE CLEAR PIECE of evidence that the medical school faculty took seriously its position and the membership within its number is a letter written in 1896, not long after the death of Carlton Frost. The "resident portion of the Faculty" sent the long missive to the nonresident members, urging them to agree to the plan to nominate John M. Gile as a member of the faculty. Despite the fact that Frost himself had initiated the idea, William Smith, Edwin Bartlett, and Gilman Frost were obviously concerned that the others might not support the idea. They made their case as strongly as possible. After detailing Gile's background and experience (which included being effectively medical director of the State Hospital at Tewksbury, Massachusetts, with about a thousand persons under his care), they went on as follows:

> We appreciate the objection that may be made that Dr Gile has neither large reputation nor experience and that it is desirable that the teacher of Science & Practice of Medicine in Dartmouth College should have both; but we must have a man who will live here & help in the work of the whole year. During Dr. Frost's time the Winter School had grown until its demands had become too great for us before we lost him. It had numbered about one hundred men this year. We needed help before & now the need is imperative. . . . The above plan we commend to your consideration as the best we can devise to meet urgent requirements.

Appended was a note from President William Jewett Tucker, making it clear that he expected acquiescence from the medical faculty.

In my last conversation with Dr. C. P. Frost the plan which is outlined in the above communication was strongly urged by him. In fact it was with a view of urging it that he called me to his bedside.

I have gone over the ground carefully with the resident members of the Medical Faculty and so far as I am competent to judge of the present situation and of the needs of the Medical School, I am altogether in favor of the appointment of Dr. Gile.

The sheet accompanying the letter was signed by the three resident faculty who had written the letter. Despite the pressure to agree, including from the president, two men nonetheless registered caveats: Tilghman Balliet insisted that Gile's appointment should be probationary, and Phineas Conner wanted there to be a "distinct understanding" that the appointment was for the coming session only and did not commit the faculty further.[2]

The point when Conner himself had been the focus of recruitment efforts offers another example of faculty concern over quality. Lyman How had written to Frost in 1877 that he thought "there must be *somewhere* in some city some prominent surgeon who would like to go to Hanover in August for what we can afford to pay him. If a contribution from other chairs was necessary to secure one I would cheerfully chip in toward it."[3] Two months later, Conner was the candidate of choice despite some uncertainty whether he could be persuaded.

Faculty members also strove to maintain good relations with each other, as excerpts from a pair of even earlier communications illustrate—though in the first instance there may be veiled humor behind the note. In late 1872, Henry Field wrote to Frost, reporting that he had "hinted to How that we *might* . . . [wish for him to give] an address at Commencement next year—as the *Salutatory* falls to you—& he took it kindly, & I judge from what he said that he would be on hand if desired. I thought we should have the better production if he had a *year's* notice."[4] Three years later, A. B. Crosby wrote to Frost expressing concern over whether plans to turn chemistry into a course that would run through the term with daily lectures might have the unfortunate effect of souring relations with Oliver Hubbard:

You know my mind as to the ultimate disposition of the chemical chair, but I do not want to take such a position as would drive Mr. Hubbard out of the chemical chair against his wishes—He has served the college many years, and my social relations with him are of the most cordial character. . . . I can see many advantages in your having a daily lecture through the term.[5]

Hubbard may have been especially prickly. Two years after Crosby wrote Frost expressing some uncertainty over what reaction could be expected from Hubbard, How wrote to Frost in a very similar tone.

We have already, as Dr. Field writes in response to a letter on this subject, imposed two changes on Prof. Hubbard for this next term. How will he stand the pressure of another and more vital one to him, because it will affect his pocket?

It has been always in our school a cardinal principle that there should be as little interfering of any or all departments with anyone as possible. Each member of the Faculty has managed his own course in his own way and there has been on this account no quarrelling and very little friction, and the school has been previously at any rate prosperous above all the rural colleges.[6]

Thus it is clear that the tensions inherent when a faculty needs to work as a group, while the professors continue to function with their wonted independence, were emerging. But there is also considerable evidence in the extant correspondence that Frost, at least, despite his status as *primus inter pares*, had good personal relations with his colleagues. Edward Dunster, for example, when he was engaged in teaching in Ann Arbor, communicated with him frequently from there. "Are you coming West this fall. Board is cheap & rum is plenty. All well," he wrote in November of 1886.[7]

Lyman How continued his special interest in curricular matters and in fitting all the pieces together, as we see from another letter he wrote to Frost around this time:

One great advantage we should obtain by Dr. Munde's resignation will be entirely neutralized by appointing Dr. Dunster to succeed him. I allude to the arrangement of the several courses of lectures. If we can choose some good man to give the course in the last half of the term it will help us all out very much—some sensitive, educated, experienced man like Dr. Chamberlin for example.[8] . . . Of course Dunster is as *good* an instructor as we can get and if he could come later I would vote for him. . . . Perhaps you have sounded other members of the Faculty and have some other opinions from them. If so would like to know how they feel about it.[9]

Of concern to us here is How's evident interest in getting "some good man to give the course."

Quality Is as Quality Does

Just how "good" the men were who taught at Dartmouth during the nineteenth century is exceedingly difficult to evaluate in retrospect. Several of them published books or journal articles; some founded and edited medical journals; some belonged to the newly forming specialty societies. Beyond that, many had fine reputations as teachers or physicians or both; a number of them had teaching appointments in more than one institution. This did not distinguish Dartmouth faculty from the faculty at most other medical schools of the time, however. With short terms, in part a result of the prevalent policy of making nonresident faculty appointments, peripatetic teaching was common. Some insight into the faculty effort to control the quality of colleagues to be hired comes from a note in the faculty minutes from 1848. When it was rumored that Joseph Roby, professor of the theory and practice of medicine as well as of pathological anatomy, was considering resigning, it was decided that preference in hiring a replacement should go to a graduate of Dartmouth Medical School.[10] (Roby did leave the next year, and his position was filled by Edward Elisha Phelps—already on the faculty.) Chauvinism reared its head on other occasions, too. Thirty years later, when a ballot was taken by mail on the election of Phineas Conner to the chair of surgery, the vote was 5 to 1 in favor. Edward Dunster, registering the sole negative, requested that the reason for his vote be recorded: "My vote is cast against Dr. Conner not because there is any personal or professional objection to him (for none such can be adduced by anyone who knows him) but solely because in my opinion the interests of the College demand the selection of a New England Surgeon. If none such can be obtained after due search then my objection is withdrawn."[11] Dunster's concern was perhaps less a matter of provincialism than simply a slowly increasing sense that nonresident faculty were less able to play the numerous roles they needed to fill than were those who lived and practiced in Hanover.

Some of those who taught at Dartmouth played a more active educational role within their own branches of medicine than was typical of the average physician. Dunster himself, for example, appears to have been a considerable credit to the faculty. Though words of praise in an obituary cannot always safely be taken at face value, the honest words in the final paragraph of the faculty's obituary statement on Dunster ("Though in the later years of his life, ill health limited his efforts and rendered him at times apparently indifferent and unsocial") incline one to trust the general tenor of what preceded:

> Of scholarly habits and cultivated tastes; well read in general literature; much instructed in matters of public policy, local and general; upright, honest and pure minded, he was an agreeable companion and a good citizen. As a physician he was attentive to his patients, ready in the detection & skillful in the treatment of disease, a safe counsellor and just to his professional associates. As a writer he was clear and concise, familiar with his subject both by reading and observation, showing himself possessed of a logical mind, as was conspicuously instanced in his well known paper before the American Med. Association at its Richmond meeting. As a lecturer he was systematic, instructive and entertaining—an exceptionally good teacher.[12]

Another who had influence well beyond Hanover was Louis Elsberg. Though foreign born, he not only founded the American Laryngological

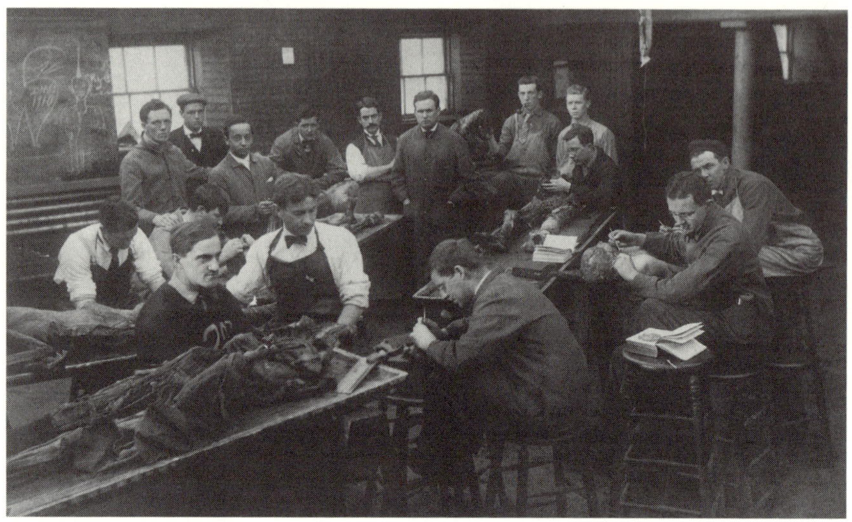

Nineteenth-century dissection class. Courtesy of Dartmouth College Library.

Association in 1878 but was the original editor (he served for two years) of the *Archives of Laryngology*, the first journal in that specialty in the United States. Earlier, his 1865 essay "Laryngoscopal Surgery" (published in 1866) had won a gold medal from the American Medical Association (AMA). Elsberg also had sufficient technical knowledge of music to make him "the pioneer medical attendant and consultant of opera singers and other high-salaried voice-users; thus he developed a specialty within a specialty [a great rarity at the time]. He was equally prominent as a teacher and inspirer of laryngologists." One of the editors of the *North American Medical Reporter* as well, he also published widely himself—books, medical journal articles, and magazine pieces. His death (at forty-nine) prevented him from completing his own textbook on laryngology.[13] His "knowledge of his specialty & his skill as an operator," according to his colleagues, "placed him in advance of his fellows in this country."[14]

Paul Fortunatus Mundé also edited a scientific periodical, *The American Journal of Obstetrics*. Mundé's 1880 textbook on surgical gynecology was important because of its unusual character. Although many books were available at the time on diseases of women, there was little or nothing on gynecological *surgery*, a point Mundé made explicit in his preface; he also expressly stated that the book was not aimed at "the gynecological expert" or "the intern at the Woman's Hospital," but rather at the student and the young general practitioner.[15] Mundé was also editor of a late edition of one of those well-known texts on diseases of women. The book's importance, as well as the significance of Mundé having been asked to edit a new edition, is indicated by the preface to the fifth edition, reprinted on page [5] of the sixth edition. There it becomes clear that one or more of the prior editions had been translated into German, French, Italian, and Spanish.

In an earlier generation, Edmund Randolph Peaslee was another long-time member of the faculty with an impressive reputation, one that led him to divide his time during the final twenty years of his career between New York and Hanover. Phineas Conner, in his centennial address, rhapsodized about Peaslee, professor of anatomy for nearly thirty years, as follows: "Of broad, accurate, critical learning in Arts as well as in Medicine, master of his subject, a genuine teacher (and he at one time or another taught in every department of Medicine and in five schools[16]), an excellent diagnostician, a successful general practitioner, a careful, skillful operator, an author of great merit . . . , a devoted son of the College [class of 1836]."

Conner went on, recounting how Peaslee reported—just weeks before he died—that one of the "last delights of his life" was that each of the professorial chairs at Dartmouth Medical School was held by "'one of his own boys.'"[17] In this expression of proprietary pride, Peaslee comes across as a kind of precursor of Rolf Syvertsen (see chapter 7). Though initially appointed as a lecturer in anatomy and physiology, Peaslee made his mark chiefly as a gynecologist and obstetrician. His fame, we are told, "extended throughout the United States and also through foreign lands, and the Obstetric Society of Berlin appointed him a corresponding fellow"; the London Obstetrical Society made him an honorary fellow. He was famous for having performed the first successful ovariotomy in New England by the large abdominal section (in September 1850); his book *Ovarian Tumors: Their pathology, diagnosis and treatment* (mentioned earlier) was the first systematic treatment of the subject in English.[18]

Strengthening the School in Other Ways

Building and retaining a faculty of high quality was only one aspect of teaching medicine more systematically. The size and quality of the student body, a more careful monitoring of the curriculum, and a general increase in standards were all part of the process as well. Among the changes made during the nineteenth century at Dartmouth Medical

School, perhaps the most significant is one mentioned in passing (in chapter 4)—the introduction by Carlton Frost of the so-called recitation term in 1870. A quick look back will show why Frost's innovation was important. In the early nineteenth century, it was still true that anyone seriously intending to become a physician would have planned to serve as an apprentice to a practicing physician for two or more years. At Dartmouth Medical School it was also expected that students would serve as apprentices—often prior to arriving to attend two or more courses of lectures. (The period of apprenticeship might also be broken up, interspersed with the lecture courses.) But the quality of education under such a system obviously varied a great deal, according to the capabilities of the mentors. The arrangement was such that "the student, for better or for worse, was exposed to a single instructor who might, or might not, take time from a busy practice to supervise the student's learning experience."[19] The first improvement began sometime after 1821, when the medical faculty at Dartmouth offered students a joint apprenticeship that ran concurrently with the lecture term.

By introducing the recitation term (also called the "recitation class") as a formal part of the medical school curriculum, Frost took a major step toward assuring that most of the students would get the same level of education. It was all still a private affair, not actually an official part of the required course for a degree. During most of its twenty-seven years, it was run by Frost himself, assisted by other resident physicians and faculty members. Because the class was conducted for a group of students at one time instead of having each individual pick up what was offered by a particular preceptor, the material taught to them was likely to be much more uniformly and systematically presented than it had been previously. The systematization led to standardization—and once in place, this mode of instruction obviously worked well; enrollment increased steadily during Frost's long tenure at Dartmouth. Not altogether surprisingly, it came to be seen as "of such great educational value that it grew almost to equal the standard lecture course in numbers, having ninety-six in it when it was last given in 1896" (the year Frost died).[20] But like many innovations, the recitation class was not initially welcomed by all, according to one historian.[21] The success of the venture can be measured in part by the fact that after Frost's death the faculty voted no longer to allow an apprenticeship to replace any of the time spent in what was from then on to be a required four academic years of study at Dartmouth.[22] According to a later account, the recitation class (in the winter term) was not the only example of the "much needed newer methods of teaching medicine" Frost introduced. He also "improved the 'summer term,' which brought to Hanover for that season a series of outstanding lecturers in most fields of medicine from all over the country."[23]

Change was a constant throughout the century, but only toward the later years do we have evidence of efforts to review the entire curriculum as a unit (like the proposal we saw How making to Frost in 1878). In the earlier years, changes were made piecemeal, as a close review of the course catalogs and faculty minutes shows. The changes in requirements (for entrance and for graduation), the courses offered—and what, if any, extra or "private" instruction was available—and the length of the term all changed a number of times. A systematic analysis would be unlikely to reveal much in the way of a predictable pattern; a few examples of what the catalogues included, taken chronologically, will have to suffice to paint a picture of the nineteenth-century curriculum.[24]

The first time the College catalogue did more than list the names of faculty and students was in 1822; from then on, a description of the medical school and its offerings appeared more or less annually, albeit in inconsistent format. The lecture term lasted thirteen weeks in 1822 and 1823; in 1824 it was increased to fourteen weeks. In 1840 the course was described as "three months" long. The fee for additional private instruction changed frequently: $40 in 1822, raised to $50 in 1826, reduced to $45 in 1828 (a further reduction was offered for payment in advance). Similarly, there were changes from year to year with respect to whether the extra tuition would be offered at all or who would do so; in 1829 private instruction was suspended because of the absence of one of the professors, in 1832 it was offered by two professors, and in 1833 it was run by Mussey alone. In 1827, surgical operations were performed gratis before the medical class during the lecture term; in 1832, surgical lectures were an extra part of the private course. In 1844 (when the course was again listed at fourteen weeks), the catalogue announced that surgical operations would "be performed before the Medical Class *gratuitously* as usual; and Patients will be treated at the Infirmary for Surgical & all other diseases, during the Term, without charge." ("Gratuitously" meant simply that the students would not have to pay for the privilege of having this kind of instruction. Patients receiving free care were, incidentally, given no choice about whether they wished to be used as "clinical material" for students.)

The course was lengthened to sixteen weeks in 1846, but two years later it was back to fourteen weeks. (Another indicator of some slippage is that the medical library was said to contain some 1,200 books in 1851—but in 1859, the figure was given as only about 1,100; in 1867 the operative figure was still 1,100.) The subjects of the lectures and their sequence were listed in the catalogue for the first time in 1866, and the lecture course was again thirteen weeks long. The faculty could not seem to decide what was optimum or practicable; twelve years later, in 1878, the course had once again been lengthened to sixteen weeks.

The catalogue of 1876–1877 eloquently pressed the advantages of medical education in Hanover, boasting of the "resources of the College," "the quiet of a country village," and "the comparative inexpensiveness of living" as reasons to believe "that this place offers superior inducements to such as wish to acquaint themselves thoroughly with the principles of a sound medical education." Moreover, it was claimed, the "extent of the field of Medical Study has been so greatly enlarged in late years, that no young man [*sic*] who would reach an honorable position in the profession can afford to forego the advantages of *daily recitations*, or the practical work of the Dissecting Room and the Physiological & Chemical laboratories."[25]

General entrance requirements were beginning to be specified by 1875. Students had to be at least 18 years old, and if they were not already matriculated at Dartmouth College or were not graduates of some reputable college, academy, or high school, they would be required to pass an entrance examination. What today would probably be called electives were added in 1879, with "special courses" in the diseases of the larynx, diseases of the eye, mental diseases, and medical jurisprudence.[26]

Graduation requirements were also changed from time to time. In 1866, for instance, natural and experimental philosophy was no longer required. On the other hand, it was another six years—1872—before a student's need to demonstrate some knowledge of Latin ceased to be mentioned. But in 1880, students were required to provide evidence that they had dissected both parts (cranium and body) of the cadaver before they were eligible for graduation. Curiously enough, however, it had not been until 1879 that explicit mention was made of the opportunity that would be provided in the latter part of the session for students to perform dissections. (To demonstrate that help in this area would be forthcoming, the 1889–1890 catalogue, finally, explicitly stated that "special attention is given during the winter to dissection, with daily demonstrations & recitations.")

In at least one way, however, requirements were reduced. In 1882, a thesis or "dissertation" was no longer required of students. (Prior to this, each student not only had to write such a graduation paper; he had to be prepared to read and defend it. In the early years, such public performances were de rigueur.) Yet written examinations were specified in anatomy, surgery, physiology, obstetrics, therapeutics, chemistry, gynecology, and practice, and it was stressed that two courses of lectures and three full years of study with a practitioner were required for graduation.

The involvement of the state medical society at examination time was amended in 1883, with written examinations being passed on to society delegates who would then conduct further oral examinations. Also in that year, participation in the recitation course (which was to last from December 12 to June 20) was urged by means of the following statement: "This work is quite essential if the student would fully profit by the lectures" (the regular lecture course, which would follow). The encouragement was even stronger in the 1889–1890 catalogue: "The plan of instr.^{n} in the College comprises work done in two terms each year. In one, the teaching is by lectures, and in the other it is done by recitation & demonstrations. The former is req^{d} of all who would gain the diploma of the College, while the latter is optional, though it is practically essential if a student would properly qualify himself for the work of the profession."

The language used to describe the 1889–1890 lecture term showed that the catalogue had become a marketing tool; no longer was it simply the announcement sheet of earlier years: "Lectures are both didactic & clinical, & will comprise full courses in all Departments of Medical Science. Coming as they do in the summer & and fall, we are able to secure the services of some of the best teachers in several of the large city schools. Upon the completion of the [hospital] now in process of erection, increased facilities for clinical instruction will be afforded. Examinations will be made & operations will be performed before the class gratuitously."

Furthermore, the unique appeal of Dartmouth's location and the putative advantages of studying medicine in such a place were also being stressed more than ever: "The quiet of this beautiful country town affords an excellent opportunity for the thorough study of the elementary principles of Medical Science, a knowledge of which is best acquired in freedom from the disturbing surroundings of city life."[27] No wonder the idea that had been floated twenty years earlier of moving the medical school to Manchester, New Hampshire (hardly a teeming city, but more nearly so than Hanover), had been discarded. Despite the assurances Professor Albert Smith once gave, in a letter to the College president, that he and Phelps were confident everything could be arranged satisfactorily "if it was the decision of the medical faculty of our school that the best interests of the school would be advanced by a removal, and no decided opposition came from the College," the medical faculty at its next annual meeting voted "that the subject . . . of a removal of the school be indefinitely postponed."[28]

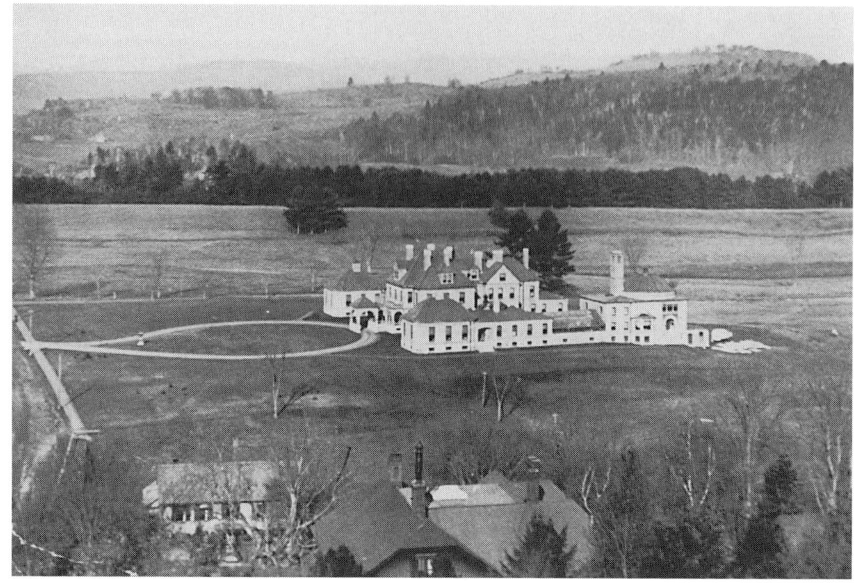

Mary Hitchcock Memorial Hospital, 1897. Courtesy of Dartmouth Medical School.

In 1885, the dates for the lecture course make it clear that the duration of the term was steadily increasing; by 1886, a lengthening to a full twenty weeks was announced. The move to regularize, systematize, and formalize every aspect of medical education was well on its way.[29] And the 1893–1894 catalogue proudly announced that the cottage hospital of thirty-six beds—the brand-new Mary Hitchcock Memorial Hospital ("constructed after the most approved modern style for such buildings") was in use, and that a "large and beautifully lighted amphitheater is provided for witnessing operations, which [would be] gratuitously performed by members of the faculty before the class." (A year later, the cover of the "Circular of Information" was graced by a picture of the new hospital, about which, more in chapter 6.) Also, students were—for the first time—to be arranged in three classes and required to complete the work of each year in regular order, passing an examination at the end of each year. They were advised that the "most desirable time to begin the study of medicine" was the opening of the recitation term. Histology and microscopy had been added to the course list (lectures to be given by a member not of the medical faculty, incidentally, but of the college department of zoology).[30] Chemistry, so long a virtual stepchild of the medical curriculum, was to be divided into three sections: experimental inorganic chemistry, qualitative analysis, and medical chemistry.

Finally, in 1895 entering students had to write an English essay of 300 words and pass examinations in Latin, physics, and chemistry—unless they possessed either a college or a high school diploma with evidence they had passed those subjects. Students seeking advanced standing had to pass all examinations already required of the class they wished to join.

Student Enrollment

A comparison of two classes twenty years apart gives us some sense of who the students in the second half of the nineteenth century were and what qualifications they brought to Dartmouth, though biographical and other details about them were not kept with complete consistency.[31] In 1855, 58 students were enrolled; in 1875, the number had risen to 79. The matriculation fee in each of those years was $5, but the 1855 course fee of $50 had risen twenty years later to $77. The increase had not come all at once; the fee was raised to $70 in 1865 and to $77 four years later. There it stayed for some time. (As late as the class of 1899–1900, when 118 students were listed, the course fee had still not changed from the $77 set thirty years earlier.)

The 1855 students came from New Jersey as well as from all the New England states except Rhode Island. In 1875, Rhode Island replaced Connecticut in the roster just as New York was represented instead of New Jersey; there was also a student from Canada. The average age of students moved from 22¾ to 24¼, and the age range increased from 18 to 33 in 1855 to 18 to 40 in 1875. In both years, the class comprised a mixture of students enrolled for the first, second, third, or even fourth time. Those in the last (and sometimes those in the third) category had their fees waived and could take the course for free. As for the time previously spent as preceptees, there, too, considerable variation was apparent. In 1855 some students were clearly just beginning, while others had been apprenticed for up to four and a half years. In 1875, the one 40-year-old had already spent ten years in practice; another student was listed simply as "practitioner," with no age given—and with the fee waived. Thus the length of time spent studying and the sequence in which formal courses and apprenticeships were undertaken were matters by no means yet standardized. One of the 1875 students was from McGill University; though only 21 years old, he was taking his fourth course. Another, enrolled in his first course, had already been in practice for five years. Although in that 1875 group there were 79 students, ten years later the total had dropped to 52. A decade after that, the number shot way up, tripling to more than 140 (roughly two thirds of whom were enrolled in the by-then-popular recitation course), a peak never reached before. The number of those receiving degrees in 1897—after two courses—was consequently at its greatest (50) that year, though not proportionately so. The number of students enrolled often differed significantly from the number graduating.

Institutional Relations

Throughout the nineteenth century, the relationship between the medical school (or "Medical Department" as it was still generally called) and its parent institution, the College, shifted and changed. As one historian put it, the "administrative relationship between the Medical School and the parent institution was undeniably a confused affair." The same writer added:

> At the start the Trustees awarded degrees and appointed the faculty but otherwise made little attempt to govern the Medical Department. In 1809 . . . [President] John Wheelock induced the Board to accept new rules concerning student discipline in the Medical School. But the Medical Department continued to function more or less independently, and relations between the two faculties were often strained. Part of the problem arose because the medical faculty was, for the most part, not dependent on College funds for its income, but this was not the whole story. The medical faculty, unlike the College faculty, was rendering a vital service as well as teaching, and their teaching from the first was service oriented. The College faculty, on the other hand, was concerned with unapplied, more abstract learning. The division between the two faculties thus had a philosophic as well as a fiscal origin.[32]

Various efforts were made to ease the tensions. We saw earlier how the trustees, at their October 1820 meeting, voted a new set of "Statutes of the Medical Institution of Dartmouth College," which—among its novelties—specified that the medical faculty "shall constitute a board for the determination of all concerns of discipline, instruction and Government, of the Medical Institution."[33] Thus, although the president of the College was still the presiding officer—not until 1873 would Dartmouth Medical School have its own de facto dean, and it was 1896 before it had a de jure dean, as we have seen—the Medical School was increasingly being recognized as an entity in its own right, which might very well have problems peculiar to it. A sign that continuity and stability were becoming hallmarks of the institution is that the published "Statutes of the Medical Institution of Dartmouth College" for 1842 opened exactly the way its 1820 predecessor did.[34]

Especially in connection with the teaching of chemistry, academic posts were sometimes joint appointments; disagreements often arose over whose treasury was responsible for salaries in such cases. Additional scattered entries in the trustees' records and the faculty minutes tell us something of how it all worked, but rarely is the reason for a particular vote given.

In 1841, the trustees passed a number of resolutions touching on matters of concern to the medical faculty.[35] The faculty in turn also passed a variety of votes concerning the management of the Medical School's affairs. Extensive notes of faculty meetings began to appear in August of 1845, for instance; new rules concerning the treasury (followed by election of a treasurer) and new "standing rules for the regulation of the proceedings of the Faculty at their regular meetings" were adopted.[36] Evidence that the faculty took its own rules seriously appears frequently. On the request of Mr. B. R. Gibson for special dispensation (he had attended two courses at the medical school in Woodstock, Vermont, and wanted to be examined after a single term at Dartmouth), it was "Voted that we cannot deviate from the rule hitherto adhered to of *actually requiring* as requisite for the degree of M.D., what we *profess* to require in our published Circular & Catalogue."[37] And when one Dr. G. Watson, who had practiced for five years but never attended lectures, sought to be granted a degree, it was "Voted that the request . . . cannot be granted consistently with our requirements."[38]

The medical faculty also began to assert itself vis-à-vis the College, telling the trustees how it wished to be treated. It was voted that "whenever any action is to be had at a faculty meeting, on any subject affecting the interests of the College beyond the current term, three weeks notice shall be given by the president of the meeting and the subject or subjects to be acted upon; and the opinions expressed in writing on the subject, by each absent member, shall be received and recorded as his vote in deciding the question."[39] Yet the relationship between the College and the medical department was often unclear. For example, the trustees' records report: "Voted, that the Board regard the salary now paid to the Professors as too small, and declare their purpose to raise it to a proper point, as soon as it shall be practicable."[40] (It is not clear whether the reference to "Professors" includes only those of that rank in the College or, more likely, those of the Medical School as well.) And on another issue: At the time of Dixi Crosby's resignation, two trustees were appointed a committee "to examine into the State of the Medical College—

and . . . report thereon." Two days later, the committee asked "leave for further time to examine and report upon the condition of the Medical Department of the College."[41] This was a critical point in Dartmouth Medical School's history. As the long resolution in the minutes of the medical faculty itself indicated when Crosby actually retired, this particular group of men had at that point been together for twenty-two years, "a circumstance probably unexampled in the history of any medical school in our country."[42]

Even when the medical faculty made financial decisions, they sought ratification from the College, though there might be—as in the case detailed in what follows—considerable delay. A memo was sent to the College Trustees, reporting a vote taken "At a meeting of the Medical Faculty of the 'New Hampshire Medical Institution,' held at the Dartmouth Hotel on Thursday, October 28th 1869." Professors Dixi Crosby, E. E. Phelps, Albert Smith, A. B. Crosby, and L. B. How unanimously voted to accept the following "action of the Medical Faculty," which was dated October 29, 1869:

> Voted, That Dr. Carlton P. Frost and Dr. Henry M. Field be appointed as Associate Professors—the former to the Chair of Theory and Practice, and the latter to that of Materia Medica—it being understood that no extra charge is to be made for the Lectures in these branches, and no new division of the fees for the other tickets: that these offices shall become vacant on the resignation of the present professors, and that they shall not be members of the faculty.

On the face of it, "they shall not be members of the Faculty" seems like an extraordinary stipulation (especially, with the wisdom of hindsight, in the case of Frost). Yet that was the way appointments were made in the first instance, and this action of the medical faculty was apparently simply accepted by the trustees, without comment—almost a year later.[43]

One of the rare occasions when something was said in the trustees' minutes about how much a particular faculty member was to be paid was in February 1878, when Edwin J. Bartlett was elected as an associate professor of chemistry (the standard one-year probationary appointment). As mentioned earlier, this move marked another effort to improve the teaching of science. Bartlett's salary was set—a few months later—at $1,500 per annum "for services in all departments of instruction"; this was, interestingly enough, the same salary granted the new professor of French in the College, whose duties also included those of librarian.[44]

Sometimes a reminder that money matters did jointly concern College and Medical School comes in an unexplained notation—for instance, of a vote in 1879 "That the $100 usually paid to the Medical School be discontinued until otherwise ordered."[45] In 1881, when there was a request from "some of the Professors" to run a "Summer Institute of Science" on the College premises, that request was granted—as long as the professors "shall be personally responsible for the use of the College property and to make good any loss or injury" to such property.[46] The stipulation was not unreasonable, but there is guardedness on the part of the parent institution about either handing out money to the Medical School or letting its facilities be used without proper compensation that anticipates a fiscal policy of requiring each part of the institution to be monetarily independent. In a complicated arrangement that nonetheless is still consistent with such a policy, it was specified—when John H. Gerould was employed by the College as an assistant in biology in 1893—that "his compensation, viz: three hundred dollars [was] to be provided from the funds of the Medical College." In an apparent quid pro quo, the professor of biology would give the same amount of instruction in the Medical College.[47] Eight months later, however, it was voted that Gerould's salary was to be paid half by the College, and half by the medical school.[48]

Money matters aside, the College was clearly willing to cooperate with the medical faculty when it came to setting and maintaining standards. At a special meeting late in 1890, the president presented "to the Consideration of the Trustees," on behalf of the medical faculty, items that it had voted at its own annual meeting. The following were voted on in turn by the trustees, and passed:

> Voted. 1. That four (4) years of Medical Study and three (3) Courses of Lectures shall be required for graduation of all, who shall matriculate after the close of the present College year. Possession of the degree of A.B., B.L. or B.S. will be accepted in place of one year of professional study.
>
> Voted. 2. That the fee for the third Course for those who have had two Courses here shall be fifty dollars and the matriculation fee. For those who have attended two or more courses elsewhere, the fee shall be the regular fee of $77. & Matriculation. Subsequent Courses free.
>
> Voted. 3. That the addition of Biology to the list of optional studies offered to the Senior Class, be referred to the Committee on the Curriculum.[49]

A more explicit indication of a sense that perhaps the trustees should become involved in the affairs of the Medical School appeared two years later, when it was voted "that the subject of the relation of the Medical School to the College be referred to a committee."[50] Uneasiness about whether the State or the College actually owned the Medical School property seems to have precipitated this action, and the committee obviously took its work seriously. After careful study, it reported as follows:

Annual Commencement
of the
DARTMOUTH....
MEDICAL COLLEGE
by the
Class of '99
TUESDAY EVENING, FEBRUARY TWENTY-EIGHTH
1899
COLLEGE CHURCH
HANOVER, N. H.

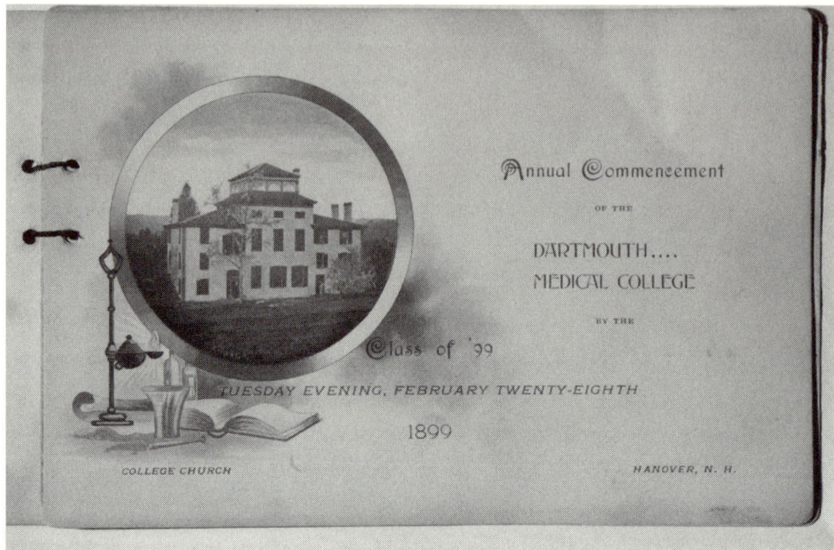

Commencement announcement, 1899. Courtesy of John Gilbert Fox.

> 1st. That the building, and probably the half acre of land upon which it stands, belong to the State. The land was probably conveyed to the State by Dr. Smith before the erection of the building.
>
> 2d. That the institution was started and has ever since been and is maintained as a department of Dartmouth College, —the Trustees appointing the professors, graduating the students, and conferring upon them the degree of M.D. —and has been chiefly supported by tuition from students, and perhaps by additional sums contributed for the purpose.
>
> It seems desirable that whatever ownership the State has in the building and land on which it is located be transferred to the Trustees, and the committee recommend that legislation to that effect be requested at the next session.

The report was accepted, the recommendation was adopted, and the committee was authorized to secure the recommended legislation.[51]

In December of that same year, the medical faculty recommended and the trustees adopted "the following regulations for examinations in the Medical College":

> 1. That at the end of one full year of the study of Medicine and one course of lectures in this College each student shall be required to pass an examination in Descriptive Anatomy, in Physiology and in Chemistry.
>
> 2. That at the end of two full years of study of Medicine and two courses of lectures, one of which shall have been at this College, each student shall be required to pass an examination in Descriptive and Regional Anatomy and a second examination in Physiology and in Chemistry.

Students entering the school in their second year and not having passed the first examination, may take both examinations at the end of the second year, together.

The examinations so passed in Anatomy, Physiology and Chemistry, if satisfactory, shall stand as final.

The fee for these examinations shall be five dollars ($5.) for the first year, and ten dollars ($10.) for the second year examinations, or fifteen dollars ($15.) for both. This sum of fifteen dollars shall be deducted from the graduation fee of twenty five dollars ($25.).[52]

In 1895, the trustees' committee on instruction reported on the terms of admission to Dartmouth Medical College, recommended by the Medical Faculty. It was then voted that in and after July 1896 those terms should be as follows:

English. Every candidate will be required to write legibly and correctly an essay of not less than three hundred words upon some familiar subject, to be assigned at the time.

Latin. To translate at sight easy Latin prose, a vocabulary of the less familiar words being furnished.

Elementary Physics. As found in Gage's or Carhart and Chute, or an equivalent text book.

Elementary Chemistry. He must have had not less than seventy hours of Elementary Chemistry, including laboratory practice, equivalent to Bartlett's Laboratory Exercises, Part I.

Persons presenting the Diploma of a college, of an approved academy or high school, will be exempted from examination, provided the subjects above required have been provided in their course of study. Candidates for advanced standing must, on admission, pass the examinations already required of the class they wish to enter. Students desiring to pass from the academical department of the college to the medical department must bring the certificate of the President that they can be allowed to do so.[53]

From the point of institutional governance, then, we see the trustees taking an increasingly detailed interest in the affairs of the Medical School as the century wore on, but doing so still largely with a rubber stamp in hand. We have no evidence that either the board or the president questioned or sought to alter recommendations made by the medical faculty. Good relations between the Medical School and the College were no doubt enhanced by Carlton Pennington Frost's friendship with President William Jewett Tucker; they were further cemented by Frost's visibility as the very effective de facto leader of the medical faculty and his membership on the Board of Trustees of the College. This dual role put him in a singularly powerful position to direct the affairs of the Medical School. As one writer has said, Frost "negotiated DMS's final transition from precarious semiautonomy to full incorporation into the Dartmouth structure."[54]

The Physical Plant Repaired

The physical plant of the Medical School concerned the trustees as well as the medical faculty, because facilities were sometimes used by both the College and the Medical School. Precedent for this existed from the very beginning. After two years of teaching in the room Rufus Graves had found for him, Nathan Smith benefited from a vote of the Board "that the room No. 6 in the lower storey in the College" (the building subsequently known as Dartmouth Hall) be "devoted to the use of Professor N. Smith for the purpose of lecturing."[55] Such shared teaching as there was, particularly in chemistry and mineralogy (and later biology), meant that students from the College and from the Medical School were in and out of each others' classrooms with some frequency. But clearly members of the medical faculty were expected to take responsibility for keeping "their" facilities in good order. A note in the trustees' records for July 1844 stated that the "Board having visited the Medical buildings[56] hereby express their appreciation of the neatness & order observable & the improvements made; also their satisfaction in the evident interest felt & industry exercised by the gentlemen having charge of the Medical department."[57]

Thomas Chadbourne's enthusiastic report on the medical school in 1845 had included the comment that the "Medical Building has been put in a state of repair, by an expenditure during the last three years of about $900."[58] Apparently those repairs were made to suffice for nearly three decades. By the 1870s, not surprisingly, the need to do something about the old building was evident. Various members of medical faculty discussed the subject in writing, mostly in letters to Frost, in 1872. Work on the building was undertaken at this time due largely to the munificent gift from Edwin Stoughton already mentioned. Peaslee, for example, writing in February, urged that "Of course we must have all the repairs on the Med. College finished before Aug. 1st Is Dr. Phelps duly impressed with this necessity?"[59]

The primary alterations that were made—which included renovating the second floor of the center section and adding a clerestory—were the first major changes in Smith's "New Medical House" in its sixty-year history. Occasional small repairs had been made through the years, but they were minor indeed compared to what was being planned at this juncture. The 1872 renovations made it possible to accommodate the pathological museum in a room that replaced the old upper amphitheatre.[60] The cupola that rose above the added clerestory on the building would become the familiar, distinguishing mark of the old Medical

School for even more generations than the original version had served. But old and new features alike aroused loyal and sometimes sentimental expressions of devotion. More than forty years after this round of alterations, when the inside was being renovated once again, a note appeared in the College alumni magazine singing the building's praises:[61]

Probably the most interesting building in Dartmouth College today is the old Medical School Building. Half hidden behind an untutored growth of evergreens, its gaunt high-shouldered exterior has something sinister and forbidding about it. . . . Yet the Medical Building is the only recitation hall in the College to retain anything of old time quality. On the first floor is the ancient lecture room much as it must have been more than a century ago. . . . Early in March 1872 the work of demolition of the central part of the building . . . [and] the work of renovating the Chemical Lecture Room commenced. . . . The brick wall of the centre front & rear was built up for 8 feet, a very pleasant arrangement of the windows above made, the inside partitions were all removed, the floors and walls "made straight" and some advance made in arranging the cases in the Stoughton Museum. . . . A new Slate Roof was put on the entire building.

In April 1873 the work on the Museum was resumed and the interior was completed by the last of June of that year. . . . The entire cost of the completed Room for the Museum was $10,000[62]. . . . The cost of the repairs on the Lecture Room and Dissecting room with the privy was $1463 80/100, which was borne by the Faculty of the College, requiring nearly or quite one half of the receipts for Lectures that year.[63]

In 1873 an effort was made to obtain from the Legislature of the State such a sum as should suffice to complete the repairs on the whole building. . . . To accomplish this end the aid of the State Medical Society was invoked, and it was most cheerfully and heartily rendered, both by reason of the general interest of its members in the cause of Medical Education and also of their special interest in this Institution of their own State. This appeal to the Legislature was based upon the special need of State aid which such an institution feels; and further upon the ground that the State holds the title to the Medical Building, and the land on which it is located;[64] that the School has been kept up by the efforts of its Faculty; and that the building had been kept in repair by their money for more than sixty years; that they had just expended $1400. in repairs, and that still several thousand dollars were needed to make it what it should be. . . . [T]he grant of $5000. was rendered. . . .

It is believed that the Building is now equal to any in the country in its internal finish and adaptation to the requirements of medical teaching— There are four suites of rooms, that can be rented to students at a price sufficient to bring in nearly $200. a year. They have been properly furnished and it is an object to keep them in good condition.[65]

Professional Matters

Part of the reason there was a concern to keep the new dormitory suites in good repair (sound property management aside) was no doubt the recognition that the handsomely renovated building gave new impetus, which needed to be maintained, to recruitment efforts for both faculty and students. In the early years of the nineteenth century, there had been very little looking over the shoulder at other institutions. But as the century progressed, tensions occasionally arose over the desire to be a New England institution that served New England, on the one hand, and a desire not to be outstripped by other medical schools—in New England or elsewhere. More than once, as we have seen, faculty minutes include an unabashed admission that a new hire should be a "New England man" if at all possible. Dunster was initially disinclined to hire Conner because "the interests of the College demand the election of a New England surgeon"—or so Dunster insisted—and Emily Blackwell, it will be recalled, was denied admission on the grounds that the faculty would "not be justified by the medical profession of New England in complying with her request." The desire not to fall out of step with competing schools also periodically manifested itself. In 1865, for example, the faculty passed a vote that the lecture fees "be raised to $75—or such a sum as may be adopted in concert with the other New England country schools."[66]

A rather different measure of the extent to which the members of the faculty had their eyes on the outside world can be found in records on whether a particular degree candidate was a "regular" physician. "No Quacks Need Apply" seems to have been the motto, certainly in the middle of the century, when the issue arose several times. In 1848, Dr. William H. Carter of Newbury, Vermont—who had attended one course of lectures twenty years earlier and had been in practice since that time—was proposed by Crosby as a suitable candidate for the M.D. degree. Objections were raised, however, since Carter's "name had been associated for some years" with a popular and widely advertised remedy called "Carter's Pulmonary Balsam." This apparently smacked too much of quackery for some members of the Dartmouth faculty. A compromise was reached: If Dr. Carter would sign a paper drafted by Peaslee publicly disavowing his connection to that "Medicine," submit to an examination, present a thesis, and pay the usual graduation fee, he would be considered eligible. In the end, Carter obviously complied; he was awarded an M.D. and is listed as a graduate of the class of 1849.[67] Four years later—whether influenced by the Carter affair we do not know—the faculty took an explicit position on the matter of "regular" medicine. At a meeting on 1 November 1852, it was voted that "No person will be admitted to an examination for the degree of Doctor of Medicine who intends to engage in any other than the regular practice of medicine, & that this be announced in our next Circular."[68]

Only occasionally do we get glimpses of how good a neighbor the medical school was, either locally or nationally. In August of 1847, Dr. Crosby was made a committee of one "to obtain information as to the expense of a fence across the passage to the Medical College," but we have no way of knowing whether this was meant primarily to keep others out or simply to mark the entrance to the school.[69]

More important as evidence of the school's position at mid-century and later are indicators of involvement in the larger medical community. In late October of 1845, the faculty discussed the meeting being planned under the aegis of the New York State Medical Society "for the purpose of adopting some concerted action conducive to the elevation of the standard of Medical Education in the United States"; it was voted to send a delegate. At the arguably much more significant meeting in Philadelphia in May 1847, at which the AMA was founded, Edward Phelps represented Dartmouth.[70] In September of 1847, Phelps and Crosby were elected delegates to the next national convention, which was to be held in Baltimore in May of 1848.[71]

Another measure of the maturity of the institution might be said to be how it dealt with students who were in difficulty of one sort or another. We have relatively little evidence, but two affairs—forty years apart—illustrate a desire to handle problems internally. In 1845, Adino B. Hall was unable to present the required certificate testifying to his two years of apprenticeship, because his mentor—Enos Hoyt of Northfield, New Hampshire—withheld it on grounds of some pecuniary disagreement between the two men. A letter was sent to Dr. Hoyt in an effort to set the record straight. The dragged-out affair finally ended when Hall appeared before the faculty insisting he had meant no harm. Perhaps it was all worthwhile. Young Hall was awarded his M.D. from Dartmouth the following year, in the class of 1846; he practiced medicine until he died in Boston in 1880.[72]

Another sort of difficulty with student behavior emerges from an unusual letter written to Frost in 1887 (marked "Confidential") by G. P. Conn, one of the nonresident faculty members. Although most faculty letters that have survived concern student grades, faculty votes, appointments, class schedules, and the like, this one throws light directly on the issue of how student discipline was handled in the nineteenth century:

Dear Doctor:

I understand three members of your class were arrested in this city [Concord, N. H.] yesterday—for being drunk and disorderly—one of whom claims to be the President of the class.

They settled yesterday and were let off and the newspapers were told to keep still. Today I hear they have been to Suncook and have come back drunk—but as they are [?] away in the Phenix—perhaps they will manage to get back to Hanover tonight.

The police came to me about it and I told them if they got sober to put them on the train for H——tonight.

Thinking you might like to know what was going on—I send you this report—

Yours truly, G. P. Conn[73]

Just how seriously this case was taken we can see from the fact that the files today still contain several letters on it in addition to Conn's. Remarkably similar stories from sixty years later show that some features of how the medical school in Hanover was run in the mid twentieth century were already in place before the nineteenth century had run its course.[74] But long before that evidence surfaced, a great deal happened both internally and externally that would change the face of Dartmouth Medical School and medical education in Hanover for decades to come.

PART III

MEDICAL EDUCATION AND REFORM: PROFESSIONALIZATION

CHAPTER SIX

The (Carnegie) Inspector Calls

Let us now speak of the inconveniences of counsel, and of the remedies.
—FRANCIS BACON, VISCOUNT OF ST. ALBANS[1]

Oh, Happy Centennial!

DARTMOUTH MEDICAL SCHOOL "has had an honorable past; may she have a yet more honorable future, and at the close of another hundred years may her sons gather about her to tell of her glories and to do her reverence." Thus wrote the anonymous author of a lengthy review of Phineas Sanborn Conner's "Historical Address." The unsigned "review" in *The Daily Dartmouth* on June 30, 1897, was actually an abstract of Connor's address, and the grand phrases that ended the article were in fact an unattributed quotation of his peroration.[2] The enthusiasm, if not the plagiarism, is to be excused. Although the program for the exercises celebrating the centennial of the school was much less elaborate than the symposium put together a century later for the bicentennial (see the preface, page 17), the affair was nonetheless a festive one. The special events to mark the "Centenary of Dartmouth Medical College Exercises in the College Church" were held on Tuesday afternoon, June 29, 1897, in the midst of Commencement activities. The program was formally opened by President Tucker at 5 P.M., following music by the Germania Band ("one of the best musical organizations in the country," according to the review); a prayer was offered by the Rev. Dr. S. P. Leeds, and then Conner gave his address, in which he took the occasion to review the history of the school.

Conner gave full credit to Nathan Smith as the founder of the institution, identifying him as a "rare man" with a "self-recognized mission to teach." He also briefly described the careers of four outstanding early graduates: Amos Twitchell, a prominent surgeon in Keene, New Hampshire; George Cheyne Shattuck, progenitor of a long line of outstanding physicians in Boston and a great benefactor of both Dartmouth and Harvard medical schools; Henry Bond, of Philadelphia; and Phineas Spalding, of Haverhill, New Hampshire. Because it laid the basis so well for some of the major questions that were to face the institution in the decades immediately following the centennial celebration, his closing warrants quoting again: "If Dartmouth is to give proper fundamental training, she must have and continue to have the right of legitimately securing ample anatomical material. . . . If she is worth saving, let her have what she needs. . . . Let the State, let the town, let the Judiciary decide which it prefers, educated physicians in whose hands may rest the life or death of the best beloved, or sentimental regard for the welfare of the animal, and half civilized worship of the decaying body."[3]

Several indications of an increased sense of gravitas about the institution emerged as the centennial year approached. Carlton P. Frost had for many years acted as de facto dean, but in 1896 the medical faculty finally undertook formally to nominate one of its own—William Thayer Smith—as dean of the Medical School.[4] The decanal position was by annual appointment; Smith served in that capacity until his retirement in 1909 and proved to be a fine choice. A DMS graduate himself (1879), he was the grandson of a doctor (Rogers Smith) and the son of Dartmouth College graduate Asa Dodge Smith (1830), who had served as the College's seventh president.[5]

A year after formally electing a dean, the medical faculty chose another of its number, Gilman D. Frost (son of the late C. P. Frost), as secretary-treasurer. The younger Frost served until 1904 as secretary-treasurer of the medical faculty; at that point, the job of treasurer was taken over by the College treasurer (Frost continued as secretary for another five years).[6]

The Hitchcock Hospital and the Curriculum

The Mary Hitchcock Memorial Hospital, still only four years old at the time of the centennial celebration, was a less-ceremonial and considerably more-tangible bit of evidence that the medical school was coming—or perhaps even had come—of age. Fifteen years after Dixi Crosby closed his small cottage hospital, Carlton Frost played another of his important roles in the local medical community by taking the initiative to organize his colleagues and a few others into the Dartmouth Hospital Association.

As luck would have it, Frost and Smith both counted among their friends Hiram Hitchcock, a semi-retired hotelier who had become active in town affairs. Hitchcock would certainly have been aware of the need for a hospital, and when his young wife Mary (only fifty-three) died in 1887, he was persuaded that a hospital named after her would be a fitting memorial. Having already paid for the redecoration of Hanover's White Church and having bought the church a new organ, by 1889 Hiram Hitchcock "had announced his intention to pay for the entire cost of constructing a hospital dedicated to her memory."[7] Construction began in 1890. The dedication ceremony took place on May 3, 1893.[8]

The town had been without a hospital for almost a quarter of a century; the new Hitchcock Hospital was the pride and joy of the local medical community when it opened. The staff comprised none other than the energetic Carlton P. Frost, his son G. D. Frost, and William T. Smith. Thus, from the start, there was a very direct connection between the hospital and Dartmouth, a fact underscored when the College's President William Jewett Tucker gave an address at the hospital dedication. Built in the so-called pavilion style, the building featured a handsome central rotunda and two domed wings that would become familiar and much loved over the decades that followed. (This was true even though patients did not exactly flock to the new hospital initially. The prevailing view of hospitals at the time was that they were places where the destitute went to die. Gradually, however, people were won over.)

In addition to making better patient care possible, the establishment of the hospital laid a basis for curricular improvements that would help medical education at Dartmouth advance "to the modern format, which combines study of the medical sciences in classroom settings with study of medical practice in clinical settings."[9] The faculty minutes for June 1, 1897, contain a report "for improving the curriculum of the college"; that record provides a useful snapshot of medical education at DMS at the time:

First—To make the course 4 years with 4 Lecture courses
Second—To ask the Trustees to permit students of Dartmouth College to matriculate in the Medical College at the end of the Junior year; to take during the first year of the Medical course the Courses in Chemistry Biology & Physics and perhaps others which are offered by the College, and to receive their degree in arts or science with the College Class, and to permit all Medical Students in their first year to recite to the Instructors in the departments of Chemistry Physics & Biology and in other departments of Dartmouth College which may be added . . .
Since Dartmouth College assumes the work of teaching during this first year, it should receive the fees for that period.
Third—The calendar for the remaining three years to be as follows: Term opens (as heretofore) about July 15, Term closes about March 1. Vacation at Christmas time identical with the College vacation
Fourth—The first two months of the term to be given up to the non-resident members of the Faculty for lectures & quizzes, with a daily recitation in Anat-

omy for the second year men, The remainder of the term to be occupied by the resident faculty.
Instruction to be given by lectures, recitations & by laboratory work. Some of the shorter courses of lectures by non-resident members may come during this period
Fifth—That we take measures to secure a resident Instructor in Bacteriology & Pathology.[10]

The proposed plan (no doubt influenced in considerable part by what was going on in other medical schools) combined the lecture and recitation terms, lengthened the lecture courses of the resident faculty, and made a more integrated whole of the lecture, recitation, and laboratory work. In so doing, the new plan took several different concerns into account. Externally, there was a new state regulation that required a longer course, as well as a need to equip graduates in a way that would permit them to be licensed in other states. The 1897 *Act to Regulate the Licensing and Registration of Physicians and Surgeons* included several stipulations—among which was that for the first time the prescribed length of time for the study of medicine was to be four years. Furthermore, the length of the school year was specified (nine months), as were the length and timing of the four required courses of lectures.[11] Additional changes in the relation between College and Medical School were also anticipated in the request to the trustees to permit students to have their final year of College studies count as the first year of the Medical School curriculum.[12] The faculty minutes for July 13, 1898, the day on which John Martin Gile gave the introductory lecture for the 102nd annual course at Dartmouth Medical School, included the announcement that the occasion marked the beginning of "the first combination recitation and lecture course under the new plan." A week later, the medical faculty voted to apply for membership in the Association of American Medical Colleges (AAMC). A new professionalism was beginning to manifest itself.[13]

Thirty students were enrolled in the fourth-year course in the first year under the new plan (1898), some evidence that prospective doctors had already begun to adjust—thanks to new rules instituted in other places—to the requirement for a four-year course that had only just been introduced in New Hampshire in 1897. (New Hampshire was no pioneer, and Dartmouth simply did what by that time was essential for its survival.)

Beginning in the 1899–1900 year, the entire four-year class-schedule was printed in a block diagram.[14] At a quick glance, the first and fourth years might look least demanding, with only twenty hours of class meetings required. First-year students would spend the bulk of their time on biology, chemistry, and physics, with the rest devoted to anatomy (human or comparative) and dissection (three hours a week). In the fourth year, twelve of the twenty hours were equally divided between "Practice" and "Clinic"; three hours a week were reserved for surgery, and two each for "Therapeutics" and "Obstetrics," the latter supplemented by one hour spent on gynecology. Bacteriology was also to be offered once a week during January and February.

In contrast, the second-year course must have looked daunting, with a full thirty-four hours of class time spelled out (spread, as in each of the years, over six days; only Sunday was free of classes). A dozen of the scheduled class hours were devoted exclusively to dissection, with several of the others alternating between dissection and histology (for two-thirds of the year) or bacteriology. Physiology, anatomy, and more chemistry filled out the second-year student's program. In the third year, students spent more time on physiology, anatomy, and dissection; they were also introduced for the first time to pathology, obstetrics, gynecology, therapeutics, and surgery.[15]

Medical Studies, Students, and Faculty

The model offered by Johns Hopkins Uniersity in the late nineteenth century for how to turn medical education into a truly *graduate* enterprise was evidence enough that the education and training of physicians could be managed differently than they traditionally had been. Years later, Abraham Flexner would emphasize the significance of Johns Hopkins as "the first medical school in America of genuine university type, with something approaching adequate endowment, well equipped laboratories conducted by modern teachers, devoting themselves unreservedly to medical investigation and instruction, and with its own hospital, in which the training of physicians and the healing of the sick harmoniously combine to the infinite advantage of both. The influence of this new foundation can hardly be overstated."[16]

Another measure of what students were being taught would be course syllabuses, but we have none. Instead, the closest we can come (with rare exceptions) is a sketchy list of the textbooks being used. Even then (as in the 1897 catalogue, for example), nothing is made of the fact that the author of more than one of the texts listed was on the Dartmouth faculty. Cases in point include: in Therapeutics, "Balliet's Notes" and "Field's Cathartics and Emetics"; in Chemistry, "Bartlett's Laboratory Exercises"; and *Diseases of Women and Children*, the textbook by Thomas and Mundé.[17] The *American Text-book of Surgery* was apparently so well known no one thought to mention that Phineas Conner was one of the eleven distinguished surgeons who had collaborated to compile the text.[18]

In fact, several of those who taught at Dartmouth during the latter years of the nineteenth century were quite distinguished and well known far beyond the confines of the Hanover plain. For example, the two faculty members who, between them, taught medical jurisprudence at Dartmouth for more than forty years, from 1857 to 1908, were part-time and nonresident, but each—Isaac Fletcher Redfield and John Ordronaux—was an extremely distinguished jurist. (They were also both Dartmouth College graduates, class of 1825 and class of 1850, respectively.) Redfield had a long career on the Vermont Supreme Court (he was Chief Justice for eight years). Ordronaux, a graduate of Harvard Law School, studied medicine in his spare time; after serving as an examining surgeon for volunteers in the Civil War, he became New York State's first commissioner in lunacy. He was the author of an 1869 text, *The Jurisprudence of Medicine*.[19]

Another member of the Dartmouth Medical School faculty who was widely known and whose talents were broadly appreciated was the surgeon Charles Nancrède. Like his mentor and friend Phineas Conner, Nancrède was a contributing author of the *American Text-book of Surgery*. His own two textbooks proved popular. *Essentials of Anatomy*, first published in 1888 in London as well as Philadelphia, came out in multiple editions; it was a standard text much in demand. *Lectures upon the Principles of Surgery*, dedicated to Conner, appeared in Philadelphia in 1899; a second edition came out in 1905 (in both Philadelphia and London).[20]

Little effort seems to have been expended to ensure that a continuing supply of non-Dartmouth students would be drawn to Hanover. In the first year of the "new plan" (1898), twenty of the thirty students who began the medical course were also College seniors. The next year, the number of Dartmouth seniors in the first-year medical school class was slightly greater: twenty-seven out of thirty-four. Thus the pattern was set that would over the years cause many to think of the Medical School as something of an exclusive Dartmouth club.

One change was that the percentage of students who had already earned a baccalaureate degree gradually increased. Those who entered with a high-school or academy diploma only were subjected to a modified set of requirements. (The 1908–1909 catalogue carried an announcement that, beginning in 1910, two years of college would be required for any student entering the medical school.)[21] One of the fullest descriptions of where things stood as the nineteenth century ended can be found in a letter from President Wiliam Jewett Tucker to Dean William Thayer Smith, written December 24, 1900. The letter summarized the meeting between Tucker and Smith, and it read in part as follows:

My dear Dr. Smith: —

. . . I have thought for some time but especially during the last year, that it would be desirable to readjust the relations between the Medical School & the College. Just what those relations were at the first it is a little difficult to say further than that the School was recognized rather grudgingly & without financial support as a department of the College. It is also difficult to say how much was meant by the action of the State when the School took for a time the name of the New Hampshire Medical College. . . . At times this system of a fee school has worked well financially, but it seems to me that the time has come when a school of this character can no longer expect steady support or assured growth. . . . I am now ready to advise the Trustees to meet the additional expense involved in an Instructor in Physiology, & in arranging suitable rooms for Bacteriological & Physiological laboratories with proper equipment, *provided* the financial management of the School is transferred to the Trustees. The Trustees would not be prepared to assume any financial obligations, such as now seem to be necessary to the growth of the School unless they can expect to gain a proper return in the increase in the school in numbers. This increase in my judgment can be brought about, by offering, through the changes proposed, greater inducements to students to enter from the outside, & also to students in the College to remain for the second year with a probability that a very large per cent would graduate from the School. . . .

I am
Very Truly Yours,
W. J. Tucker[22]

Ungreased wheels turn slowly. More than four months later, at a meeting of the trustees in May 1901, the president was authorized to appoint a committee "to act with him in reference to the suggestions contained in his annual report concerning the relation of the Medical School to the College."[23] A year after that, the committee reported at the May 1902 meeting, and the trustees voted to accept Tucker's various suggestions.[24]

Early Calls for Reform

Reform of medical education was in fact closely allied with a move toward reform in higher education generally; this was the period when the modern university was being born. Contrary to common impressions, interest in standards for medical practice did not spring full-grown from the brow of Abraham Flexner or the American Medical Association.[25] A number of initiatives—such as the formation of the Rockefeller

Institute for Medical Research—had been undertaken even before "agitation for the reform of medical education [came] to a head within the American Medical Association," and "Abraham Flexner and the AMA leaders did not originate reform; they only routinized it."[26] For example, in 1900 the AMA had begun collecting and publishing statistics on various matters having to do with medical education; in 1904 the AMA formed a Council on Medical Education (CME). Annual conferences of the CME began in 1905 (at the first of which "a minimum standard of medical education was formulated"), and by 1907 the CME was ready to present the first of several reports of inspection and classification of medical schools.[27]

Public concern about physicians' qualifications was at an all-time high, both cause and effect of laws like New Hampshire's 1897 statute to regulate the licensing of doctors. Nor was only the public concerned. A large number of American physicians studied abroad in the late nineteenth century (some 15,000 in Germany alone, for instance, between 1875 and 1914), and they typically came home "increasingly disturbed by low-grade education and by the lack of effective licensing" in their native land, very ready to do battle with the proprietary school graduates who actually benefited from the existence of inferior schools.[28]

Despite the CME's vigorous efforts at collecting information, formulating standards, and grading medical schools, the organization "was handicapped in these activities because its members hesitated to pass judgment on colleagues in other institutions."[29] The problem is common enough; self-policing, one of the hallmarks of a profession, is always fraught with the possibility that the power will be abused.[30] What was needed was an independent survey, directed by someone outside the profession. It was to be provided, to a remarkable extent single-handedly, by the talented, energetic, and relentlessly determined inspector underwritten by the Carnegie Foundation, Abraham Flexner.

Editors of the *Journal of the American Medical Association* (*JAMA*) understood the value of both investigations. The mid-August issue in 1909 carried an article by the CME's secretary, N. P. Colwell, on why an "inspection" of medical colleges was needed. There was also an unsigned editorial titled "The Influence of the Carnegie Foundation on Medical Education." "According to current reports," readers were told, "the medical work is investigated with the same thoroughness as other phases of the institutions in which the foundation has become interested," and "as a result undesirable conditions and shortcomings have been brought to light which call for change and improvement . . . If the results of expert work along these lines were given full publicity much good would surely come of it to medical education in general. The actual facts would be more helpful in the end than the poetry of the medical school catalogues and advertisements."[31]

The Flexner Report

The introduction to the document that would come to be called the "Flexner report"—formally its title was *Medical Education in the United States and Canada, A Report to the Carnegie Foundation for the Advancement of Teaching*—was written by Henry S. Pritchett, president of the Carnegie Foundation.[32] In it, he gave the rationale for undertaking the study in the first place by reviewing the status quo in medical education. Too often, medical schools had been empires unto themselves (each an "*imperium in imperio*" was how he put it), with the parent institutions taking no responsibility for standards and giving little support. The stiffer requirements for beginning medical study that many institutions had recently introduced, coupled with the growth of science and—with that—greater importance than ever of the laboratory, meant there was a new reason to define the relationship between medical education and general education.

For a quarter of a century, there had been an "enormous overproduction of uneducated and ill trained medical practitioners," a function of the large number of commercial medical schools. It stood to reason that there should be fewer schools—and that they would need to be better equipped and better conducted. Not surprisingly, the for-profit schools incurred the most vigorous censure: "Our hope is that this report will make plain once for all that the day of the commercial medical school has passed." And finally, Pritchett expressed the additional hope that "this publication may serve as a starting-point both for the intelligent citizen and for the medical practitioner in a new national effort to strengthen the medical profession."[33]

The choice of Abraham Flexner to head the study was not so strange as has sometimes been thought. The fact that he was not a doctor was part of a deliberate strategy on Pritchett's part. Precisely what he wanted, Flexner recalled Pritchett saying, was for professional schools to be studied from an educator's rather than a practitioner's point of view. In Flexner, Pritchett concluded, he had found a kindred spirit who was also a medical layman and an independent thinker. Looking back years later, Flexner affirmed the principle behind Pritchett's decision: "Dr. Pritchett was right: . . . the proper person to study medical education was a layman with general educational experience, not a professor in a medical school."[34] Another reason Flexner turned out to be such a happy choice was his close association with the faculty at Johns Hopkins (he was himself a graduate of that university). Years later, he wrote, "I had a tremendous advantage in the fact that I became . . . intimately acquainted with a small but ideal medical school. . . . Without this pattern in the back of my mind, I could have accomplished little."[35] Thus from the outset of Flexner's investigations, the medical school at Johns Hopkins was the standard against which all others would be measured.

Where Flexner found the time and energy to do the work he undertook for the Carnegie Foundation is beyond fathoming. He personally visited all 155 medical schools in the United States and Canada.[36] The bulk of his work on the report was presumably already done at the point in 1910 when he wrote to Ernest Fox Nichols, the still relatively new president of Dartmouth, on how to evaluate a medical curriculum. "[T]he proper procedure," he wrote, "is, I think, to study the science and practice of medicine as it is now carried on, to ask what schools and teachers ought to provide on that basis, and to confront the schools as they are with the criteria thus arrived at."[37]

What Flexner himself acknowledged as his own "utmost frankness" still has the capacity to startle today.[38] He was not one to mince words; the shock with which the faculty at Dartmouth—to say nothing of those who taught at other schools that received even sharper criticism—read what he had to say about their beloved school must have been considerable. Even in part 1 of the *Report*, in which the history of medical education in the United States and its then-current status were laid out in general terms, Dartmouth was the subject of some uncomplimentary asides. But it is in part 2, where each medical school is reviewed individually, that DMS received the severest criticisms. In a section on New England schools, Flexner wrote, "A more critical attitude on the part of the state boards and the student body" would have the following salutary effects:

> A thoroughly wretched institution, like the College of Physicians and Surgeons of Boston, would be at once wiped out. The clinical departments of Dartmouth, Bowdoin, and the University of Vermont would certainly be lopped off; *there is no good reason why these institutions—colleges all of them—should be concerned with medicine at all* [emphasis added]. The mere fact that they are all old schools is a poor reason for continuing them if they fail to do justice to the student, and thereby fail to subserve the public interest. . . . The argument that these small schools train all-round doctors who go out into the country, prepared to do everything, is refuted by the obvious fact that schools, unable to command obstetrical cases, contagious diseases, and the ailments that throng dispensaries, are not really sending out the type of practitioner which, by their own admission, the rural districts need.[39]

Notice that of the four medical schools associated with Nathan Smith, only Yale escaped Flexner's sweeping indictment; New Haven was no longer rural (even in Smith's day it had been more nearly a city than Hanover, Brunswick, or Burlington). Elsewhere Flexner remarked that "let never so many low-grade doctors be turned out, whether in Boston or in smaller places like Burlington or Brunswick, that are supposed not to spoil the young men for a country practice, these unpromising places . . . will not attract them."[40] (Hanover's absence from this list may be explained simply by its having lacked alliterative value here.) The implicit question was whether Nathan Smith's vision remained relevant at the beginning of the twentieth century.

When the physical facilities at Dartmouth were described, there was a pronounced sting in the tail: "*Excellent working laboratories* are provided for pathology, bacteriology, histology, physiology, and for the medical subjects cared for in the academic department. Every student serves four weeks during his second year as an assistant in the pathological laboratory, *and thus gets an admirable practical experience*" (emphases added). But then: "Anatomy, taught by a practitioner, has not as yet been developed on modern lines."[41] In an undated letter to President Nichols, Colin C. Stewart sputtered indignantly that Dr. Gilman Frost "is the best teacher of Anatomy I have ever known" and insisted that "Dr. [Percy] Bartlett gets more thorough work out of the men in the dissecting room than any of the rest of us can get in our laboratories. To pick on Anatomy as a weak spot is to imply a weakness in the whole criticism."[42]

That was by no means the worst of it, for next came the assessment of the clinical facilities at Dartmouth, which the CME had already identified as a problem:

> These [clinical facilities] are very limited. The college controls a hospital of 40 beds, of which 24 are in wards at reduced rates. . . . Still further to weaken the teaching value of the hospital [it went without saying, that this number of beds was far too low], surgery predominates to the extent of 80 per cent of all cases. Students are employed to assist in surgical operations, but the backbone of clinical instruction—an adequate clinic in internal medicine—is lacking. . . .
>
> There is no dispensary [outpatient clinic].[43]

In the section headed "General Considerations," Flexner praised what he found praiseworthy, but his sober conclusion was clear enough: Dartmouth should not expect to—could not—survive as a four-year school:

> The development of its clinical work presents a serious difficulty. The village is rather inaccessible; the surrounding country is thinly populated. . . . Surgical

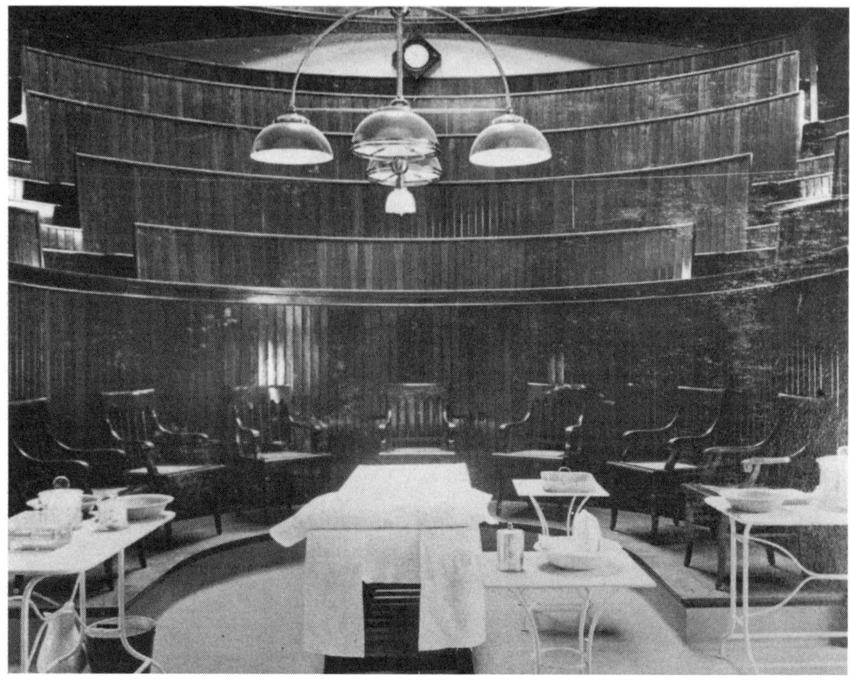

Operating room at the Mary Hitchcock Hospital, 1893. Courtesy of Dartmouth College Library.

cases are attracted easily enough. Can medical cases be attracted too? Certainly not without a very large outlay in the form of professional salaries and hospital expense. . . . That the school cannot much longer continue in its present stage is clear.[44]

What was written in those opening pages of the *Report* explicitly about Dartmouth made for a bleak picture, not least because Flexner took issue not only with the current situation but with the very arguments Dartmouth had traditionally used to explain its mission:

It is alleged in extenuation that "our graduates pass state board examinations, get hospital appointments, and succeed in practice." It is quite true: what of it? The argument if valid would commit every school above the lowest to deliberate deterioration of its facilities. Bowdoin makes light of a wretched dispensary on the grounds above cited; Dartmouth men succeed by the same tests without any dispensary at all. . . . So much for the worst. It may be, however, that in the case of some schools with weak hospitals and no dispensaries, the didactic instruction is vigorous, clean cut, in its way effective. Such is the claim made at Dartmouth and at Bowdoin. Let us concede its justice: what of it? Logically, the position of these institutions would be stronger if they stuck to didactic instruction altogether. The moment that they offer a course in clinical microscopy, they are committed to an entirely different scale of values. For that they require patients whom they can observe closely and continuously.[45]

Given New England's population, Flexner concluded that 125 new doctors were needed. To produce such a number, he said, "two schools, one of moderate size and one smaller, readily suffice." In other words, all except Harvard and Yale could be dispensed with. Lest anyone misunderstand, he clarified: "It is unwise to divide the Boston field; *it is unnecessary to prolong the life of the clinical departments of Dartmouth, Bowdoin, and Vermont.* They are not likely soon to possess the financial resources needed to develop adequate clinics in their present location. . . . *The historic position of the schools in question counts little as against changed ideas*" (emphases added).[46] This last remark was fully in keeping with the overall theme of Flexner's *Report*: "The improvement of medical education cannot . . . be resisted on the ground that it will destroy schools and restrict output: that is precisely what is needed." Indeed, what the country needed, Flexner insisted, was "fewer and better doctors." Thus the doctors at Dartmouth were not being singled out for especially harsh treatment. Yet it was hard not to feel implicated in remarks of Flexner's like the "truth is that existing conditions are defended only by way of keeping unnecessary medical schools alive."[47]

Though Flexner never suggested that Dartmouth belonged to the class of "thoroughly wretched" institutions, there was no denying the direct relevance to DMS of Flexner's general discussion of the third and fourth years of study: "The backbone of the structure is the clinic in internal medicine. . . . The sufficiency of the school's clinical resources depends at bottom on its medical clinic; the value of its training depends on the systematic thoroughness with which it is in a position to use an adequate supply of medical cases."[48]

Dartmouth's Own Reform Agenda

Reform had been happening at Dartmouth, too, initially quite independently of anything proposed by either the CME or Flexner. The 1905–1906 DMS catalogue gave evidence that Dartmouth was among those inspired by the success at Johns Hopkins in using the hospital as a genuine teaching resource for upper-class students in particular. DMS followed the trend to make the third and fourth years of medical school explicitly "clinical years."[49] For a six-month stretch, the third-year students spent three afternoons a week "in laboratory and wards," while the fourth-year students were divided into "sections" for "clinical work in wards" at the hospital. The fourth-year curriculum included such special topics as ophthalmology, otolaryngology, dermatology, diseases of children, and diseases of the nervous system.[50] A "Report of the Dean" (at the annual meeting of the medical faculty in 1905) took up the issue of just how well Dartmouth medical students had done on their examinations. Although Dartmouth's results were far from stellar, the dean seemed for the most part satisfied. The percentage of Dartmouth candidates who passed in 1903 was 85.5; in 1904, it was 85.7. In both years Dartmouth fell just above the median, with 74 of 152 schools having a better record. Dean Smith was even more pleased to report that figures for those two years from the Massachusetts State Board of Registration showed only Johns Hopkins students with a higher average mark (five candidates averaged 78.8 percent). Tied for second place were Dartmouth with eight candidates and the University of Pennsylvania with three; their average was 78.1 percent. "Harvard, McGill, Jefferson, Columbia and many other first class schools were lower on the list," he reported with understandable pleasure.[51]

At a September 1906 DMS faculty meeting, it was voted "that the Council on Medical Education of the American Medical Ass'n be informed that this Faculty is in sympathy with any forward movement, but is not now ready to accept the recommendations of the Council."[52] Then, in 1908, the medical faculty forwarded several recommendations to the trustees aimed at further tightening and clarification of entrance requirements and courses of study:

1. That in and after 1910 two years in College be required for admission to the Medical School.
2. That a two year course be arranged in Dartmouth leading to the Medical School.
3. That students in Dartmouth College be permitted to matriculate in the Medical School at the beginning of Junior year, and to receive the degree of A.B. or B.S. at the end of four years, and the degree of M.D. at the end of six years.[53]

President Tucker endorsed these recommendations.[54] Nonetheless, when the trustees voted on the recommendations in August of that year (1908), they did so with qualifications. Among other concerns, the trustees clearly did not want benefits for the Medical School purchased at the cost of lowered (or even altered) standards in the College. A faculty committee was appointed "to join with members of the Academic Faculty in planning for new arrangements of courses." Its amended report was accepted at the faculty meeting in October of that year.[55]

This was the context in which President Nichols received the following letter from N. P. Colwell of the Council on Medical Education, in early 1910:

> Dear Sir:
>
> . . . We have just gone carefully through our data regarding the Dartmouth Medical School and regret to say that owing to the extremely limited clinical and hospital facilities, we cannot list as satisfactory the last two or clinical years of the course. . . . On account of the limited population in Hanover,[56] we do not see how any satisfactory increase in such facilities can be obtained. It seems also that if the money at present expended toward the work of the last two years were used to further develop the work of the first two, it would enable you to strengthen to a great extent that portion of the medical course. Although we find your school weak in its clinical end, we feel that you should be complimented upon the good work being done during the first two years. . . . Has the subject ever been considered whether it would not be advisable, . . . to discontinue the last two or clinical years of the medical course? We are presenting these matters to you frankly and should like very much to obtain your views in regard to the points mentioned.[57]

The faculty minutes give no indication whether the practitioners who had worked so hard to make Dartmouth Medical School a place of which they could be proud—not least by organizing the hospital and erecting a new building (named "The Nathan Smith Laboratory" when it was completed in 1908)[58]—were prepared for the dire judgment rendered by the CME: "[O]wing to the extremely limited clinical and hospital facilities, we cannot list as satisfactory the last two or clinical years of the course." Anticipated or not, the indictment must have been a blow, softened only slightly by the complimentary remark Colwell inserted about the quality of the work being done in the first two years.

E. J. Bartlett was given the task of investigating and preparing a response. He went quickly to work and reported a plan whereby he "might obtain from . . . some of the larger New England hospitals personal expressions of opinion as to the qualifications and training of the Dartmouth graduates whose work they had observed."[59] In retrospect, the hope that writing letters to such individuals would produce data of the sort the CME was seeking (and that would impress the CME) seems a rather weak, even somewhat desperate, effort to bolster reputation. The letters that arrived in response were encouraging, however. John Nichols, superintendent of the state infirmary at Tewksbury, Massachusetts, testified to the "high standards" of the DMS graduates on his staff. He also reported that the work of those who had prepared at DMS "stands out in point of efficiency" when compared to others on his staff from Tufts, Harvard, Johns Hopkins, the University of Vermont, McGill, and Ann Arbor. Regarding the performance of DMS alumni at Carney Hospital in Boston, Henry M. Christian wrote, "I have found these Dartmouth men were capable of doing good work in their various duties as house-officers." A letter written on behalf of Dr. Harvey P. Towle at Boston City Hospital quoted him saying that "During [the past fourteen] years the two best men I have had at all were both Dartmouth men."[60]

President Nichols sent these (and two other) testimonial letters to Abraham Flexner, only to have Flexner return them in a letter of May 4, 1910, commenting that "the number of men involved is not large, so that I should be slow to arrive at any conclusion on the basis of these letters alone. I should also eliminate at once the men who made good as surgeons, because your training in surgery is not in question. Our criticism touches only your medical clinics."[61] Flexner's blunt and crisp tone, as it turned out, was mild compared to what was to come in the formal report. But even that, excerpts from which we have just seen, did not deter Dean Gile from writing an optimistic column in the alumni magazine fifteen months later. There he insisted that the increased number of patients treated annually at the hospital had "provided ample clinical material for students, and the close proximity of school and hospital has rendered it so easily available that it has been used to most excellent advantage."[62]

Yet the opportunities for Dartmouth students to engage in clinical work at the Mary Hitchcock were restricted to what amounted to class sessions being held for groups of students seeing patients together at the hospital. While this was better than no exposure to patients, it was not adequate when compared to true clinical clerkships of the sort offered, not surprisingly, at Johns Hopkins, as well as Michigan, Pennsylvania, and Jefferson. A small community hospital like the Mary Hitchcock was simply not equipped to allow Dartmouth Medical School to do likewise.[63]

Although members of the Dartmouth Medical School faculty were concerned about the CME's negative judgment, they did not yet think—or want to believe—that the indictment was really serious. The minutes of the medical faculty meeting in October of 1910, for instance, reflect very much a "business as usual" approach to life at the Medical School. Thus the faculty voted to accept a new "Code of Regulations for the administration of the school,"[64] but made no mention of Flexner's just-published report.

In the August 1911 issue of the College alumni magazine, Dean John M. Gile briskly explained away decreases in enrollments and then devoted himself to explicating the benefits and outstanding features of the school: the six-year program, improvements in the library room of the new medical building; the "entirely remodelled" operating room at the hospital, and the fact that graduates "almost without exception, secure excellent outside hospital appointments." When he closed by saying that in "steadily raising the standard of admission and curriculum the faculty and trustees have taken the step that they believe the future of medical education demands," no one would have guessed that Dartmouth Medical School was being pressed so hard by the independent inspection teams.[65]

In the autumn of 1912, there was further "informal discussion" about the curriculum. The continuation of the combined academic and medical program leading to both a bachelor's degree and an M.D. does not appear to have been up for debate.[66] Nonetheless, the full force of the publicity generated by the Flexner report would soon make it essential for the faculty to focus less on the details of course schedules and more on how they might improve clinical opportunities for their students. In January of 1913, the nonresident faculty gathered in Boston to discuss a proposal that arrangements should be made "for the clinical teaching of our students in the Boston hospitals, this teaching to be given by faculty members holding appointments in such hospitals." A letter was sent to Dr. Arthur Bevan, chairman of the CME, in an effort to ascertain whether that committee was likely to view such a plan favorably.[67]

Bevan's response was prompt. The CME had earlier suggested to Dartmouth that they should consider making an affiliation with Harvard. If DMS students were to be sent to Boston for clinical work anyway, Bevan argued, they ought to be given "the benefit of the well organized clinical department of Harvard." He also proposed that graduates defined as "Dartmouth-Harvard men" might find the label "a mark of peculiarly excellent medical training."[68] In so doing, Bevan utterly failed to take Dartmouth pride into account. Furthermore, although he again stressed "the difficulties in the Dartmouth situation and the really excellent work that has been done handicapped as you have been for the lack of necessary clinical facilities which can be secured only in a large center of population," his remarks were hardly calculated to please the Dartmouth Medical School faculty, the members of which apparently believed they were doing a good (not merely adequate) job.[69]

Swimming Against the Tide

Looking back, it is difficult to see how any institution could have withstood these withering attacks as long as Dartmouth did. The explanation can hardly lie in the fact that the Dartmouth faculty did not believe or take seriously the criticisms; they had been hearing them for some time. N. P. Colwell had (on October 2, 1911), for instance, sent to President

Nichols a copy of the five-page CME report on Dartmouth Medical School from its 1909 visit, in anticipation of the announced visit for October 31, 1911. Granting that the "preliminary standard of DMS is up to the ideal set by the AMA in 1905," Colwell nonetheless noted that the real problem was "the work of the clinical years." In contrasting the ideal with the actual situation at DMS, Colwell had noted "how little is available at Hanover." So there had been preparation for Flexner's harsh conclusions.[70]

In November 1912, a lengthy unsigned "Report drawn up for use of the Special Trustee Committee and of the President" was released, which also spelled out the recommended standard as the CME had published it that July.[71] A reminder of how Dartmouth had fared was also included. We learn that E. J. Bartlett had been delegated to attend the 1910 conference in Chicago, prior to the announcement of the ratings of the schools; his task had been to forestall Dartmouth's losing its "A" rating. That he had succeeded seems quite astonishing, for he apparently did so on the basis of precisely the kinds of arguments Flexner so disdainfully dismissed.

In yet another indication that Dartmouth had underestimated the influence Flexner would wield, little was said about his assessment in the faculty's own "Report." Flexner's criticism of the Department of Anatomy was mentioned, and one of his paragraphs ("It is unnecessary to prolong the life of the clinical departments of Dartmouth . . .") was quoted. But these were asides. The author(s) of the faculty report dwelt much more on all that had been done at Dartmouth recently to improve the teaching of medicine. There was much of which they could be proud.

Dartmouth's ranking by the CME was then considered. Here there is evidence of the kind of kid-glove treatment Flexner implied the doctors of the CME were bound to give their medical colleagues, a standard of gentleness to which he did not need to be held. For a medical school to be rated "A+" required simply receiving a mark of 70 percent or better in each of ten categories (equipment, faculty, curriculum, etc.); an "A" rating could still be earned even if the school fell below the 70 percent mark in three categories. When we learn that of the existing 116 medical colleges, only 50—among them Dartmouth—earned an "A+" or "A," we may be less impressed than the author of the report probably wanted his readers to be.

The Effects of Outside Influence

Yet right around the corner, so to speak, was the reality that the CME itself had also issued a call for Dartmouth (despite its "A" rating) to dispense with the clinical years. Minutes of several faculty meetings in the early part of 1913 record efforts to avoid reaching Flexner's conclusion. Various reform efforts were reported. There was Dr. Bevan's proposal that Dartmouth affiliate with Harvard and much talk on the merits of affiliating with the State Hospital in Tewksbury.[72] The March 10 meeting consisted largely of Gile's report to his colleagues on the meeting he had attended on their behalf in Chicago. He painted a full picture of the influence of outside bodies on medical schools in 1913, which included his assessment that the Carnegie Foundation could be ignored—that its views were irrelevant—on the subject of medical education.

> The organizations holding meetings in Chicago were: The Council of the American Medical Association on Education and Legislation, the Association of American Medical Colleges, and the Federation of State Medical Boards.
>
> In general the influence of these organizations appears to be working more or less harmoniously and very definitely in the same direction.
>
> The [CME] seems to be able, independent, and unprejudiced. . . . The [AAMC] seems to me to be little more than an instrument in the hands of the Council for whipping certain recalcitrants into line. . . .
>
> The Federation of State Medical Boards is another matter. Here, though the Council may endeavor to and doubtless does, have some influence, it cannot sufficiently control the personnel of the Federation to be steadily certain of the trend of its action. . . .
>
> I do not mention the Carnegie Foundation, first because it did not appear to any extent in the recent meetings, and secondly because it seems to me that in the matter of medical education its judgments have been so largely discounted, both by the medical profession and the general public, that its views and influence but little affect us.

Gile's view is surprising, if not naïve. Already in 1909, the *JAMA* editorial in the education issue cited earlier had stated that the Foundation was "a factor of great importance to medical education," one that—if "wisely managed"—might "exert a powerful and growing influence for good on the development of medical education in this country."[73] Whether Gile had not read this, had forgotten it, or had dismissed it as in-house puffery is unclear. He continued:

> First and most important, that a fifth year of clinical work will be urged on the medical schools as a regular part of their instruction, . . . a well defined rotational service in a large institution or institutions where all branches, both general and special would be both seen and taught under the definite guidance of the school authorities. . . .
>
> This fifth year in the hospital would bear hardest on the smaller schools that do not control large enough hospital facilities for their fifth year work. . . . In our own case many of the hospitals that we now depend on would doubtless be closed to us and many of the smaller ones would not be accepted as offering the required facilities. . . .
>
> I was instructed to endeavor to secure a favorable decision on our application

for membership in the Association of American Medical Colleges, and to see in what way the Council would look upon a course which included a year at Tewksbury. . . .

You may fairly charge me with constantly suggesting the inference in this report that the outlook is not favorable for the continuance of the medical degree at Dartmouth. I admit this impeachment as far as these outside influences are concerned, and it is only with them that this report deals. So far as they affect us, it is necessary for us to see them as they are and not to minimize their importance. . . . I see no chance that we shall . . . succeed in securing students for the last two years of the course. Influence at times becomes so strong as to amount to authority and I have the premonition that a situation where that is true now confronts us.[74]

One senses a feeling of resignation in the votes that followed at the faculty meeting a week later. First the Tewksbury plan was voted down, five to three. Then a decision on whether to suspend the M.D. degree was tabled, as was the question of whether to continue with a fifth clinical year. Three documents were to be sent to the nonresident faculty. The first was Gile's report; the second was a letter explaining the vote on the Tewksbury plan written by the secretary of the medical faculty, George Sellers Graham; the third was an emotional appeal by Stewart proposing that the school be continued as it was. The point of sending all this material, made explicit by Graham, was to inform those colleagues of "the progress of the discussion" and "to enlist . . . assistance" as well as to solicit "any suggestions, criticism, or new proposals."

In his letter, Graham soberly pointed out that if DMS graduates could not be licensed in other states, that would be reason enough to cut the last two years. He closed with the reminder that the "future attitudes of the Board [of Trustees] will presumably depend upon their evaluation of the remedial measures which we may take in the meantime looking toward the betterment of our clinical resources." All members of the faculty were urged to respond.[75]

Stewart advocated forcefully against "any proposed action leading to the withdrawal of the third and four year courses in medicine and to the cessation of the conferring of degrees." The first arguments he put forward were the sentimental ones that both Bevan and Flexner had waved aside: the "history of the school," the "obligation of the Faculty to maintain that history," and the "duty of the school to its constituency and to its alumni." Then Stewart undertook the more difficult task of arguing in favor of Dartmouth's educational program.

There seems to be little difference of opinion as to the excellence of the methods of instruction and the nature of the finished product. The admitted defect in our opportunities in Hanover is a lack of medical clinical material of sufficiently varied and extensive character. The result of that lack, from the standpoint of the School, is that men are graduated who, though thoroughly grounded in the fundamentals of Medicine and Surgery, have yet not seen a sufficiently wide range of cases to be in a position to begin the practice of medicine—in brief, to diagnose their cases. . . .

The whole problem as it must be decided by the governing board of the School resolves . . . into a question as to whether we can . . . continue to draw a sufficient number of students to justify the continuance of the School.

Stewart finished with a dramatic flourish: Giving up the clinical years without a fight was tantamount to committing suicide, an act, he reminded his colleagues with rising vigor and enthusiasm, that is "in almost all systems of morals . . . a sin, in all systems of law . . . a crime."

The emotional appeal did its job. The minutes of the next month's meeting recorded the following vote: "Upon motion of Dr Stewart, there was adopted the Resolution—that the medical faculty express their confidence in the general methods and results of the School as at present constituted; and recommend that, if possible, steps be taken to provide for the continuance of the School."[76]

Some basis for Stewart's expression of confidence did exist. Just a few months earlier, Graham had been able to include in his regular column for the College alumni magazine this upbeat report:

The record shown by the graduates of the school continues at its former excellence. The men just graduated have been able to secure coveted positions in some of the best hospitals in New England, including the City Hospitals of Boston and Worcester, and the Rhode Island General Hospital of Providence. . . . [O]f a total of twelve Dartmouth graduates . . . examined by the licensing board of five states during the past year, none of the candidates failed to pass the examinations. This record was equalled by only thirteen others from the total of 119 medical schools in the United States.[77]

Finis

It was not, however, enough. In a five-page committee report to the Board of Trustees, probably prepared shortly after the CME's most recent visit to Dartmouth, President Nichols reviewed for the trustees the various options studied by the committee appointed "to Consider the Present Status of medical Education and the Medical School." The work of DMS had been, he was able to tell them, "above criticism"; the rating of the school by the CME was A, with A+ being the best possible. But, he had to add, "we have been officially notified that next year the school will be dropped to the B grade." In addition, the New York State Board of Regents—which had earlier said it would approve DMS graduates up to 1914—was now saying it would debar "our future graduates . . .

Medical School, report of Com. as to status of.

The Committee appointed to consider and report upon the status of the Medical School made a report which, upon motion of Mr. Chase, was accepted and placed on file; and in accordance with the recommendation of the Committee, it was,—

Medical School, last 2 yrs of course discontinued.

Voted, that after the year 1914, instruction appertaining to the two last or clinical years of the course in Medicine be suspended for the present; and that the resources of the School, in teachers and equipment, be concentrated upon the first two years of the course, which may be elected by undergraduates of the College.

Trustees minutes from April 26, 1913, handwritten, showing the text suspending the four-year program. Courtesy of Dartmouth College.

from practicing" in New York. DMS had been "sharply criticized by the Council for the limited amount and variety of clinical material available for purposes of instruction," and the judgment had been made that the "clinical requirements cannot possibly be met in Hanover." Despite a resolution—the only one "upon which [the DMS faculty] could unite"—to the effect that the current "methods and results of the School" have their "confidence," a "considerable majority could see no other course open to the Trustees than to discontinue the last two years of clinical instruction and strengthen the first two laboratory years of the course." Others, unable to come up with anything novel, could offer only "a counsel of despair." In the end, President Nichols felt compelled to recommend to the trustees "that after the year 1914, instruction in the last two or clinical years be suspended for the present, and that the resources of the School in teachers and equipment be concentrated upon the first two years of medicine, which may be elected by undergraduates of Dartmouth College."[78]

The trustees met on April 26, 1913, a week after the committee's confident assertion reported by Nichols that "the general methods and results of the School as at present constituted" were reason enough to recommend continuing the school. Each resident member of the DMS faculty was invited to meet with the trustees' Committee on Medical Education, since it was known that there were "differences of opinion among the members of Medical Faculty concerning what steps should be taken . . . toward the future of the School."[79] Against this background, the trustees took the following action:

The Committee appointed to consider and report upon the status of the Medical School made a report which, upon motion of Mr. [Charles P.] Chase, was accepted and placed on file; and in accordance with the recommendation of the Committee, it was—

Voted, that after the year 1914, instruction appertaining to the two last or clinical years of the course in Medicine be suspended for the present; and that the resources of the School, in teachers and equipment, be concentrated upon the first two years of the course, which may be elected by undergraduates of the College.[80]

Four days after the vote, a memorandum went out "To the Alumni of the Dartmouth Medical School," explaining why the Board of Trustees, after most careful consideration, had "come to feel that it is wise, temporarily at least, for the institution to discontinue granting the degree of Doctor of Medicine." (For the complete text of the letter, see Appendix C, pages 298–99.) The statement departed from its matter-of-fact tone only once, briefly, with an aside implying that the CME had perhaps not dealt altogether fairly with Dartmouth (but acknowledging that the damage done by the CME's criticisms was too massive to overcome). Once again, the Flexner report was not mentioned. The memorandum ended with an expression of hope that the alumni of the medical school would agree "as to the wisdom of the action taken."[81]

Hope was nourished by in the words "for the present" in the faculty resolution, and in Nichols's cautious "temporarily at least," but the forces arrayed against the status quo were overwhelming. In June, the

schedule committee reported the results of its correspondence with other medical schools relative to the transfer of our men. Letters were read from sixteen of these schools, seven having thus far failed to answer the committee's inquiry. . . . The secretary was instructed to continue the correspondence with such schools as make conditions upon the transfer of our men into them, also to write in the matter to the Council on Medical Education of the American Medical Association and to the New York State Board of Regents.

Thus quietly, amidst considerable debate over the addition of a department of pharmacology, the whole discussion of whether the clinical years should be dropped from the program at Dartmouth Medical School came to an end. Concern shifted—appropriately and importantly—to where second-year students might continue their third- and fourth-year studies.[82] Gile, in his regular dean's column in the College's alumni magazine, reprinted the announcement (which had been mailed to DMS alumni) and an explanation of why the trustees decided to eliminate the final two years.[83] The following summer, in the June 1914 issue of the magazine, the headline "Associated Schools Hold Commencement" alerted readers to a simple, unsigned notice: "The degrees granted by the Medical School are the last which will be conferred in that department."[84]

Looking Ahead

However hard the medical faculty members at Dartmouth may have had to swallow in taking the steps they did, by August of 1914 they were ready to put a good face on it all. For the Dartmouth public, this took the form of an article by Frederic Pomeroy Lord in the *Dartmouth Alumni Magazine*. His apologia propounded themes that would be heard many times in the years ahead. Among them was a familiar appeal to Dartmouth tradition and pride: "In continuing the teaching of medical courses at Dartmouth there is the strong impetus given by the knowledge and influence of 117 years of an honorable and highly successful record, with its wealth of tradition and inspiration."

Lord described the future course of medical study at Dartmouth in terms that sounded much more like what had been heard earlier from the CME, and from Abraham Flexner in his report, than like what the Dartmouth faculty had previously insisted. "[T]he first two years of a medical course are concerned with the fundamental sciences that underlie the practise of medicine," he wrote, "while the last two years take up, in addition to a continuation of these scientific principles, their practical application." His explanation of the consequences of these two different kinds of education constituted a major capitulation. No longer was there the stubborn insistence of just a few years earlier that with hard work and good faith the school would get a good rating. Instead, the emphasis was all on what was good about the way things stood in 1914 and on why one should be optimistic about the future.[85] His confident tone was not unjustified. A month later, N. P. Colwell sent President Nichols a copy of the CME's pamphlet No. 85, "Choice of a Medical School," reprinted from the August 22, 1914, issue of *JAMA*, rating medical schools across the nation. DMS was one of the seven two-year schools (out of nine) to receive a grade of Class A, which indicated it was an "acceptable" school but one that "could make certain improvements to advantage."[86]

A year after Lord's magazine article had appeared, Colin C. Stewart—then secretary of Dartmouth Medical School—wrote a comparable piece to report on the first year of the school's experience with the two-year format. He began by outlining "two notable advances" that had nothing as such to do with the school as a two-year institution. One was the establishment, under Walter L. Mendenhall, of a department of pharmacology. (Mendenhall added prestige; he had formerly taught both in the medical school at Drake University and at Harvard University.) The other was that the modifications in the Nathan Smith Laboratory made to accommodate the new department had resulted in improvements to the library. He ended with a spirited defense of the new status quo:

> Dartmouth Medical School is in a particularly favored position to offer the courses in the fundamental sciences of the two pre-clinical years in Medicine. With classes of such a size that the men are always under the direct supervision of the instructor in charge of the course, with ample equipment for the work, and with a freedom from distracting interests not found in large medical centers, we believe that we are able to turn out a type of man whose training will be a guarantee of later success.[87]

That these words should appear over Stewart's name is remarkable, given his strong letter only two years earlier in opposition to ending the third- and fourth-year classes. If Stewart's language can be taken as indicative of the mood on campus, he and the rest of the faculty and the trustees had determined to support wholeheartedly the project of turning DMS into a first-rate, two-year school. To do so made a great deal of sense. By 1915, "the prospects for [medical] education and licensing were promising. 'Medical reform' had at last been achieved in the United States." In other words, the Flexner report and the CME's rating scheme had largely achieved their goals. There were fewer schools (many merged or were closed); a small number—like Dartmouth—had retrenched and become two-year schools; and the National Board of Medical Examiners (founded in 1915) was on the way to solving the peculiar problems that arose from having independent examining boards in each state, most of which did not offer reciprocity.[88]

For members of the Dartmouth medical faculty, the question always present in the background was whether they should expect to remain a two-year school or whether they should work to reestablish DMS with its "honorable and highly successful record" as a full-fledged, degree-granting institution. Whatever other concerns might come before the faculty, over the next few decades the issue of whether to reinstate the clinical years as part of the curriculum at Dartmouth Medical School would keep recurring.

CHAPTER SEVEN

Reassessing the School's Identity

Give the buried flower a dream. —ROBERT FROST[1]

A CERTAIN IRONY lay behind Flexner's judgment about Dartmouth Medical School. The faculty consisted of doctors who were experienced medical practitioners. To have the basic science program of the first two years praised and yet be pressed to give up the clinical training of the third and fourth years must have seemed passing strange to the dedicated physicians who had done so much to improve medical education at Dartmouth. Thus it is hardly surprising that the possibility—the desirability—of restoring what had been eliminated was a recurring topic in faculty discussions year after year.

The Lord Report

The first time after the capitulation that the debate over reintroducing a four-year curriculum surfaced in a formal way was 1923. The previous October, the trustees had voted to ask President Ernest Martin Hopkins to appoint a committee "to consider the condition of the Medical School and the Thayer School."[2] Professor Frederic P. Lord was chair of the committee of medical school faculty that submitted its lengthy report on the "Future Status of Dartmouth Medical School" (the "Lord report").

The report carefully reviewed the history of the school, laying emphasis on the curriculum changes over the years and the steady increase in requirements for matriculation as well as graduation.[3] One effect of thus belaboring the institution's history was to establish how closely intertwined College and Medical School were by 1923. Implicit in those close ties was responsibility for the welfare of the Medical School on the part of the College and its trustees.

Mentioning that DMS had ceased being a four-year, degree-granting school in 1914, the report spelled out the requirements in place since 1920 and stressed that the AMA had since 1914 rated Dartmouth as a "Class A" school. "In fact," the Lord report emphasized, "the high pre-medical requirements of this school, the small size of the classes, and the general spirit of hard work and interest that pervades the students, make it possible to turn out men unusually well prepared in the first half of their medical work." How DMS had coped with the main findings of the Flexner report about inadequate medical training was summarized. There followed a review of the then-current situation, with respect to the number of faculty, number of buildings, and operating expenses. Finally came the crux of the matter—the reasons for considering "possible change" at DMS. There were not enough physicians in rural New Hampshire, and too many of them were elderly. Post-Flexner, the report continued, too few good medical schools were left; national authorities were "calling for an increase in the number of medical schools."[4]

The Lord report presented three options: discontinuing the school altogether, continuing it as a two-year school, and reestablishing a four-year school. Reasons in support of each option were given, with five pages being devoted to a careful discussion of what returning to a four-year program would mean. While granting that the severest problem was still "obtaining . . . clinical material, sufficient for the needs of the school," it was proposed that this could be overcome by the creation of a "medical center, which . . . would attract more and more patients."[5]

The committee scattered through its report several sentimental points indicating that a restoration of the four-year school would be welcome: Having DMS return to its prior status as a degree-granting institution would be widely received with favor. The students and alumni wished it to happen (95 percent of 78 letters said so), and a factor not to be overlooked was "the desire to bring back to its former status a school founded 125 years ago and having such an honorable history, and carrying the imprint of so many able and widely known physicians."[6]

The report at first seemed to have been persuasive. At its May 4, 1923, meeting, the Board of Trustees gave the Medical School a vote of confidence, believing that "the continuance of the medical school is essential to the welfare of the College, and that the restoration of the last two years of the medical course is desirable."[7] But the trustees' records suddenly go silent; there is no further mention over the next five years of the condition of the Medical School, or of the committee that was supposed to be undertaking "further examination." No "later report" appears to have been made. Even what the medical school faculty itself thought about restoring DMS to its former status is obscured. A curious gap in the minutes of the medical school faculty occurs between September 20, 1917, and June 17, 1923, and nothing about the Lord report appears in the minutes once they resume.[8] In 1928, the alumni weighed in. It was reported that they were "heartily in sympathy with the oft-time expressed hope that the trustees of the College would, when the proper time arrives, re-establish the final two years in medicine."[9]

The Hitchcock Clinic Is Born

The complex and symbiotic relationship between the Hitchcock Hospital and Dartmouth Medical School began to be exposed in a new way once the two clinical years were no longer part of the DMS curriculum. Without those clinical years, the clinical faculty obviously had less to do, and the lack of a clinical program at DMS made the medical scene in Hanover considerably less desirable from a professional point of view. Not surprisingly, the hospital began to have "difficulty in attracting an adequate group of well-trained men to practice in the area and to serve on its staff."[10]

As fortune would have it, a Dartmouth faculty member conceived of a way to stop what amounted to a brain drain. John Pollard Bowler had graduated from Dartmouth College in 1915, just too late to do his entire medical training at DMS. After completing the first two years of medical school in Hanover, he earned his M.D. at Harvard in 1919. Following further work in surgery in Boston, he spent three years on a surgical fellowship at the Mayo Clinic in Minnesota (1921–1924). He then returned to Hanover to open a practice and was promptly made an instructor in pharmacology. Up to that point, there was little reason to suspect the profound influence Bowler would have on medicine in the region. In 1927, however, he not only became dean of Dartmouth Medical School—a position he held until 1945—but also joined with four colleagues to form the Hitchcock Clinic.[11]

The four others who aided Bowler in this pioneering effort were already Medical School colleagues: John (Jay) F. Gile (not so incidentally Bowler's brother-in-law), Harry French, Percy Bartlett, and Harold DesBrisay. Bartlett was the oldest, both in age and in years of service on the DMS faculty, having been there since 1904 (four years after earning his M.D. from DMS). French had joined the faculty in 1916, five years before finishing his medical studies at Rush. Gile had taught at DMS since 1922, and DesBrisay had joined the faculty in 1925, a year after Bowler. Just how unusual this new organization was—it amounted to a group practice—we can appreciate only with difficulty today, when solo practices are rare and groups are the norm. Though Bowler and Gile certainly had been influenced by their experience at the Mayo Clinic, Bowler's letter to the trustees of the hospital asking them "to consider the advisability of sanctioning the group of the staff as a general medical and surgical clinic" makes no mention of it.[12] The members of the new Hitchcock Clinic, explicitly constituted as a multi-disciplinary group, were also the staff physicians at the hospital and would continue to serve as such.

From the point of view of Dartmouth Medical School, it may be that the most important service rendered by John Bowler was to prepare the ground (whether he realized it or not) for the reestablishment of a full-fledged medical school at Dartmouth. Without the Hitchcock Clinic, there seems little doubt that the trickling away from Hanover of doctors would not have stopped when it did; soon new and talented physicians were being attracted as additions to the local medical population. The growth in the clinical population—the primary missing element in the mix necessary for the sustenance of a four-year medical school—was notable. In an address given at the DMS sesquicentennial in 1948, Frederic P. Lord observed: "Among the changes that have affected the School none has affected it more profoundly and advantageously than has the coming of the Hitchcock Clinic. . . . [I]ts existence has meant an extended instruction to its students, an added stimulus to its faculty, as well as a general increase in the quality of medical care given every one in this community."[13] The essential connection of the Clinic to the Medical School from that time forward cannot be denied.

Some sense of just how new the whole idea of a group practice was can be seen from remarks made by John F. Gile, in a paper presented on behalf of the Hitchcock Clinic to members of the Hospital Corporation at its annual meeting in 1931. He defined for his audience what it meant for the staff of the Mary Hitchcock Hospital to have been organized into a "group clinic" (no definition would have been necessary had the concept been a familiar one): "an organization of physicians engaged in cooperative and contiguous medical practice using facilities, personnel, office space, laboratories and medical equipment in common; covering as well as it may in its own instance and as completely as possible the entire scope of medical practice; providing a free discussion, consultation, and combined service to the patient into whose hands the patient first comes, and to the extent that is required by the nature of the case."[14]

Gile was then at pains to explain that this organization in no way has to lead to "the loss of intimacy of contact with the family doctor"—a common complaint. He was even more discursive in explaining how

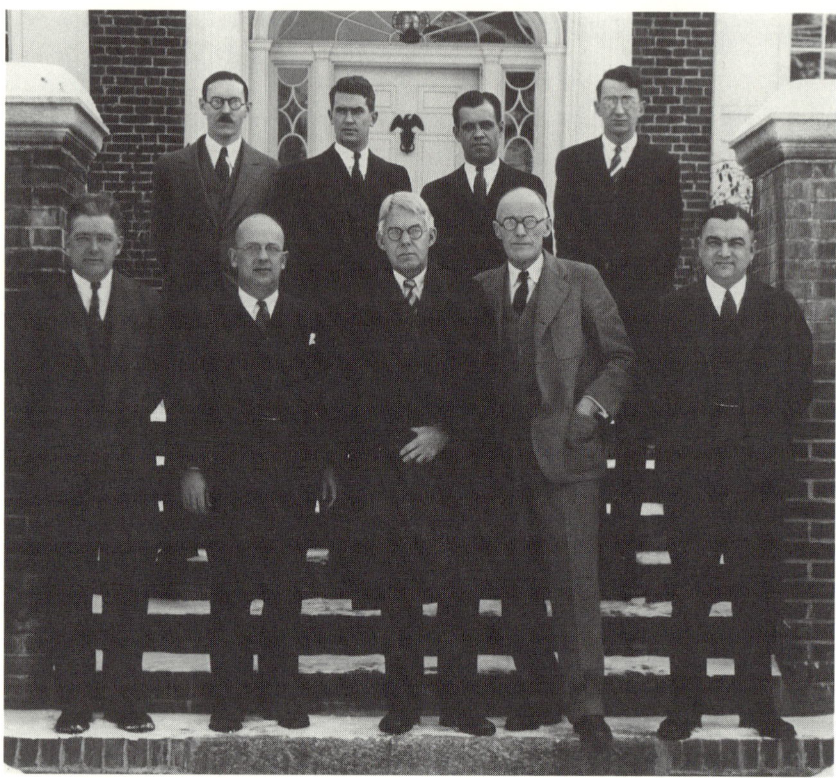

Hitchcock Clinic, four of the five founders and additional colleagues in front of the site, 1932. Front row, from left to right, Drs. French, Bowler, Bartlett, Carleton (not a founder), Gile. Courtesy of Dartmouth Medical School.

the members of the Clinic not only engaged in general practice within Hanover, but also took care of "the rural work in the back sections of our town and neighboring towns where physicians are not available." Anticipating the possibility that "the places of . . . older rural practitioners [would not be] filled by younger men," he proposed hiring a junior member specifically to hold office hours on an itinerant basis in those towns otherwise bereft of medical care. He was, he acknowledged, eager to demonstrate that this particular group at least was in no way engaged in "competition with individual practitioners."

Strikingly, Gile said nothing at all about the relationship between the Clinic and the Medical School. Later, the issue of which medical school faculty members would be welcome to join the Clinic would become as sensitive as the refusal of the Clinic to endorse any "rural practitioners" as members. Nor did he say anything about the highly unusual principle of equal pay for members of the Clinic regardless of specialty, a principle that stayed in operation until 1979. This was a radical notion indeed, and just one of the ways the Hitchcock Clinic revolutionized medical care in the Hanover area.

Gile's explanation of the still-new Clinic's advantages and the way it worked ended on a high note: "After four years of life it is our opinion that this form of organization . . . has established its own justification." Certainly Gile's long association with the Clinic (as well as with Mary Hitchcock and the Medical School) brought great benefit to the people of the area who needed medical care. For all his Dartmouth connections, Gile is a prime example of those who might very well not have stayed had it not been for the Clinic. At the time of his death in 1955, a *Boston Herald* article made explicit Gile's importance to clinical medicine in the Hanover area: "The resident portion of this village was sad today and it seemed that even the students were walking more softly. The community was saying its final farewell to Dr. John Fowler Gile, '16, noted son of a noted father, and a Dartmouth son in the finest tradition. A great surgeon and prime spirit in the founding of the now impressive Hitchcock Clinic."[15]

Focus on Enrollment

The faculty was not oblivious to ongoing discussions about its future in the media and in professional circles. Minutes of the medical faculty meeting on March 27, 1935, included a long report from Dean Bowler based on discussions at an AMA meeting he had attended the previous autumn. His account was an attempt to respond to questions about how calls for more doctors would affect the familiar old issue—whether Dartmouth should remain a two-year school teaching only the preclinical, basic sciences.

In the meantime, however, throughout the 1920s and 1930s the faculty minutes reflected more than anything a preoccupation with how well Dartmouth Medical School students were doing—both with respect to their work at DMS and in relation to students at other schools. Students who failed in courses amounting to six or more semester hours would be automatically "separated" (expelled) from the school—unless there were exceptional extenuating circumstances; a student who lied to the admissions officer and was also failing in course was expelled; a minimum standard of scholarship was to be required for admission, and this was to be published in the school's annual bulletin. But rules and regulations could be bent. When Joseph Greeley Pollard was failed in accordance with the rules of the faculty, a discussion ensued resulting in a vote to interpret the rules of automatic separation to exclude comparative anatomy (*why* is not clear)—and the new interpretation was made retroactive, thus rescuing young Pollard.[16]

Discussions of how to handle transfers—both into and from the medical school—also appear in the faculty minutes. It was voted that a committee should undertake to make arrangements with Bowdoin College and the University of New Hampshire for seniors in those institutions to be admitted to the first year of Dartmouth Medical School on the same basis as Dartmouth College students were. Rolf Syvertsen, secretary of the medical faculty, articulated a more cautious approach in 1927, saying that "the working policy . . . had been to admit, from other institutions, one-half as many students as were admitted from Dartmouth College and that usually not more than one student had been admitted from any single institution." The Committee of the Faculty, as Secretary Syvertsen's notes reported it, saw no reason to alter this policy.[17] At that same meeting, "The Secretary mentioned that twelve men took the National Board examinations, and that eight men passed all examinations; that two men failed in part; and that two men failed all examinations"[18] and that "all members of the Second Year Class had been transferred to the third year class in some other Medical School."[19]

The New Shape of the Faculty

In 1925, John Martin Gile had stepped down as dean and Colin C. Stewart—who had been secretary—became acting dean; Rolf Syvertsen, who had been carrying out secretarial duties, took on that position officially. Gile had also concluded he was no longer able to perform the duties of instructor in physical diagnosis; his son John F. Gile was appointed in his place, and Bowler in turn took over from the younger Gile as instructor in anatomy. A changing of the guard was slowly taking place once more.[20] Around the same time, a "Committee of the Faculty" was created, which kept its own minutes—frequently more revealing then the minutes from meetings of the medical faculty as a whole. The Committee was to consist of John Pollard Bowler (as dean—he had been appointed in1927) and Syvertsen (as secretary), automatically; there were three appointed members as well.

Various shifts in policy had the effect of slowly but surely giving a remarkable degree of status to Rolf Syvertsen. Beginning already in November of 1924, meetings of the medical faculty were called to order no longer by the president of the college or by the dean of the medical school, but by the de facto secretary—Syvertsen. In addition, when he began to keep the minutes, they took on a rather different character. Since he was also a member of the Committee of the Faculty—effectively the admissions committee—Syvertsen held an increasingly important and powerful position at Dartmouth Medical School from late 1924. Even with the rise to prominence of John Bowler, the charismatic Syvertsen remained the central and dominant figure in the minds of most students. Bowler had a profound impact on the school and on the medical scene in Hanover and beyond; after 1927, he constituted a veritable triumvirate in his own person. Syvertsen, on the other hand, moved into prominence in a less conventional manner. Exactly how it came to pass is unclear. His Dartmouth credentials were fine: He had a Dartmouth bachelor's degree and he had finished the two-year Dartmouth medical curriculum. But he was made a member of the medical faculty long before he had earned his M.D. degree (which he did not do until 1936), and he seems to have more or less slipped into his first position of special status—secretary of the medical faculty.

Looking closely at Syvertsen's minutes (he kept them for faculty meetings and for meetings of the Committee of the Faculty) is the most effective way to become acquainted with faculty preoccupations and to get a sense of the students and student life in the first decades of the twentieth century. Which students to admit, how to evaluate student work, and how students fared when they transferred were regularly discussed in his minutes. Syvertsen reported in October 1927, for instance, that the fifteen-year average enrollment had been 31.8 students, 26.6 of whom came from Dartmouth College, and that the 1926–1927 enrollment of 36 represented a 20 percent increase. He also had figures for the whole period of the two-year curriculum, to the effect that "186 men have completed the two-year course and have been transferred to 23 different schools. Sixty percent of the graduates of this School have received the degree of Doctor of Medicine from Columbia, Harvard, or Pennsylvania, or are now candidates for this degree at those institutions."[21]

The statistics showed consistency over several years (between twenty and twenty-four students in each class, with the vast majority coming from Dartmouth—of whom almost all were seniors in the College). In 1935 the first-year class consisted wholly of Dartmouth College seniors—twenty-three of them.[22] This was not chance so much as it was policy. Already in 1928, shortly after becoming dean, John Bowler reported on the policy of admission, saying that Dartmouth men have a preference and then, other things being equal, "applicants from schools with no medical schools of their own come next."[23]

Syvertsen's careful records also make it possible to explode the myth that has grown up concerning where students went after completing their two-year stint at DMS. Although there were periods during which a majority transferred to Harvard, by no means all of them did—and in some years Harvard was not even in first place. In 1929, students transferred to nine different institutions; McGill accepted more (five) than any other school.[24] The 1930 crop of students transferred to a total of ten schools.[25] Of the twenty-two students who were voted two-year certificates in June 1932 for having passed all requirements, the record shows their dispersal as follows: five to Harvard; four to Rush and three to McGill (two other perennial favorites in those years); Johns Hopkins, Columbia, and Penn each took two; and one each to Jefferson, Cornell, Washington University, and Stanford.[26] Two years later, transfers once more went to ten different schools; Harvard led again, with four students. But three went to McGill (again) and Cornell; two each transferred to Penn and Bellevue; and one each went to five other schools. In 1935, as in 1929, transfers went to nine different schools; this time, five (of nineteen) went to Harvard.[27] Thus although many students did move to Harvard from Dartmouth, that was not everyone's first choice. Nor was there any guarantee of acceptance by Harvard of the Dartmouth transfers—persistent repetitions of this myth notwithstanding.

Student enrollments and transfers, and then the standing of individual students, were of course not the only topics at faculty meetings. Curricular changes—such as whether there should be a requirement of embryology for all pre-med students, whether more or less time should be allowed for one course or another, what modifications (if any) should be made in the chemistry requirements, and what the sequence of courses should be—were all discussed. In the spring of 1928, for instance, as various changes were being proposed, the faculty requested Syvertsen to prepare possible schedules to show how each could be accommodated. Less than three weeks later, he was ready; he presented three separate plans of curricular organization, after which he was empowered to incorporate the results of the discussion into a "Plan D" that would "be the schedule for the coming year." But in August, a special meeting was held to consider whether to approve the plan. After "careful consideration of the various points involved, it was Voted: to accept the schedule for the year 1928–1929."[28] Whether the special meeting and discussion were merely pro forma or whether the rest of the faculty really did want to exercise authority over what Syvertsen had set out must remain a matter for speculation.

The Regulators Come Knocking Again

These administrative matters were not the only concerns of the faculty. In October 1930, Dean Bowler reported from a meeting of the AAMC that "a simplification in the matter of the number of boards, committees and agencies exercising supervision and responsibility for the curriculum in the medical schools" had taken place, and that there was, in his view, an "evident swingback toward the older, definitely specified and rigidly fixed curriculum." Two years later, the dean reported from another such meeting of the AAMC that "some discussion had taken place as to the reason for two-year schools and as to the transfer situation."[29]

Then in 1934, another report on medical education in the United States was undertaken by the AMA's Council on Medical Education. Visits to Dartmouth were made on September 24 and 25, 1934; the inspection team consisted of Herman G. Weiskotten of the AMA's CME and Harold Rypins of the Federation of State Medical Boards. An abstract of the portion of the report having to do with DMS was sent to Dartmouth at the end of December 1935.[30] But even before the report was in hand, the faculty became agitated about moves the CME had made that year. A special meeting was called in October to consider a September 27, 1935, letter from William Cutter, secretary of the CME. The Council, he reported, had "'Resolved, That after July 1, 1938, the Council on Medical Education and Hospitals will no longer publish a list of approved two year medical schools.'" That decision seemed tantamount to saying there *were* no "approved two year medical schools"; Dartmouth's position was that this was unwise and unfair, because it indiscriminately lumped DMS together with other less-worthy two-year schools. The faculty, having worked for more than two decades to turn DMS into an outstanding two-year school, was outraged. Considerable discussion ensued—about what the CME was trying to accomplish and what the effect would be on DMS.[31] The story is recounted in a six-page document sent by Dean Bowler to DMS alumni on December 27, 1935.[32] Bowler began by saying how gratifying it had been to have "evidence of interest" expressed by a number of alumni in what had by then become a very public affair. He reprinted both the letter from Cutter announcing the infamous resolution and the Dartmouth faculty's response to that—a letter over his signature—which ran to more than three single-spaced, typed pages.

Bowler's communication to the alumni had two very different elements, skillfully woven together. One was his scathing criticism of the Council's decision: "This resolution is entirely without discrimination and thus impresses one as being of that type of executive action which results from a combination of high-handedness and lack of courage." The second was a ringing defense of what Dartmouth was doing for medical education:

> For [our] contribution to the medical profession—in both stock and quality—we offer no apology. To state to us that Dartmouth Medical School contributes nothing to medical education because such applicants would be admitted to any other school only begs the larger question of the functions of a medical school; to answer the immediate question that they could receive a better or fuller training under mass methods, we disagree. . . . For twenty years, the program has been definitely one of the creation of the best two year school that could be developed.

Loyal DMS alumni must have loved the letter—especially the melodrama of Bowler's penultimate paragraph: "if we read the implications of your notification correctly, Dartmouth Medical School" could respond by "locking the doors on July 1, 1938, after taking the portrait of Nathan Smith over to the Library to repose in perpetuity beside the Seal of the College on which the inscription reads, 'Vox Clamantis in Deserto.'" That possibility, he stated flatly, "can be eliminated."

Bowler's letter to Cutter had obviously caused something of a stir. When Bowler returned from the meeting of the AAMC in Toronto (shortly after the letter went out), where the resolution on two-year schools was passed, he was able to report that "the two-year school question was the unofficial topic in the meeting and out, and that our letter was in the air all the time. Dartmouth seemed to have been the only school to have made a definite organized move. . . . Our letter appeared to set the position of the two year schools in the meeting." Having talked with "almost all deans of schools to which we transfer," he found that "hardly anyone had a question, and that there was no question about our positive position. . . . Dr. Cutter did not appear pleased that our letter had gone around but made no direct statement." With some satisfaction, Bowler went on to report that "it now appeared that in all probability no other school was in a position to have written a letter such as ours." Faculty members were aroused and annoyed. The minutes from this particular meeting are among the fullest ones we have.[33]

Also included in the communiqué to the alumni were the texts of three other documents: the resolution passed unanimously at the October AAMC meeting asking the CME "to reconsider its action upon the two-year medical schools" (apparently inspired by Dartmouth's strong stand), Bowler's brusque response turning down Cutter's invitation to appear before the CME, and—the triumph—Cutter's mid-December letter (received on December 15, 1936), which amounted to full capitulation. The Council had voted to reconsider its September resolution, and from henceforth "two year medical schools [would] be considered individually instead of collectively." It was all over in three months; Dartmouth had won the round.

The lengthy account of this victory put Bowler in a perfect position to alert the alumni that he intended in the spring to ask for funds. Plans were afoot for the Mary Hitchcock Memorial Hospital to be expanded. The message was clear: DMS was a force for the good in medical education, and it was just going to get better—but alumni help would be needed to make it happen.[34]

The February 1936 faculty meeting was then devoted in part to a discussion of the abstract of the CME inspection committee's interim report that had arrived at the end of December. The opening affirmed that "Dartmouth Medical College is unique among American Medical Colleges." This was exactly what Dartmouth claimed and liked to hear. Yet that was followed immediately by a less-satisfying remark: "The factors underlying its uniqueness are the basis of both its weak and strong points." The same old song ("limited clinical facilities") was being sung again. New minor-key tunes had, however, also been composed and inserted. "The weak points," the report went on, "with notable exceptions," were "an inbred, provincial and relatively unproductive and small faculty; an inbred and consequently provincial student body; insufficient influence of productive research. . . . Too much of the teaching appears to be didactic, academic and uninspiring. . . . There is little evidence of any premium upon scientific curiosity or investigation."

Flush with their recent success in bearding the CME lion in his den, the faculty must have chafed under these criticisms. The report was not exactly damning, but the praise was certainly faint: "From the viewpoint of its unusual student body and their achievements in medical school, Dartmouth should be given a good rating. However, the quality of its faculty, its limited clinical facilities and its comparative scientific sterility strongly indicate the wisdom of its limiting itself to the first two years of medical education." This interim report made the equivocal nature of the CME's overall assessment of DMS all too clear: The Medical School may have been doing well what it was doing—but it was not doing enough.[35]

A Closer Look at DMS Students

Who were these former students, that they could be expected to help? What was life like for students at DMS in the first half of the twentieth century? A few scattered indications from a variety of sources will give us a partial picture, and that must suffice. For many years the students came largely from Dartmouth College, as has been noted. The intensity of the desire to keep it that way is exemplified by the minutes of the Committee of the Faculty in the autumn of 1927, when a special meeting was held with undergraduate deans and "those who are acting as advisors to students." The advantages of staying at Dartmouth for medical school were stressed. Once again, the desirability of keeping the Dartmouth Medical School student body and faculty alike as strictly "Dartmouth" as possible—where everyone and his attributes and accomplishments were known quantities—was emphasized.[36] The CME had found this policy something to criticize rather than praise, but this chauvinism may itself have been a factor in the kind of intensely personal interest that the faculty as a whole seems to have taken in the welfare of individual students. Many discussions about the academic standing of particular students were primarily directed at trying to maintain high standards to impress the outside world. One example, in 1934, provides us with interesting evidence of the faculty resisting pressure from a physician-father "prominent" in a county medical society in another state, on behalf of his son with a poor academic record. Even though the Dartmouth faculty was virtually certain transfer could be arranged for the young man after two years, "[i]t was finally decided by the Committee that neither of these candidates [another with a similarly poor record was also under discussion], when considered on an absolute basis, was particularly desirable; . . . it was Voted: to decline admission."[37]

But when we read that a "possible explanation of [Clifford] Mills' standing was his illness, and a possible explanation of [Richard] Potter's absence was his difficulty at home which had required at least two absences to attend court," we see also a faculty that knew its students personally, and well, and that was prepared to make allowances for extenuating circumstances when warranted.[38] The dean's observation about the poor effect of numerical grades on competition and morale also seems indicative of a genuine concern for the students' welfare.[39]

The frequency with which applicants were denied admission is of interest, because of what it tells both about admission standards and about the popularity of Dartmouth's two-year program. For instance, in 1927, admission was being denied to eight applicants (two from Cornell, three

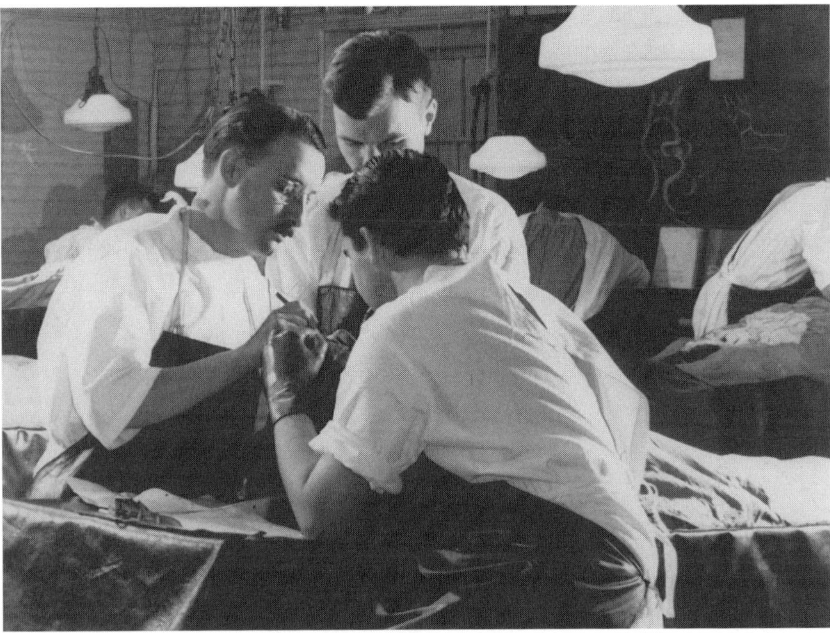

Professor Rolf Syvertsen and students doing dissection, c. 1940. Courtesy of Dartmouth Medical School.

from Columbia, one each from New York University, CCNY, and Providence) while being granted to four (one each from Bates, NYU, Cornell, and Penn). Two weeks later, admission was denied to another twenty-eight applicants (including one from Dartmouth), while two were admitted and four were left pending.[40] In August 1928 it was noted—presumably because it was unusual—that one student who had been admitted decided to go to Rochester instead of Dartmouth.

The Jewish Question

Only rarely are hints (other than a vague report of "low scholarship") recorded of the reasons for denying an application. But given the history at Dartmouth of a quota system for Jewish students and a sometimes-blatant anti-Semitism (manifested at DMS, it has been hinted, in Syvertsen's picking and choosing whom to admit), a few entries in the minutes beginning in 1927 seem significant.[41] We have seen that large numbers of students were sometimes denied admission. Two lists of students rejected in September 1927 are typical of the period as far as the numbers are concerned, but the rejections bear some striking features. Six of nine denied admission on September 14 had names that hint strongly at the candidates having been Jewish (Camins, Cantarow, Cline, Levine, Rothman, and Rubin); the same is true of nine out of ten rejected on September 19 (Flaxman, two Goldbergs, Goldstein, Gordon, Kaplan, Keizler, Rabinowicz, and Schrek). Carl Adolph Weiss, on the other hand—a Dartmouth College graduate who equally possibly was Jewish—was reconsidered and admitted after having been earlier denied admission.[42]

In 1929, Dean Bowler reported that the Moss-Hunter Medical Scholastic Aptitude Test had been given to all pre-med students in the junior and senior years; each applicant would be interviewed by the Committee of the Faculty and rated on a scale of 1 to 5 on "general acceptability" before his scholastic record was even considered. The dean added that "more emphasis should be placed on the applicants from D.C. [Dartmouth College] and that no student should be admitted from any school on the basis of requirements and scholarship alone."[43] Perhaps it is reading too much into this remark to think it indicates concealed anti-Semitism, though when it is coupled with the somewhat ominous remark of the secretary two years later that it had become "quite apparent that scholarship alone is no longer the deciding factor in the acceptability of our graduates at other medical schools," the suspicion is fueled. What *were* the deciding factors? We are told Syvertsen "cited several recent cases to establish the point"—but not what those factors were or which Dartmouth students had been seen as less acceptable than others.[44]

In 1934, we have something closer to genuine evidence of a prejudice against Jewish students. At a March meeting that year, Harold Bertram Orenstein and Jules Harrison Bromberg were moved to be admitted; the motion was promptly amended so that each case could be considered separately. "After considerable discussion during which it was discovered that Mr. Orenstein's *personality and physiognomy* did not meet with the unanimous approval, it was Voted to grant [him] tentative acceptance" (emphasis added here and in the next sentence). As for Bromberg, "considerable discussion . . . disclosed that Mr. B similarly did not meet with the unanimous approval because of faults of *personality, appearance, and speech*, [and] it was Voted to grant [him] tentative acceptance."[45] The Committee was apparently somewhat uneasy (or at least not done with considering these two cases), however, for on April 17, there was a vote to waive the Latin requirement for Orenstein. Then, on June 21, the tentative nature of the acceptances for both Bromberg and Orenstein was reconfirmed (along with those of several others).[46]

To the Committee's credit, Bromberg and Orenstein were eventually admitted. This emerges from Dartmouth College alumni records, however, rather than from the Committee of the Faculty's minutes. Both, it turns out, had been exceedingly strong members of their Dartmouth College class; both graduated Phi Beta Kappa (after having taken the option of having the senior year count as the first year of medical school). Orenstein finished at Rush and Bromberg at Northwestern; each earned an M.D. in 1938 and ended up practicing in Brooklyn. There is no reason to think they were not a credit to Dartmouth Medical School as they had been to the College.[47]

Another trio of cases that tells a mixed story begins with that of Mortimer Stewart Mintz, a Dartmouth College graduate (class of 1936). His application was noted—with several others—on March 1, 1935. While his classmate Charles Albert Lehman was accepted, on March 12 (from DMS he went to Penn for his M.D.), Mintz and another classmate—Nathan Leo Leavitt—were denied admission, a year later, on March 26, 1936.[48] Neither became a doctor; Mintz went into the grocery business.[49]

That Syvertsen, at least, saw trying to find transfer slots for Jewish students as a problem emerges from a letter he wrote to Harry French in March of 1938, when he reported on recent admissions decisions. Of Morris Jacob Seligman, Sy commented: "There were a number of reasons for accepting Seligman. He is a New Hampshire boy; he has a good record; he has a high aptitude rating and faculty recommendation; it removes a little of the stigma from the Committee [presumably for its less-than-welcoming attitude toward Jewish applicants]; it helps Mr. Hopkins [perhaps in the same way]; and it will give the Secretary a two year headache planning for his transfer."[50] Seligman—a Phi Beta Kappa graduate of the class of 1939—was accepted and completed two years at DMS; he earned his M.D. at New York University School of Medicine.[51]

Subtle (and perhaps not so subtle) anti-Semitism was not the only kind of hidden prejudice that raised its ugly head in the Committee of the Faculty. One of the rare occasions when any policy about admitting minority students was explicitly raised came in 1931, when there was discussion about the admission of "Negroes." The conclusion was reached that since Dartmouth College's "own students of negro birth" had to be admitted, there could be no "possibility of extending this privilege to graduates of other institutions." The rationale seems to have been that it would be too difficult to find a school to which the student in question could transfer, but it sounds like an "enough is enough" attitude if not an outright invocation of a quota system.[52]

DMS and the Great War

A letter from the medical school's alumni association dated October 10, 1917, announced there would be no reunion because of the war. The following June, the secretary of the association sent out a questionnaire to all 481 of those who had graduated from DMS since 1890, in order to "find out how many of the men are engaged in the Service of the United States." The 247 responses received showed the following results: From the classes of 1890–1900 there were 107 replies, of which 28 were from officers—whether they were serving as doctors is not specified; 70 were not in service; 5 had applied for commission; and 4 were state employees. Replies from the classes of 1900–1917 indicated there were 37 officers in uniform, 64 not in service, 8 applying for commission, and 2 state employees. It was observed that these data show "approximately 25 per cent of all the graduates of the DMS since 1889 are now enrolled in the service of the United States."[53]

Percy Bartlett, professor of surgery, was one of ten faculty members granted leave for war service.[54] Correspondence from the National War Work Council of the Young Men's Christian Association (YMCA) in 1918 to President Hopkins expressed appreciation that Professor Frederic P. Lord would be allowed to "remain abroad throughout the next year." Earlier correspondence indicates that the trustees had granted Lord a "sabbatical year" so he could serve in France.[55] As a result, back at DMS, anatomy was entirely in the hands of Harry Tapley Johnson French (1913), still not finished with his own medical studies (though he had earned an M.S. in physiology in 1918). A June 1919 letter from Dean John Martin Gile to Lord, still in France, makes clear how Lord's service there had required some juggling of teaching assignments just as it hints that—in young French—a new Dartmouth star was in the ascendance: "The more I see of [French]," wrote Gile, "the more I am satisfied that he is the sort of man we want to keep and I felt that it was up to us to do something to bring that about." (French would in the end spend most of his adult life in Hanover, associated with Dartmouth, where he taught anatomy for more than forty years and was a mainstay of the Hitchcock Clinic, of which—as we saw earlier—he was one of the founders.[56])

But Lord was much missed: "Shall be very glad indeed to see you back," Gile began the final paragraph of that letter.[57] Gile himself, during the war, was a reserve medical officer; he remained in Hanover, one of the few physicians at DMS (and, indeed, in the area) during the war. Dean from 1910 and a life member of the board of trustees from 1912, both until his death at home in July 1925, Gile had also been a member of the governor's council in 1911–1913.

In the meantime, the faculty was growing and apparently being better paid—though the discussions over faculty salaries are sometimes difficult to follow. In 1916, Harry French was offered $1,000 per annum to be an instructor in anatomy. Two years later, Frederick S. Page was to be paid $1,300 to an instructor in biology, while at the same time, Colin C. Stewart—professor of physiology and secretary of the school—had his salary raised from $1,000 to $1,200, and French (now listed as a professor) was raised to $1,400. An assistant professor of modern languages in the Tuck School was raised from $1,900 to $2,200. Why these medical professorial salaries were so much lower than those in the College—$2,700 (raised from $2,500) for John H. Gerould, an associate professor of biology, and $2,200 (raised from $1,900) for Leon Burr Richardson, an assistant professor of chemistry—already a year earlier, is not explained. (There may have been an assumption that doctors could earn additional money from medical practice or that they did less teaching.)

Legendary Faculty

Some things money can't buy. Among the most thoroughly Dartmouth-connected members of the faculty was Frederic Pomeroy Lord, whom Dean Gile so warmly and eagerly expected back from France. Lord's Dartmouth lineage is unusually long. Born in 1876 into a family that has provided twenty-three Dartmouth alumni, he was a member of the College class of 1898 and earned his M.D. at Dartmouth in 1903. His great-grandfather Nathan Lord had been president of Dartmouth College, and his father taught Latin in the College for almost half a century. He, his father, and his son (class of 1936, the fourth consecutive generation of Dartmouth men in the family) each graduated Phi Beta Kappa.

Frederic Lord also taught at Dartmouth Medical School longer (thirty-five years) than all but a few others. He was emblematic of the institution in a number of ways—typical, for instance, in being a dedicated and outstanding teacher who loved his students and worked hard to impart both his knowledge and his enthusiasm to them. Having begun his teaching career at the University of Iowa, he returned to DMS in 1911 and taught Anatomy until 1946. He stepped down then—in part because of ill health—in the year during which he would in any case reach a worthy age for retirement (he would turn seventy late that December). One former student expressed what was likely the sentiment of

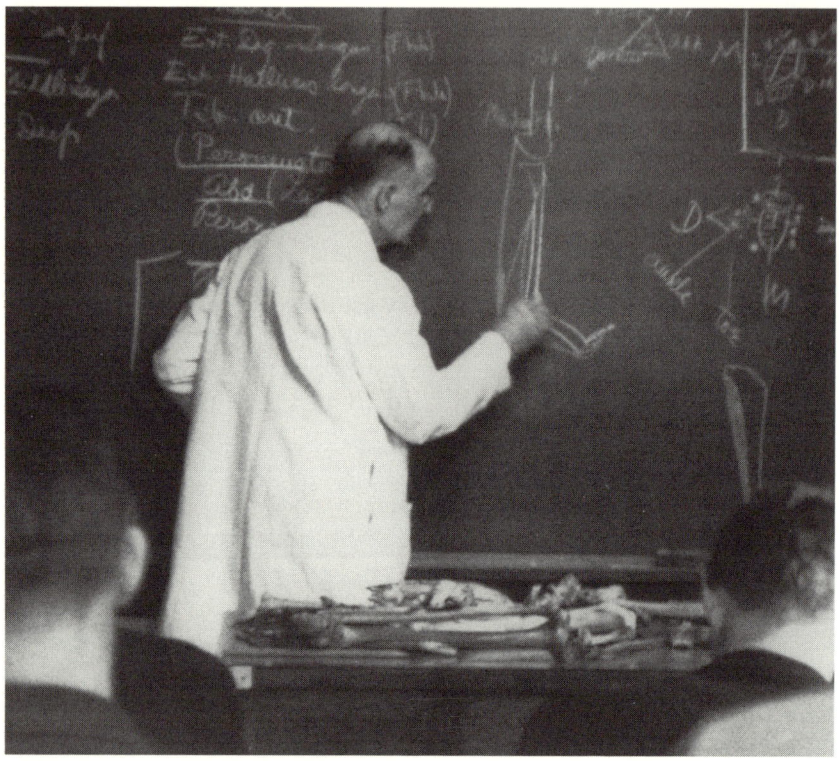

Professor Frederic Lord in anatomy class. Courtesy of Dartmouth Medical School.

many when he said that "spending a year studying anatomy with Lord was simply one of the beautiful things of life." Lord was "simply marvelous," and his students emerged knowing anatomy "better than most surgeons."

Almost twenty years after a faculty resolution had been read in recognition of Lord's retirement, his long service to Dartmouth Medical School was further celebrated at a meeting of the Nathan Smith Medical Society, on October 16, 1965—fittingly designated "Frederic P. Lord Appreciation Day." Professor Harry Savage, who had been a student of Lord's forty years earlier, read a testimonial that was then presented to Lord along a book of letters from more than 185 of his former students. The standing ovation accorded Lord lasted "several minutes."[58]

One former student, Arthur Ecker (DC 1931, DMS 1932), reminisced from a distance of sixty years about how class began: "After 15 minutes of our mid-morning game of touch football (in autumn) or soft baseball (in spring), Dr. Lord would lean out of the window and ring a cowbell to call us back to class."[59] The cowbell and its use were recalled by several students from that era; one of them claimed direct responsibility for its appearance on the scene. Writing that the medical students were disinclined to attend chapel and that they instead "engaged in a daily touch football game," which often "became sufficiently spirited that a call to the next class, physiology, went unheeded," Joseph Placak (DC 1930, DMS 1931) said that he and Warren Parish (also DC 1930, DMS 1931) "bought a cowbell, which was ceremoniously presented to Dr. Stewart. Thereafter, he used it to announce the end of the chapel period."[60] These stories mesh well enough to both be true; there is no reason to think either Stewart or Lord had a monopoly on cowbells.

Lord's ability to mix the serious with the humorous seems never to have deserted him. Following the "Frederic P. Lord Appreciation Day," Lord sent a postcard to then-Dean Gilbert Mudge, with a photo of himself and his ancient bike. His own typed caption on the postal card begins: "Dear Dr. Mudge I am sending on this card the picture of 2 relics, one already in a Museum (that of the Hanover Historical Society), the other on the way to whatever it may be." More seriously, he added: "You expressed a very real understanding of what this anatomist tried to do—to teach, to instill a love of anatomy for its marvellous [*sic*] condensation of myriad functions, made from relatively simple early structural units, each having been fitted into a complex whole and each perfectly adapted to its purpose. . . . I loved teaching and had a rich reward in the exercise of my profession and in the students I had."[61]

One whose career at Dartmouth might well have matched Lord's for longevity had tragedy not struck was Ralph English Miller, a Dartmouth College graduate in the class of 1924. Serving as an instructor in anatomy immediately after earning his M.D. at Harvard in 1928, he then turned his attention to pathology. In 1934, as medical referee (examiner) for Grafton County, New Hampshire, he played the lead role in the gruesome task of sorting through the rubble and bodies when nine Dartmouth fraternity students died of carbon monoxide poisoning in what came to be known as the "Theta Chi disaster."[62]

Miller's early death (he was sixty, at the peak of his career) came after his private plane crashed in New Hampshire's Pemigewasset Wilderness on February 21, 1959. (Robert Quinn, the colleague with him who also died, was only thirty-two.) The accident was riddled with ironies, among them that the two men survived the crash and then died of exposure, even though there was a well-stocked cabin only about a mile from the crash site.[63] The drama of that event has tended to overshadow some of what made Miller's death so tragic, namely his profound influence on the careers of many students and colleagues and his great abilities in a wide range of fields. He was an accomplished sportsman—pilot, skier, sailor (and cook), hiker—and outdoorsman generally, as well as an "enthusiastic and inspired teacher and . . . very likeable," according to John Lyle. "For example," Irving Kramer wrote, "one beautiful early spring day, we came into pathology lab and Professor Ralph Miller said, 'You know, fellows, it's much too nice a day to be cooped up in a lab. Why don't we go up to my cabin and relax?' We piled into some cars, picked up a couple kegs of beer, and off we went for one of the most enjoyable and memorable days at Medical School."

Miller was, however, an extremely dedicated and serious pathologist. His absolute belief in and insistence upon the usefulness of post-mortem examinations for medical education profoundly influenced several student generations. Lewis Chipman recalled Miller's tutelage this way: "Professor Ralph Miller can be remembered not only for his fine lectures in pathology but for his supervision of the students on duty in the autopsy room. . . . Dr. Miller's fetish was to be in the autopsy laboratory before the ink had dried on the permission certificate."[64] Other former students have recalled how he proved autopsies needn't be messy by once performing one in his tuxedo when called away from a formal dinner.

Dartmouth's President John Sloan Dickey, in his eulogy at the service for Miller and Quinn on May 9, 1959, said of Miller, in part:

> [A]ll who knew [Dr. Miller] also know that here was a life with dimensions and reach and variations utterly beyond any formula of measurement. The memory of such a life must not be suppressed into any summary of words. It is itself a living part of each of us: the hundreds of doctors he helped to educate; the specialists in pathology throughout northern New England who were reared under the rigor of his intellect and self-imposed standards; his colleagues in the Mary Hitchcock Clinic whose diagnoses so often rested on his reliability; the countless Dartmouth men who learned enjoyment of the out-of-doors, especially the fun of good skiing, under his unobtrusive aegis; and the host of others who in nameless ways through him touched the pulse of life's adventure.[65]

Finding Cadavers

To teach anatomy and pathology fully and properly, as Lord and Miller did, required a steady supply of cadavers—an old problem that had by no means been eliminated by the 1930s. An extensive correspondence spanning the years 1929 to 1937 deals in a variety of ways with the problem of access to and receipt by DMS of unclaimed cadavers from public poor houses or the like.[66] For example, there is a letter—dated August 17, 1927—to Thomas A. Carr, Clerk of Committee, in Manchester, New Hampshire. It concerns bodies from Hillsborough County Farm that had been sent, as the law then permitted, to Dartmouth Medical School. DMS had paid expenses for shipping and embalming, which typically amounted to $40 for each body. Dates and costs for receipt of bodies from the County Farm are also attached.

In a letter of April 29, 1934, Lord addressed the chairman of the Sullivan County commissioners in Claremont, New Hampshire. Once again he raised the issue of reimbursements for costs and referred to "our state laws" that accorded DMS the right to receive unclaimed bodies. The letter was forwarded to L. M. Grant, superintendent of Sullivan County Home, who wrote to Lord on May 18, 1934, agreeing to accept $20 for the body, plus $5 for transportation. Inked in the margin, presumably by Lord, is "OK 26 May." A carbon copy of a note from Superintendent Grant to DMS announcing receipt of $25 for "one body" sent "about March 1, 1934" provides evidence that some such transactions did get carried through.

A letter to Dean John Bowler a couple of years later (March 30, 1937)—no name given, but it must be from Lord—begins plaintively:

> The cadaver situation in the Department of Anatomy has, since the first of this year, reached such a condition that I feel myself unable to carry any longer the responsibility for the proper teaching of anatomy. . . . We shall be next October without another body for the incoming class; certainly would not have the extra bodies which any respectable anatomy department should have for special use, and of which we have been deprived for the past years. . . . The school has suffered from this lack . . . and it bids fair to suffer more in the future, if not actually to be put out of business on any suitable basis for the teaching of anatomy.

Just as the lack of "clinical material" was said to hamper the teaching of clinical medicine at DMS, the relative paucity of cadavers ("subjects") was hampering the teaching of basic science and eliminating the chance for at least some kinds of research. More than half a century earlier, in a long letter almost certainly to Carleton Frost (it is headed simply "Dear Doctor"), Professor L. B. How had written with concern, "I think it would be better if we could have a *whole* subject for any dissecting class that may be formed this Fall. I would order one. Some years we have not had enough. The material was so bad last year no one would touch it."[67] On the other hand, just how much of a problem this still was in the 1930s is open to debate.[68] No doubt some years were better for bodies than others.

And Then There Was Sy

Among the many fondly remembered stories about Rolf Syvertsen are ones that have to do with the teaching of anatomy and the cadavers requisite for that purpose. One "invention" of Syvertsen's was "the ancient and honorable Secret Society of Sextons" (sometimes also referred to by the name given to the initiation ceremony, "Eight by Eight by Eight"). The aim was to dispose of the cadavers that had been used in anatomy classes in a manner that would impress upon the medical students that such cadavers "were to be regarded with respect and buried with reverence." This was accomplished in part by making the whole procedure deliberately "formal and rather mysterious"—complete with a letter announcing the election to the society of the chosen students and a midnight run to a burial site out of town. There "a large grave measuring eight feet wide, eight feet long, and eight feet deep" (hence the name "Eight by Eight by Eight" for the society) was dug. The students "would return after dark to carry out the burial service conducted by Sy with appropriate prayers and readings." Afterwards, the Sextons were generally treated by Syvertsen to lobster dinner at the Hanover Inn.

Sometimes it was difficult to maintain the solemnity of the occasion, as an account of a particularly bizarre episode in October 1943 makes clear. But Edward (Ted) Mortimer (DC 1944, DMS 1944), who as one of that year's four chosen Sextons was a witness on that occasion, has also related soberly why there was the (perceived) need for secrecy: "The cadavers were, sadly, paupers or prisoners from New Hampshire. . . . [B]urial . . . had to be done rather surreptitiously to keep New Hampshire citizens unaware 'out-of-staters' were dissecting the remains of their neighbors."[69]

Syvertsen in fact did many things in a way quite unlike anyone else's. He interrupted his studies in the spring of 1917 to enlist in the U.S. Army and was discharged in 1919. Then, with his B.S. degree barely under his belt, he began teaching biology and evolution in the College while working as an assistant to both the registrar and the dean.[70] When he finished the DMS course in 1923, he did not transfer but stayed on as an instructor in anatomy and histology. Already in 1923 he started recording the minutes of the medical faculty meetings (he was not officially made secretary until 1925, as we saw). He was, it would appear, a general faculty factotum, willing to do whatever needed to be done.

Granted a leave of absence for 1931–1932 to continue his studies at

Chicago's Rush Medical School, he was awarded his M.D. degree only after he finally found time to do an internship in 1935–1936. Dean Bowler apparently "could not [further] spare him from his teaching duties" after his time away at Rush, according to John Moran (DC 1954, DMS 1955).[71] Thus except for the time spent in Chicago, Syvertsen was a fixture on the Dartmouth Medical School faculty from 1921 on—progressing steadily (perhaps in part on the strength of his original position as assistant in biology at the College) to instructor in biology and anatomy (1921–1923), assistant professor in anatomy (1923–1938), and full professor in 1938. He was secretary of the school from 1924 to 1945; after serving as assistant dean for a year, he was made dean. Already as secretary of the school, he was "in effect, the admissions officer, admissions committee, financial aid officer, registrar, and librarian." Once he became dean, "he continued to run the School largely single-handedly until the mid-fifties."[72]

This last statement hints at a degree of ambivalence about Syvertsen's legacy. Those with the fondest memories talk about how "he had his own way of dealing with academic and disciplinary matters" and recall the many stories of "Sy's 'rescues'" of students ("It seems to have been generally accepted on and off the campus that Sy was to be the first person called on any matter involving a medical student").[73] Other recollections include an observation on how remarkably Sy "kept track of students at Dartmouth Medical School and their future peregrinations."[74] He is remembered by hundreds of DMS graduates spanning more than three decades as the central figure in the early period of their medical studies. We have already seen evidence of Sy's strong hand on the admissions process; much more of the same, sometimes including what seems to have amounted to nearly unilateral decision-making power (long before he became dean), can be found in the minutes of the faculty and, especially, minutes of the Committee of the Faculty.[75] And there are undeniably many grateful and fond memories from those who benefited by being admitted ("I think that Sy handpicked the class . . . and the Committee simply applied the rubber stamp. . . . If the right person does it, it works," according to one student who was thus "handpicked").

Unfortunately, however, the School overall did not fare consistently well under Syvertsen's leadership, as will become clear in the next chapter. But he was certainly instilling in his many, many "boys" great devotion to him. The entire student body is said to have attended his funeral service at St. Thomas—"one of the largest ever held in Hanover."[76] Those students fostered by Sy seem to have been a mostly happy lot, pleased to be at Dartmouth and confident that they were learning what they needed to learn (and having fun in the process). Furthermore, they were by and large being well taught; they were transferring successfully to the schools of their choice for the final two years of medical studies. “Sy’s boys” did well.

CHAPTER EIGHT

Fading Fortunes, Facing Facts

Nor honest human impulse underrate.
—EDNA ST. VINCENT MILLAY[1]

Stark Realities

THE RELATIVE SUCCESS of the Dartmouth medical students in the middle of the twentieth century—still being accepted as transfers to top schools, including Harvard—concealed something else. Bit by bit, in the later years of Syvertsen's deanship, Dartmouth Medical School itself was not doing so well. Even prior to World War II, medicine and medical education were changing dramatically. "Typically regarded as a quiet time in American medical education, the interwar period was in fact highly dynamic," according to a recent study. "Medical research advanced and medical schools grew in size, wealth, and complexity—particularly the commitment of medical schools to research."[2] Yet precisely these things were largely missing at Dartmouth. Simply put, DMS was not moving with the times medically speaking. This continued to be true in the post-war period.

In fairness, it has to be said that some at DMS were aware of this, though they were slow to do anything about it. Significantly, it was left for external evaluators both to notice and take action. Dartmouth's hand was forced when the joint accreditation team of the AMA's CME and the AAMC (one representative from each) issued an extremely negative report following a site visit in March 1956.[3] The report distressed and embarrassed everyone who cared about the venerable school. Many also thought the external review was again quite unfair, given the steps that had already begun to be taken by the College administration to improve the situation. Although students from those years typically recall their time at DMS with great warmth and enthusiasm, it is now possible to see that—despite the best efforts of many able and earnest faculty members—the 1930s and 1940s were hardly the brightest ones in Dartmouth Medical School's history.

Bowler and Syvertsen

Both John Pollard Bowler and Rolf Christian Syvertsen were already playing major roles at Dartmouth Medical School in the 1930s. Though each would be dean for an extended period, the two men exhibited very different personalities; the Medical School was also faced with very different challenges (not to say crises) during their respective deanships. Both men experienced DMS as a small and "incomplete" (that is, two-year) school, and as one suffering from somewhat uneasy relations with the trustees of its parent institution. But in the period leading up to and following the appointment of Syvertsen as dean in 1945, DMS increasingly became Syvertsen's school. This is in no way to denigrate the significance of the multiple roles played by Bowler. Without a doubt, in the period between his return to the Dartmouth community in 1924 and his retirement in 1960 (also the year of Syvertsen's death), Bowler was the more seminal figure of the two in determining the overall shape of the medical firmament in Hanover. Yet the uniquely personal grip Syvertsen had on the young men who came to think of themselves as "Sy's boys," and the huge array of colorful "Sy stories" that have been passed down orally and in writing, leave one with the distinct impression that DMS in the 1940s had become a special place run in a very personal manner by Syvertsen. The Medical School in those days was "sort of like a family enterprise"; everyone got "the most personal kind of parental handling you can dream of, and very pleasant," according to one student at the time. Syvertsen, it has been said, would have been an outstanding "Dean of Students."

This popular view makes it easy to overlook the importance of Bowler, who was more in charge and in more frequent behind-the-scenes consultation with Syvertsen than is sometimes acknowledged or assumed. Positioning Syvertsen as the central figure at the medical school also tends to obscure the part Dartmouth played in medical history under Bowler's leadership. The firm stand he took against the AMA's Council on Medical Education in the 1930s marked a turning point in how medical schools were evaluated; that alone guarantees him a position on one of the pedestals reserved for the giants at Dartmouth Medical School.

But as we have seen, that is hardly the whole story. Bowler was also *primus inter pares* of the group that founded the Hitchcock Clinic. It was he who initiated the idea and developed the concept on the basis of his experience at the Mayo Clinic. He frequently served as either chairman or secretary of the Clinic group during the first fifteen years or so; when in 1942 it was decided the Clinic should have a president, Bowler was named and held the position until he retired eighteen years later. As the Clinic expanded, he served as chairman of its Board of Directors. He was also president of the Staff Board of Governors at the Mary Hitchcock Memorial Hospital (MHMH) from 1942 to 1960, on the hospital Board of Trustees from 1949 to 1960, and dean of Dartmouth Medical School from 1927 to 1945 (where he began as an instructor of pharmacology, later taught anatomy, and then was appointed professor of surgery). Thus he basically ran the medical world in Hanover. Barely imaginable then, it would be totally unmanageable today. Even after Bowler gave up the deanship, he retained his dual leadership roles in the Clinic and at MHMH until he retired; he was also on the board of directors of the Dartmouth Eye Institute, and his initiative led to the establishment of the Hitchcock Foundation. His name was indeed one to conjure with for many years, though colleagues (and others who knew him) often chafed under his style—variously described as "arrogant," "autocratic," or "controlling."

Yet it was Syvertsen who seems to have treated the School like a private fiefdom, and top administrators at Dartmouth were apparently quite content to let him do so. A medical school is always a headache from an economic point of view. When Syvertsen, once he was dean, repeatedly assured those in charge that everything was just fine and that there were no problems at DMS, the administrators were happy to take him at his word.[4] Nor was Syvertsen dissembling; there is every reason to believe he thought everything *was* just fine. He was in charge, he knew what he was doing, and what he was doing had met with considerable success for a number of years. If an occasional *quondam* student or former colleague has had the temerity to insist that Syvertsen was not a great teacher—criticism of any sort sounds heretical to the faithful acolytes—no one denies that the students were enormously fond of him. One student insisted that Syvertsen "was without doubt the most beloved of our teachers. He was remarkably well versed in the anatomy of the human body but was also intimately conversant with the individual psychology of each of his students and could chide any one of us regarding eating habits or amorous propensities. We were extremely fond of Sy."[5]

Small Is Beautiful

Such an intensely personal feel to the place under Syvertsen added to the whiff of provincialism that Dartmouth has always seemed to outside observers to have about it. Indeed, the school began to play its role in the history of American medical education for the most provincial of reasons: The foundation stone of the school was Nathan Smith's belief in the importance of having a rural medical school in northern New England to train local students to become physicians who would serve the area's rural patients.

In the interwar period and well into the 1940s, the Medical School at Dartmouth continued to be a tight-knit—even ingrown—community. Of the twenty-four members of each medical school class, there was rarely more than one who had not been a Dartmouth College undergraduate. Most had taken advantage of the opportunity to make their senior year of college the first year of medical school, effectively majoring in medicine and reducing by one year the time required to become a doctor.[6] In the process, the tie between College and Medical School was strengthened. A number of courses, notably chemistry, were taught to the medical students in the College classrooms—part of a concerted effort to avoid duplicating courses.

On the other hand, the College administration was by no means convinced at all times that maintaining the Medical School was in the parent institution's best interest. During the Great Depression, for instance—in 1935—President Hopkins informed Dean Bowler that "the Trustees seriously questioned the propriety of using $50,000 of general funds each year" for an enterprise that was not part of the original mandate of the College charter. This despite the fact that, a short time earlier, Hopkins had hotly defended DMS to the secretary of the CME, William Cutter, in response to the severe criticisms of the Dartmouth Medical School in the report issued by the inspectors. It is as if Hopkins believed no one outside Dartmouth could possibly understand it; only such internal criticism would be tolerated.[7]

Hopkins and Bowler each in his way took great issue with what accrediting agencies said or implied about Dartmouth Medical School. There was, for example, a "Current Comment" *JAMA* editorial in August 1935 that reviewed for the journal's readership just how much similarity existed between the situation of American medical education then and the situation when the Council on Medical Education was founded thirty years earlier. The rallying call was based on a conviction that "the factors that caused such deplorable conditions then are evidently again at work." The long paragraph headed "Incomplete Schools" that followed would have been impossible to miss. Arguing that the recent (positive) trend was in the direction of "bringing the clinical subjects into closer coordination with the preclinical," the author of the editorial condemned the "schools which, because of their limitations, offered only two years of medicine." They were "unable to participate in this development because, located as they were, clinical facilities were nonexistent. It has become increasingly difficult for the students of such institutions to make the transfer that is necessary to enable them to complete their training. The present status of these incomplete schools is therefore unsatisfactory."[8]

Dartmouth students did *not* have difficulty transferring, but it would have been hard to argue that the barb in this paragraph was aimed only at all the other two-year schools (of which there were several). Visits were already under way from the inspectors who would eventually produce the "Weiskotten Report" (recall chapter 7); DMS was on the agenda for September 1935 (the next month). "Incomplete school" indeed! Despite the conviction locally that a good job was being done, the president, the dean, and much of the faculty felt they were on the defensive.

In addition to being "incomplete," as a basic-science school lacking the clinical years, DMS was also notably small. Even a decade and a half later, in a report on medical education, Dartmouth stood out as the smallest by far—with a total enrollment of forty-six—among the seven "Approved Schools of the Basic Medical Sciences" (two-year schools) listed.[9] The faculty was also small, the full-time contingent numbering only six members (clinicians who taught were part-time). Nor was Syvertsen the only person at DMS who had close personal relations with the students. One member of the class of 1943 recalled that it was precisely "the smallness of the class, the intimacy with the faculty, [and] freedom to do it at your own pace" that turned the two basic-science years at DMS into "such a wonderful experience of learning"; the students, he stressed, found themselves in a "splendid learning atmosphere." A member of the same class once wrote that there "probably wasn't and isn't another med school in the country that had such small classes and such a high faculty-student ratio," and that he and his classmates "were extremely fortunate, and most of us didn't appreciate it until we had moved on to our third year into classes five times larger than we had enjoyed at DMS."[10] Of course everyone at DMS knew everyone else well. Students were to a remarkable degree unpressured; the pace was pleasant. "We worked very hard," says one student from the period, but "we had a good time." Another noted that the "common denominator in everyone's experience," the anatomy lab, was memorable partly because of "the wonderful coffee and donuts that we enjoyed out on the rocks."[11]

Explanations and interpretations in class could be (and were) done in a very personal sort of way. Colin Stewart, tall and dignified and slow-moving, had a dry humor that could catch students off guard but captivated them. Frederic Lord used colored chalk to draw on the board elaborate diagrams that were works of art in themselves. Ralph Miller was a dramatic and sometimes intimidating instructor, but a wonderful person, not averse to calling off class on a beautiful day to take students on a cook-out. He instilled in his students a sense of the "importance of autopsies in the understanding of disease."[12] Ralph Hunter had "a patrician, somewhat austere, but friendly manner."[13] In Harry Savage, Syvertsen (as dean) had the "perfect front man" (according to one student at the time who says he never met Syvertsen until later). He was a "kindly doc, completely non-threatening." Educationally, too, Savage made a lasting impression. "There was no such thing as 'continuing medical education' at that time, but Harry Savage . . . kept advising us: 'We are not so much teaching you facts—though you have to learn a lot of them—as trying to educate you on how to learn.' "[14] Another student, writing down his memories of more than forty years earlier, corroborated this view: "My earliest recollection of [him] was his lecture on opening day, when he tried to allay our apprehensions about facing the enormous amount of material that we knew we were going to tackle. . . . His gentle nature and hospitality . . . will not be forgotten." What "made medical school memorable," he continued, "wasn't so much the academic content as the wonderful attitude of Sy and Harry Savage. There were other heroes there as well, but I think most of us will agree that those closest to us were Sy and Harry, particularly Sy." That same former student also said, of himself: "I am absolutely certain that without Sy I would not be a physician today."[15]

Clearly, in matters of personal relations, a strong sense of community, and Dartmouth spirit, DMS earns high marks during this period. But if a medical school dean is to be judged on his ability to lead a strong faculty dedicated equally to research and teaching (never mind patient care), the verdict on the Syvertsen years is less clear. Despite Syvertsen's uncontested contribution in making DMS what today is often called "a student-centered institution," the lack of progress in other areas came to haunt the institution later. But other phenomena also had profound effects on DMS in the early 1940s. One was global, the other local.

The Campus in Wartime

Dartmouth was not the only institution of higher education dramatically affected by World War II. But "with two thousand Navy and Marine trainees on July 1, 1943," the College had "the largest [Naval officer training] unit in the nation."[16] Altered policies and a compressed academic calendar changed things for faculty and students alike. Both College and Medical School began to operate on a year-round schedule almost as soon as war was declared. Even before Pearl Harbor, Lewis Chipman (DMS 1941), for example, was quoted as recalling "the gathering clouds of war that hung over his last year at DMS. Like many other students, he wasn't making any firm plans for his future."[17] Lots of things were soon different. There was a large contingent of "converted faculty" at Dartmouth, who began "teaching in new fields" or who were "enrolled in 'refresher' courses which [would] enable them to carry some of the heavy teaching load in the new program." Then, in May 1943, President Hopkins announced special arrangements for granting a Dartmouth B.A. degree in absentia (after the satisfactory completion of one year in a "professional medical course"), to students who left the College to enter medical schools elsewhere. The new arrangement was "immediately applicable to men in the Classes of 1943 and 1944," and it was to be "effective for the duration of the war."[18]

A notice appeared in the *Dartmouth Alumni Magazine*, reporting that the "[t]wenty members of the second-year class of the [DMS], all enlisted in the medical corps of the Army or Navy, received diplomas on February 6 [1943] prior to continuing their studies at other medical schools. . . . Fourteen hold the commission of Ensign in the Naval Reserve, while the remaining six have been commissioned 2nd lieutenants in the Army Medical Corps Reserve."[19] The twenty-five members of the first-year class also signed up, bringing enlistment at the Medical School to 100 percent. (One of the oddities that resulted from this fast-paced course of study was that some students ended up as members of the same College and Medical School classes—Charles Regan, DC 1944 and DMS 1944, for example. There were even some—like William R. Schillhammer, Jr., DC 1946 and DMS 1945—who graduated as members of a *College* class later than their two-year Medical School class.) In November of 1943, the alumni magazine carried a photograph of twenty-four DMS graduates, all in uniform.[20]

One DMS class secretary recalled the mood and style of the educational scene in Hanover during that period this way:

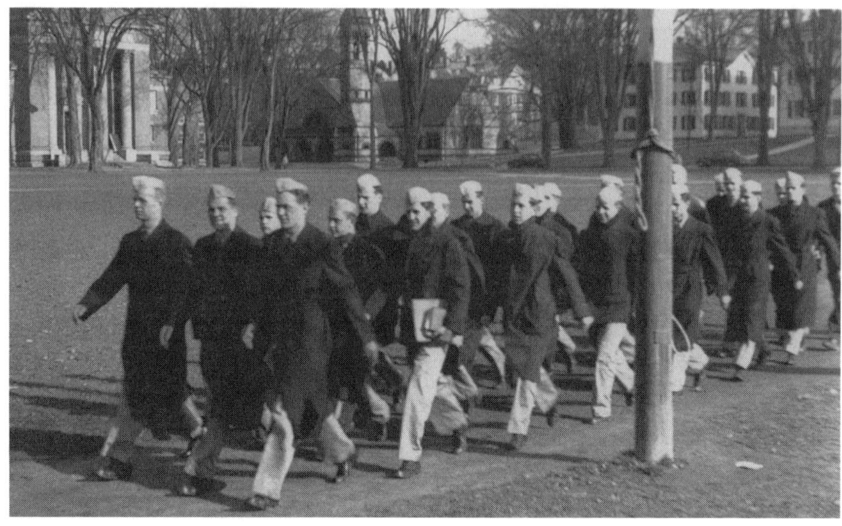

U.S. Navy medical students marching to class during World War II, 1943. Courtesy of Franklin H. West, DMS Class of 1943.

WWII increased in intensity daily. The College, through the V-12 program, assisted in the military education effort. Fraternities closed, curriculum went year-round with no, or barely any, breaks. Long grinds, sudden death for *any* failure, separation of students into Navy and civilian groups, including in the dorms. Then came our passage from [Leslie Ferguson] Murch's physics and [Joseph Greeley] Pollard's smut class [Pollard taught physical education] for those who were fortunate enough to be accepted to DMS. Class of '45 had 24 students, '46 had 24, but only 23 showed up (one was A-12 and the Army sent him elsewhere). . . .

Remember those unannounced exams—you walked into the classroom and there were those abominable blue books. . . . Do you remember Dr. [William] Ballard's New Year's Day exam in parasitology? Who expected that? One student didn't recognize there was no eyepiece lens in the scope (he became a pediatrician).

. . . Once Sy escorted some navy brass around, and I think their stomachs rolled when they saw us in gross anatomy dissecting with one hand and eating lunch with the other (when else could you do it?).

. . . Those were long days and nights, but there was lots of fun along with the drudgery. Then it was over, the formal educational part of it.[21]

This account treats the impact the war had on life at the College (and no doubt in Hanover generally) rather casually. Recollections from a member of the class of 1944 stressed the effects of the war rather differently and in somewhat greater detail:

And of course the war was ever in the background, or foreground, in those days. It colored just about everything we did, from our finances (what a help!) and our clothes (who can forget the olive drabs and the midshipman uniforms), to how we ate (mess at Thayer cafeteria) and where we slept (Crosby Hall and North Fayer). . . . What a change! And the parades, with Charlie Regan leading the Navy contingent (once we finally got our uniforms!)? And the officer trainees counting cadence at 6:00 a.m. outside our windows after some of us had been up till all hours observing deliveries?[22]

The Broader Impact of World War II

In addition to wartime changes on campus, the school was affected by those who were *not* present. Enough Hanover physicians served in the war to leave both the Hitchcock Hospital and the Clinic badly understaffed. Hanover was of course not so dangerous a place to be as the battle zones where numerous Hitchcock physicians, recent interns, and DMS graduates found themselves. But in the dozens of letters written by these men (and women—nurses who had worked or trained in Hanover were also in the armed services) to Bowler from literally all over the world, one of the most frequently repeated observations is that the writers realized Bowler and his remaining colleagues were working extremely hard.

In early 1943, Captain John Grindlay, after first insisting that those on the home front probably had no idea how fortunate they were to be at home, added, "I realize that home is not what it used to be, that rationing has cut the comforts & amenities to a minimum, that people are working longer & harder (particularly the doctors). You don't get any medals or promotions but I know you'd do more just as willingly."[23] A few months later, Captain Henry Heyl echoed the sentiment. "You & J[ay Gile] & George [Lord] must be having a stiff time of it, infinitely harder than battle service because it is apparently so unrecognized by the world at large. The community you serve must be unendingly grateful however. Actually it is you who are making the sacrifice and there are few in the service who would trade with you."[24]

Among those absent from Hanover for an extended period was Ralph Hunter (DC 1931, DMS 1932), who spent more than four years on duty—fifty-three months in all. Thirty of those months were spent in Londonderry, Ireland; the final thirteen found him working in neurology at the Naval Medical Center in Bethesda, Maryland.[25] In March of 1943, he wrote to Bowler from Londonderry: "I often think of the [Hitchcock] Clinic work in Hanover. . . . My own lot seems very easy compared to yours."[26] Later, he expressed his distress over "the sad news about Dr. Gile.[27] Knowing him I'm sure that he carried on long after he should have stopped."[28]

DMS graduates no longer directly connected with the institution also played their part in the war, too. An example comes from a journal kept by a young Dartmouth graduate, Bruce Lemmon (DC 1938, DMS 1939), in September of 1944, while he was on board a ship off the beach during the invasion of Peleliu Island in the Philippine Sea. His vivid description makes clear that the doctors on duty did at times have occasion to use all their medical skills. Just when Lemmon and his colleagues were beginning to feel some pride in the fact that they had had no deaths among their patients, despite having as many casualties to deal with as any of the transports, four of their patients did die. "It was depressing, of course," he wrote, "but inevitable that some wouldn't make it. A couple of the men I had come to know rather well." Almost sixty years later, Lemmon said his "most memorable event of the war" was that first burial at sea:

> All four of the men I had come to know, and I could not help thinking of their expressions of gratitude (how much more we owed them!) and confidence, their speaking of home and family, their young but tired and battered bodies. I am fairly stolid, but I felt like crying. And I seemed to feel the smack myself when their bodies slid from beneath the flag and, pitching on over as they fell, hit the water full in the face. I know we should pay those heroes homage, but that kind of military funeral is hard to take.[29]

Another theme that echoes through virtually all the letters was homesickness—for Hanover, the Clinic, the Hitchcock Hospital, and the College. But the strongest thread running through them all was gratitude. John Feltner (DC 1931, DMS 1933) wrote from North Africa: "I have been doing orthopedics exclusively and there hasn't been much in the books I haven't yet had—I believe I've had a fracture or comp. fract. of almost every bone in the body & have dug out shrapnel or bullets from every conceivable locality. Dr. Lord's anatomy teaching never proved sounder than here for me—One can't mention figures—but our medical staff of a number equal to Mary Hitchcock—but no internes—is now handling a number of patients equal to about 10 × the mileage to Littleton from Hanover—in truth. I have about ⅓ of these."[30]

Back in Hanover, the war made a greater difference to the hospital than to the medical school. Between 1938 and 1943, we are told, "the work of the hospital doubled, while shortages of personnel and materials became acute." With salaries in war-related industries escalating, "the hospital had a difficult time competing for staff to provide some of its most basic requirements." Moreover, the medical staff was just as "severely affected by shortages as the rest of the hospital; seven of the clinic's twenty-two members [clinical and associate staff] served in the armed forces. Those who remained became accustomed to long hours and seven-day work weeks." On the other hand, there were side benefits. Both the Clinic and the Mary Hitchcock experienced increases in revenue as demand for charity services declined and "area residents, finally enjoying full employment and steady incomes, paid their outstanding debt," giving the hospital an unprecedented degree of self-sufficiency.[31] Educationally speaking, also, the staff shortage at the hospital "turned out to be a boon for medical students," giving them greater and earlier exposure to clinical work than they would otherwise have had.[32]

The Dartmouth Eye Institute

Another important development that took place during the war years was the gradual unraveling of the carefully woven fabric of what had come to be known as the Dartmouth Eye Institute (DEI). The story of the Institute begins much earlier, but during the early 1940s, the struggle over what kind of a position a post-graduate institute could or should have at a college like Dartmouth began to be sharply defined. The ramifications of this debate—and the decision to let the DEI fade into oblivion (or die an ignominious death, as some would have it)—were far greater than anyone could have suspected at the time. The DEI plays a relatively small part in the overall history of Dartmouth Medical School; yet to the extent that the central issues in the controversy over the Eye Institute foreshadowed the rise and fall in the 1960s of the first graduate program at the Medical School, in molecular biology, it is a story worth telling in brief.

The only attempt to provide a thoroughgoing account of the development, accomplishments, and eventual demise of the DEI—a much-heralded and once-important feature on the Dartmouth landscape—is David C. Bisno's book *Eyes in the Storm—President Hopkins's Dilemma.*[33] The central thesis of Bisno's analysis is that President Ernest M. Hopkins was caught on the horns of a dilemma. On one side were Hopkins's pride in the honors bestowed on the eccentric and creative Adelbert Ames and several colleagues in physiological optics for their innovative research, and enthusiasm for the very promising clinical implications of that research. In this he was supported by John Bowler, who according to Bisno "welcomed" Ames's anomalous group "as a department under the medical school's umbrella." The group moved into quarters in the basement of the hospital in the early 1930s, certainly an indication of the close ties between the Hitchcock Clinic (which largely controlled space) and the DEI. Tellingly, however, the "exact relationship between the clinical division, the department, the college, and the medical school . . . remained vague." On the other side was Hopkins's commitment to the ideals of Dartmouth College, which included a deep and abiding "dedication to undergraduate education." Bisno insists that Hopkins "had never been fond of any of his graduate schools," that he was "torn between serving his undergraduate college and supporting Ames." Dartmouth itself "had a history of discouraging graduate studies on its campus."[34]

Part of what makes these tensions of particular interest in the context of a history of Dartmouth Medical School is what Bisno refers to as the "predominant question"—then and later—namely, "whether big science can thrive on the campus of a small college." The DEI, he claims, "forced the Dartmouth Medical School to consider whether big, new science could, and should, be pursued at a professional school on a small, but prestigious college campus."[35] A second point of interest in the DEI story for historians of DMS is that when Bowler sought funding for Ames from the Rockefeller Institute in the early 1930s, their "appointed evaluator of medical and research grants . . . would play a significant role in the development of the Dartmouth Eye Institute." The evaluator was Alan Gregg, who would later become a critical figure in the unfolding drama at Dartmouth Medical School itself.

The astonishingly original work on aniseikonia—"discovered" or "invented" (depending on the degree of one's skepticism)—at DEI brought flocks of eye patients to the Institute. Yet that began to be a problem for Bowler, who saw the clinical side of the Institute's work as competition for the Hitchcock Clinic. Furthermore, Ames's interests began to shift to areas like aesthetics that were harder to see as having any plausible relation to either the Clinic or the Medical School. Even Gregg could not keep Rockefeller money flowing to Dartmouth in support of the DEI. Hopkins grew increasingly uneasy about the need for the College to support the Institute. In a January 1, 1945, memo to the Board of Trustees, he argued that support of the DEI should cease. That summer, just prior to his own retirement, Hopkins effectively closed the Dartmouth Eye Institute by separating it from the College.[36] That solved what Bisno called Hopkins's dilemma, but the old tensions remained, between the insistence that Dartmouth should be a (mostly) undergraduate College and the vision that Dartmouth would evolve as an institution to embrace graduate programs.

The Veterans Administration Hospital

This is not the place for a complete history of the VA Hospital any more than what just preceded is the whole story of the Dartmouth Eye Institute. Still, the institutions with which Dartmouth Medical School has been and is connected—the College, the Mary Hitchcock, the Clinic, the Hitchcock Foundation—cannot be wholly ignored, either. They belong in the picture. How DMS became involved with the Veterans' Administration Hospital in White River Junction, at a point when DMS was not strictly speaking itself directly involved in patient care, is a curious tale that illustrates the complex relations among the medical institutions of the Upper Valley.[37]

Happily, not all affiliated institutions created problems for the Medical School as large and significant as those that hovered over the DEI. The formal connection established between the Veterans' Administration Hospital in White River Junction (WRJ), Vermont—which had opened in 1937—and DMS went into effect in 1946, when the VA officially became an "affiliated teaching unit" for the Medical School.[38] (The close ties continue beneficially to the present time; see chapter 11.) The opportunity for affiliation of some sort presented itself because the government was trying to upgrade the hospitals in the VA system. The idea was to arrange for medical schools located near VA hospitals "to use their faculties to augment and improve staffs at the veterans' hospitals."[39] The words "augment and improve" are key. The affiliations (for which the door was opened with a new chapter in the Federal Regulations—Title 38 USC) were never intended to give authority over the care of veterans to the medical schools. Rather, the idea was to give the schools oversight of education and research programs as well as a strong voice in patient care. In the case of Dartmouth and the White River VA hospital, it is clear that "[c]omplying with the government's request would have been impossible for DMS without the resources of the Clinic."[40] John Bowler once again played a leading role in the region's medical drama. By arranging for Clinic physicians to have consulting and attending appointments at the VA, he further strengthened the links among the separate medical entities that would eventually make up a true medical center.

Almost as soon as the affiliation between the VA and DMS was established, however, things began to change—initially, at least, not for the better. New VA hospitals were opened in Manchester, New Hampshire (1950), and Albany, New York (1951); combined with other demographic factors, this led to a decreased patient census in WRJ. The reduced patient load had economic consequences, leading in turn to a shortage of equipment and personnel as well as in surgical residents (though this was not a problem in the medical residencies). The loss of the director of research at White River led to a major gap in the academic program. Members of the professional staff in WRJ were isolated by distance and found it difficult to attend conferences at the Hitchcock

Hospital and at DMS; they lacked "the stimulating effect of daily contact with other faculty members."[41]

Howard Green (DC 1956, DMS 1957)—whose DMS credentials are as complete as they come: student, resident, fellow, faculty—was recruited by Thomas Almy to help build the Department of Medicine at the Medical School in 1968. This was very much a matter of institutional relations, because the recruitment and the desire (or need) to establish such a department at DMS were in the minds of some a direct response to tensions between the School and the Clinic. Reasonably enough, the Clinic's ethic was centered on clinical practice. The Medical School, on the other hand, had by the late 1960s—this is getting ahead of the story that will be told in later chapters—firmly embraced a position that good teaching and medical practice were both dependent on research, preferably in the basic sciences. Though Clinic staff members were accorded Medical School faculty status, they had little in the way of teaching responsibilities, and the Medical School faculty were by no means automatically granted Clinic membership. The Clinic was still a closed institution, and one that harbored some suspicions about what was going on at DMS. Some of the unease was no doubt based on the clear sense that what little *clinical* investigation was being done by Clinic members stood much lower on the ladder of academic value than research in the basic sciences. Suspicions were, in other words, mutual. The wonder of it all is that cooperative efforts continued to be made until it could quite correctly be stated (in 1993) that "the VA affiliation has clearly been integral to the evolution of [the Dartmouth-Hitchcock Medical Center]."[42]

Green became chief of staff at the VA Hospital in 1973. There he set out to shore up the teaching component, especially, in what he believed was already a good clinical program with a strong research tradition that had been maintained by a number of good people. He had invaluable support from William Yasinski, who had assumed the position of hospital director the year before. Green's focus, no doubt showing the influence of his work with Almy (and as a research fellow under Heinz Valtin), was on academic medicine. Since the Hitchcock Clinic largely controlled the Hitchcock Hospital (Clinic patients made up the bulk of the MHMH patients), despite the supposed independence of the latter, the parallel growth of clinical and academic medicine at the VA Hospital and Green's close ties to the Medical School provided a useful model for how hospital and school could work together. The VA, in other words, provided DMS with a kind of clinical identity that it badly needed, given that it was still only a two-year basic-science school.

Even when the clinical setup at the VA had improved, its main value was tied less directly to the Medical School itself than to the expanding program in residencies. First to be board certified were the residencies in internal medicine and surgery; others (including orthopedics, urology, and dermatology) followed within a few years. These Dartmouth residencies became enthusiastically sought after; at the VA Hospital, residents had more responsibility for direct patient care (and thus more opportunity to learn) than in some other residency programs. The Dartmouth affiliation worked precisely as the government proposal had intended: Patients at the VA began getting top-notch care, which had not always been the case prior to the time when Dartmouth stepped in.

What made this possible (as indicated in the earlier quotation) were the resources of the Clinic. Dartmouth Medical School, willingly or not, was very dependent on the Hitchcock Clinic and the Hitchcock Hospital alike. Those two institutions in turn could conceivably have continued to exist (though not in their then-current form) without any academic connection, and there is reason to think Hospital and Clinic alike were at times inclined to ignore the School if they could. The Clinic had increased enormously in size and power throughout the 1950s and 1960s (by the early 1960s there were ten times as many physicians in the Clinic as there had been at its founding); the Mary Hitchcock also continued to grow (the Faulkner building, four stories and a basement plus a three-story wing with a basement, was completed in 1952). Thus those two players may well have underestimated *their* dependency on the School. (In chapter 11, we will learn more about the struggles before the model of an academic medical center won out.) Only when DMS became a full four-year, degree-granting institution was it able to carry its own weight in the ever-more-complex world of medicine—and medical education—in the Hanover area. The more integrated and collegial whole that would eventually emerge was still some years in the future. The realization developed only slowly that no single one of the medically related institutions could stand entirely on its own. Considerable distrust existed between what amounted to two separate power centers—Clinic and Hospital (including some features of the programs at the VA) on the one hand, and the School (with some claims on the educational aspects of what was going on at the VA) on the other. The unease had to be overcome before further shaping of the medical center could take place. Given what was at stake, it is understandable that it took years to convince all parties of the value of a unified organization. Even then, more years would pass before implementation was achieved. All the parties concerned needed to make adjustments in their expectations and their view of their own roles.[43]

The Hitchcock Foundation

Another pair of changes that took place in 1946 signaled further maturing of the Hanover-based medical establishment. The Hitchcock Clinic, originally a partnership, became—"under the guidance of attorney Robert Reno"—a professional corporation. Once again, the Mayo Clinic served as a model. Then, in December, responding to the requirements of the then-current New Hampshire laws that such a professional corporation had to be a for-profit organization, the nonprofit Hitchcock Foundation was created. (Reno had the Articles of Agreement for the Foundation, signed by the sixteen senior members of the Clinic, drawn up in a manner that anticipated the eventual evolution of the Clinic into a non-profit organization.)[44]

Once again John Bowler was in the thick of it, helping to make things happen. The new Foundation, he believed, would be "a way of coordinating research and educational programs." He saw it "as an arch connecting the Clinic, Hospital, and Medical School." And it was under his leadership that the "seed money to establish the Hitchcock Foundation came from the Hitchcock Clinic and Mary Hitchcock Memorial Hospital."[45] Absent the infusion of cash, the Foundation might never have come into being, and the history of the Clinic would have been very different. For one thing, the Foundation was able to receive donated funds, the classic gifts from "grateful patients," which the for-profit Clinic could not accept. More generally, its purpose was to foster research. On that agenda there were four objectives: aiding and advancing the study and investigation of human ailments and injuries, and the causes, prevention, relief, and cure thereof; studying and investigating problems of hygiene, health, and public welfare; promoting skill, education, and investigation in medical, surgical, and scientific arenas; engaging in and conducting, and aiding and assisting in, medical, surgical, and scientific research in the broadest sense.

These aims were deliberately broad, and the confidence of those who established the Foundation (still today run by a volunteer board and a minimal paid staff) has been vindicated. Several different research funds, a couple of fellowships, an annual lectureship, and a revolving loan fund for residents attest to the value of the enterprise. Of particular import in the context of the history of Dartmouth Medical School is the evidence that already in the 1940s concern was being expressed about the need for *clinical* research, not just the more obvious kind of research in the basic sciences. Twenty years later the need was still great. (As we will see in chapter 10, the mid to late 1960s were the absolute height of the conflicts over whether DMS's primary task was to train physicians or to educate researchers.) The Hitchcock Foundation's ability to fund clinical research helped DMS enter a new era. Options were kept open for clinical faculty members not engaged in major bench-science research projects during years of disagreement and high blood pressure.

The Sesquicentennial Milestone

Thus even in the midst of disappointment and confusion over the Dartmouth Eye Institute, there were reasons to celebrate. The affiliation with the VA and the establishment of the Hitchcock Foundation both heralded important opportunities and initiatives; the Hitchcock Clinic was growing in prestige and success. On top of all that, 1947 marked the 150th anniversary of Dartmouth Medical School's founding—though in fact the celebration was not held until July of the following year. A news item in the *New Hampshire Morning Union* of July 22, 1948, announced the opening of the three-day sesquicentennial event; other publicity appeared in the *Hanover Gazette* and the *Manchester Leader*. Dean Syvertsen had sent a letter to all DMS alumni announcing the event. The elaborate program included exhibitions and demonstrations open to the public on Friday and Saturday mornings. Set up in the Rotunda of the Mary Hitchcock Memorial Hospital was an exhibit emphasizing efforts to coordinate basic science teaching with clinical work; it was proudly titled "Our New Teaching Hospital." There were also clinical rounds—both medical and surgical—at the Hitchcock and VA hospitals.

At the opening reception, Syvertsen extended a welcome to all in attendance. The recently retired and much-loved Frederic P. Lord gave a charming retrospective ("Fifty Years of Teaching"), which was followed by Leon B. Richardson's "Dartmouth Medical School: A Historical Sketch." At the Friday night banquet, Creighton Barker (DMS 1913), then secretary of the Connecticut Medical Society, "impressed the gathering with some hitherto unknown details concerning Nathan Smith" (according to Harry Savage's later report).[46] In between, there was a symposium titled "Dartmouth Medical School Today," which—following the dean's presentation ("The Medical School")—comprised ten presentations, ranging from topics like "The Cytologic Diagnosis of Lung Cancer" by John B. Holyoke, to a talk on the Hitchcock Hospital by its president, John P. Amsden. The whole, happy celebration ended with a Saturday barbecue under a tent set up in front of Butterfield Hall on Tuck Drive; in all, 323 people were officially registered for the program.[47]

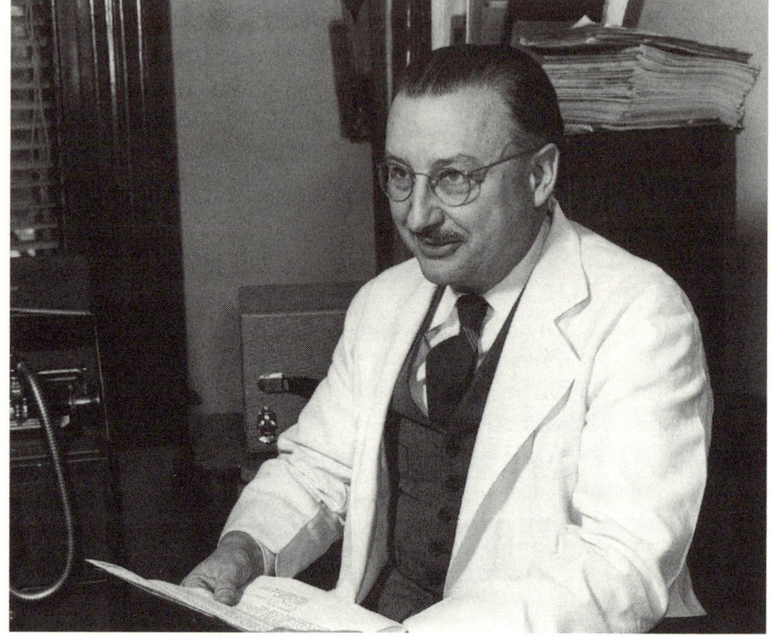

Rolf Syvertsen as Dean. Courtesy of Bull and Ewing.

Real progress in several areas topped off by a grand celebration could not hide the growing problems at DMS, however. For all the good feelings, all the well-trained students about to become physicians, all the pride in the institution's history, there is no escaping the simple fact of geography—Hanover in the late 1940s still counted as a remote area—and the complex facts of what might be called Dartmouth Medical School's geopolitical stance (or lack thereof). In the aftermath of World War II, DMS had been growing more insular—not just isolated—than ever. There was, according to one who knew the Hanover of the 1940s and the DMS of the time, looking back forty years later, "a pervasive naiveté in Hanover about medical schools in the nation in the 1950's and how anomalous Dartmouth Medical School really was in this company. It survived in a not so splendid isolation and for decades had maintained [a] pretense of professional stature without ever testing reality by self examination."[48]

The "place was fifty years out of date," according to one researcher who spent several years on the DMS faculty in the 1960s and then left. A student from the post-war period (also later on the faculty) used almost the same words: "DMS was fifty years behind." The school suffered during World War II and "sort of muddled along" in the words of a faculty member at the time; it was "a little school in the backwoods," according to another later member of the faculty; "the postwar explosion of physical and biological knowledge had passed it by." Medicine and medical education had moved into new territory, where investigation and scientific research filled the near horizon and was increasingly acknowledged to be a critical part of medical education. Dartmouth seemed slow to recognize the importance of the shift in focus that this necessitated. As later dean Carleton B. Chapman once put it, the medical school at Dartmouth "in general remained aloof from the activities and trends in medical education" that had for years been taking shape "in some of the country's larger medical schools."[49]

A student from the war years acknowledged retrospectively that one way "DMS was behind, or becoming so, was . . . [in] the size of the faculty." A single professor was generally in charge of each subject—and it was "no longer possible for one person to handle all the complexities" of a given discipline. Another student, from ten years later, said he realized only ex post facto that there were "some tremendously exciting things happening" in science—Watson and Crick were working on the structure of DNA at the time—that DMS students simply missed out on. We were "oblivious," he said. "Nor did we have the language to describe [what happens] in virology," he added, just one more example of being out of it.

How medicine was changing and the explosion in scientific knowledge were not the only issues. More immediate, in a way, was how Dartmouth College viewed its Medical School. How the College decided to deal with the financial and other challenges entailed in keeping the venerable school alive would determine its future. A dramatic story was about to unfold, one that in its own way is as remarkable as the story of what Nathan Smith had accomplished 150 years earlier. Under the inspired and inspiring leadership of Stephen Marsh Tenney (DC 1943, DMS 1944), Dartmouth Medical School was soon to be put on an altogether new footing. Accomplishing that was a considerably more complex enterprise than the bold and single-handed establishment of the school had been—not surprising, given the more complex times in which the later event took place. Furthermore (equally unsurprisingly), the sequelae of that action and the way the first years of the new era in DMS's history played out were to have ramifications and subplots that would shape the school for years to come. We turn next to follow the sometimes-rocky road that eventually led Dartmouth Medical School back to a more visible and honorable position on the landscape of medical education in the United States.

PART IV

THE REFOUNDING PROJECT: STABILIZATION

CHAPTER NINE

Rising to a New Challenge

> If you are a leader, take the long view in the governance of what is entrusted to you, that your accomplishments may be distinguished.
>
> —PTAH-HOTEP[1]

FROM THE TIME Daniel Webster made his impassioned plea before the United States Supreme Court on behalf of Dartmouth as "a small college," the institution of which Dartmouth Medical School was a part had an uneasy ambivalence about what came to be known as its "associated schools." Anything that made the College look like a university—as the Dartmouth Eye Institute did—was cause for concern. Nonetheless, pride as well as concern enveloped these affiliated professional institutions; an understanding that a periodic review would be needed was implicit. In 1954, anticipating a development campaign that would be connected with the College's 1969 bicentennial, the Trustees Planning Committee (TPC) undertook just such a review.

The Triumvirate: Morrison, Gregg, and Tenney

The Thayer School of Civil Engineering and the Medical School seemed in particular need of prompt action plans. Despite the fact that the very existence of the Medical School had been called into question ("Consideration was even being given to closing it down," according to one historian of the period), in the end the Thayer School proved so vexing that recommendations about *its* future had to be postponed.[2]

A hint of just how little attention was being paid to the Medical School can be found in the pages of the *Dartmouth Alumni Magazine*—even in its intermittent "Associated Schools" column—which made no mention of DMS from 1949 to 1956. But by the early 1950s, it had begun to be "apparent that basic decisions concerning the Medical School had to be faced." By the middle of the decade, President John Sloan Dickey was no longer able to ignore the problems or simply accept Dean Syvertsen's assurances that all was well. He began "to explore various alternatives concerning the School's future by seeking the counsel of the country's leading authorities on medical education."[3] Among those tapped for advice were George P. Berry, Dean of Harvard Medical School; Robert F. Loeb, Professor of Medicine at Columbia; W. Barry Wood, Vice President at Johns Hopkins University; and Alan Gregg of the Rockefeller Foundation.

A key member of the TPC was Dickey's most trusted lieutenant, political scientist Donald H. Morrison. When the committee began studying the "situation" at DMS, Morrison promptly demonstrated his aptitude for handling complex administrative problems; he would prove to be an exceedingly quick study. He may have been the perfect person for the job, though the path of his ascent to a position of such prominence was hardly the usual one. In 1948, disappointed after three years on the Dartmouth faculty (he had arrived from Princeton thinking all faculty members at Dartmouth were true "teacher-scholars" but soon concluded that reality did not match reputation), Morrison went to Dickey to explain why he was planning to leave. This was a bold move for a young faculty member, not yet tenured, but Dickey responded with boldness of his own: He asked Morrison to stay—making him Dean of the Faculty on the spot. Morrison, then only thirty-four, accepted.

The brilliant young dean's efforts on behalf of DMS, especially beginning in 1954, were notable. (In 1955, Morrison became the first incumbent of the newly created position of College Provost.) From the moment he joined (or chaired) the various special committees and subcommittees associated with a review of the Medical School, he was instrumental in securing DMS's future.[4] Everyone agrees that Morrison played a key role. Particular testimony to that fact was given by none other than later Dean of the Medical School S. Marsh Tenney, generally credited with having accomplished the "refounding" of the institution, at the time of DMS's bicentennial celebration. On that occasion, Tenney publicly stated that it was Donald Morrison, an "articulate, persuasive advocate of the Dartmouth Medical School," who "sparked the renaissance known as the refounding of DMS. It was he who gave us what we have today."[5]

Morrison chaired a "Schedule Committee," appointed at a June 1954 DMS faculty meeting "to study curriculum and present for consideration such changes as [were] thought indicated." The "Initial Report of the Schedule Committee" was made in September 1954; its "Second Report"—much more extensive, including two fully worked-out programs of study for the school's two-year course (one was for the "most desirable program regardless of available facilities," the other outlined the "program possible with the facilities at hand")—was made in February 1955.[6]

A month earlier, on January 6, 1955, Morrison had completed a memorandum titled "Dartmouth College Hitchcock Medical Center," a working paper on which he had collaborated with Dean of the Medical School Rolf Syvertsen for the TPC's "Medical School Study." In this ten-page document, Morrison attempted four tasks: to "indicate some future trends and problems in medical care and education"; "inventory the resources that may enable Dartmouth to make a distinctive contribution in the field of medical education"; "identify changes in personnel and facilities necessary in order to make such a contribution"; and "indicate some developments in program that will be possible with the necessary facilities and personnel." No one reading the memo could doubt that Morrison had, in a remarkably short time, superbly grasped the nature and scope of his assignment. (That he was also prescient in some details can be fully appreciated only in retrospect. A case in point is his observation that there "may be in Hanover the opportunity of developing a unique center for medical education and care.")[7]

Nor could anyone reading the memorandum seriously doubt that Dartmouth was well under way with an evaluation of its medical school that would determine what needed to be done and balance that against what could be done. Even as he listed the "favorable institutional and environmental factors [in Hanover]" for responding to the challenges and problems facing the future of medical education nationwide, Morrison mentioned that Dartmouth Medical School's "principal strengths have been the quality of its students, the intimacy of the teaching program, the willingness of dedicated teachers to work with inadequate facilities, and the availability of the personnel and facilities of the Hitchcock Hospital and Clinic." He also acknowledged the existing shortcomings:

> But the Medical School is seriously handicapped by obsolete and crowded buildings. Although the laboratories were designed for a class of 18, the entering class now is set at 24. Lack of space has made it difficult to maintain and impossible to augment a full-time medical faculty of competent teachers who are also active in medical research. Any increase in the size of the student body has been out of the question with existing facilities.

Most of the remainder of the memorandum was devoted to explaining what remedies needed to be taken. The first tasks were to upgrade facilities and personnel, after which it would "be possible to establish other parts of the plan" (which was, overall, both visionary and expensive).

Morrison and three other members of the TPC constituted a subcommittee on the Medical School that met with former Dean John Bowler and then-current Dean Rolf Syvertsen in preparation for a visit from the chief among the outside consultants, Dr. Alan Gregg, Vice President and former Director of Medical Sciences for the Rockefeller Foundation.[8] The choice of Gregg made good sense. Not only was he experienced in matters of medical education and familiar with the situation at Dartmouth (recall his involvement with the Dartmouth Eye Institute); he was also known personally to Dickey, who served with Gregg on the General Education Board of the Rockefeller Foundation.

Gregg visited the campus from January 10 to 13, 1955. Among his encounters was a dinner at the president's house to which the entire second-year class was invited. "Everyone in the class recognized the school was in trouble," recalled one of those students; they were anxious about possibly not meeting standards in the schools to which they would be transferring. But Gregg impressed them with a kind of parlor trick that demonstrated clearly how clinical tasks (like taking a patient's temperature) are grounded in science and—simultaneously—left them feeling reassured, because they understood him. Gregg, in turn, seems to have concluded that the students were by no means out of their depth.[9]

A three-page "Memorandum for the Medical School Study File" (undated and unsigned, but presumably written by Morrison) reviewed in brief an oral "progress report" given by Gregg on the Dartmouth Medical School; it was accompanied by a more fully fleshed-out memo (which *does* bear Morrison's initials) that appears to be a draft of the final "Gregg Report."[10] Gregg's official provisional assessment is found in the much-longer report put together by Morrison a week after Gregg's visit, on January 21, 1955. That this should be referred to as the "Gregg Report" despite having been written by Morrison is perfectly reasonable. In addition to summarizing very effectively the conclusions Gregg reached during his four days of conferences with students and with various officers of the College, the Clinic, and the Hitchcock Foundation as well as the Medical School, it carried Gregg's imprimatur. Inserted at the head of the report is a note indicating that Gregg had approved it "in a letter of January 25, 1955, which said: 'I have read Dean Morrison's memorandum and I find it excellently reflects my views. You are at liberty to use it in any way you please.'"[11]

The first part of the Gregg report, "Factors Affecting Trends in Medical Education," mirrors much of what Morrison himself had said in his report of January 6, 1955. He went on to consider the school's future quite optimistically: "The school is not in a crisis state." He made three recommendations: "Continue the school as a two-year school"; "Concentrate on the basic medical sciences and on a physiological approach in teaching"; and—more complexly—take advantage of Dartmouth's "liberal arts mission and the intimacy of teaching which small classes permit" to emphasize "competence in observation," "reasoning," "critical reading," and "compassion." Morrison reported that Gregg also "listed three conditions which should be met to justify the very great effort required to maintain a medical school": Make the experience at DMS one that "measures up to the quality of [the] exceptional students"; add new facilities; and strengthen the faculty. (These same conditions appear in the "Memorandum for the Medical School Study File" mentioned earlier, though their sequence is not the same in the two documents.)

Gregg followed this less than a month later—on February 12, 1955—with a letter to President Dickey, in which he boiled his "numerous impressions . . . down to the essentials," while also stressing once again that "Morrison's digest of our conversations is excellent and misses none of the points I wanted to convey." The letter addressed the issue that was surely uppermost in the trustees' minds if not in Dickey's, namely, that the warnings and recommendations he was making would call for "a considerable sum of money"—the demand for which should not "be met at the expense of the resources of the college." The need for money could hardly be news to anyone. What was rather more important in the letter, for those weighing what to do about the Medical School "situation," were Gregg's repeated insistences that Dartmouth should not give up its medical school.[12] Paramount for Gregg was the quality of the students. On that ground alone, he said, "the record . . . corroborates my optimistic estimate of the logic of continuing your medical school." But he also saw at Dartmouth an opportunity to implement what he considered a key to reducing the shortage of doctors in the country, namely, cutting the length of time required to become a physician. He clearly liked the two-year school idea, especially when—as at Dartmouth—the first year could be coincident with the last year of college. With such a model, he said, "Dartmouth might draw attention as a pilot plant in the evolution of American medical education. In this sense Dartmouth may accomplish something of national significance."[13]

How important Gregg's visit was can be judged from the fact that one day later (January 14, 1955) the TPC voted and reported to the Board of Trustees:

That the Trustees Planning Committee believes that the Dartmouth Medical School is making an important contribution to society, that it contributes positive values to the undergraduate college, and therefore that long-range planning should proceed on these assumptions: (1) that it is desirable for the Dartmouth Medical School to be continued; and (2) that further planning with respect to Dartmouth's role in medical education be directed toward the dual objective of providing the facilities and personnel believed desirable for a two-year school and of establishing the Medical School on a more nearly self-supporting basis.[14]

This was the central part of a memorandum that ran more than three pages. Four documents were appended (the first was called "Views of Dr. Alan Gregg on [DMS]"; it would frequently be used thus as an "Exhibit") when the TPC made its April 1955 report to the full Board of Trustees on the numerous steps that had been taken subsequent to that all-important visit from Gregg. And, we are later told, "It is a certainty that Alan Gregg's judgment was absolutely crucial in persuading President Dickey and the Trustees to take the necessary steps to revitalize and restructure its moribund medical school."[15]

The excitement in the air must have been palpable—not least because, although not reported in that April memorandum, other steps had also begun to be taken that would eventually bring Stephen Marsh Tenney back to Hanover. Particularly in light of the way academic appointments are made today, Tenney's description of his recruitment helps show how differently things were done in 1955. Tenney was then on the faculty of the University of Rochester School of Medicine and Dentistry. When Gregg traveled to Rochester to check on initiatives made possible by Rockefeller monies, Tenney had made his acquaintance. "During my conversations with him in Rochester," Tenney later wrote,

I had no reason to mention Dartmouth but almost immediately following his visit to Hanover (of which I was unaware) I began to get inquiries about when I was going to return to Dartmouth. [Tenney had spent a year's leave from Rochester at DMS in 1950.] The way it was phrased caught me by surprise, but I subsequently learned that I had been appointed an Assistant Professor in the Medical School and was on a "leave of absence"! All of this was completely unknown to me. Such were the oddities of the place. In any event, I felt at ease in writing Alan Gregg to solicit his opinion, and he promptly replied at length on February 7, 1955, essentially repeating what the Morrison memorandum on his views had contained, except that he dwelt . . . on the excessive and burdensome length of time required to educate a physician. Dartmouth, he was sure, could trim one year from the process without compromising quality, and this would be a very great contribution. His letter concluded with a familiar scrap of attenuated encouragement: "there is a challenge and an opportunity at Dartmouth."[16]

That final comment was just the sort of thing calculated to whet the appetite of a bright young scholar like Marsh Tenney. Morrison pressed the issue, writing to Tenney on February 25, 1955, in anticipation of a visit:

> I think that I can explain the situation, which is understandably confusing to you, when we have a chance to talk about it. In essence, it is simply that, since your visit here, the College has decided that it must try to develop a first-rate two-year Medical School in Hanover.[17] Without such a decision, I believe you would have no interest in coming back . . . to the Dartmouth Medical School unless we could accomplish something close to a revolution. We have been working very hard on this and have, I hope, made some considerable progress.

Morrison's use of the word "revolution" is interesting; the ground was being prepared for truly restarting the Medical School. As he spelled out the matters to be discussed, he also seemed clearly to be laying the basis for Tenney to be appointed as full professor with tenure. "I shall be glad to fill in this outline," he went on, "when I see you on the 14th."[18] The letter and visit from Morrison, coupled with Gregg's observations, had the desired effect. A few months later, when Tenney was offered a position as Chair of the Physiology Department and the title "Associate Dean for Research and Planning" (to begin in the autumn of 1956), he accepted.

Meanwhile, another committee chaired by Donald Morrison developed a proposal for a "Medical Science Building." The initial report, issued on July 13, 1955, acknowledged that even if financing for the building were to be settled, the Board of Trustees would still face decisions about the direction for Dartmouth Medical School. A hint about one feature of "the overall program" came in the introduction to the report: "The Board of Trustees has 'accepted' the conclusion of the [TPC] that [DMS] has a fine future as a two-year school."[19] Thus it is clear that the focus of the refounding efforts was to shore up the two-year program—no more and no less—that had been in place since 1914. (On other points, Morrison and Gregg were not in full agreement on what DMS should look like. This became evident when, despite Gregg's having discouraged too much emphasis on the College's "Cold Regions Research," the plan for the new building included a whole floor for a "Department of Environmental Physiology.")

In September, the ad hoc committee's report went to Tenney for comment. (Having agreed to accept Dartmouth's offer, Tenney began serving as a consultant to Dartmouth while still in Rochester.) The report perpetuated some "deeply entrenched ideas" that Tenney saw as "misguided"; in a reply to Morrison on September 28, 1955, he "explained in a long argument" why he thought continuing to emphasize environmental physiology was "inappropriate." Later he also "challenged the tactic of amalgamating three departments—Biochemistry, Physiology,

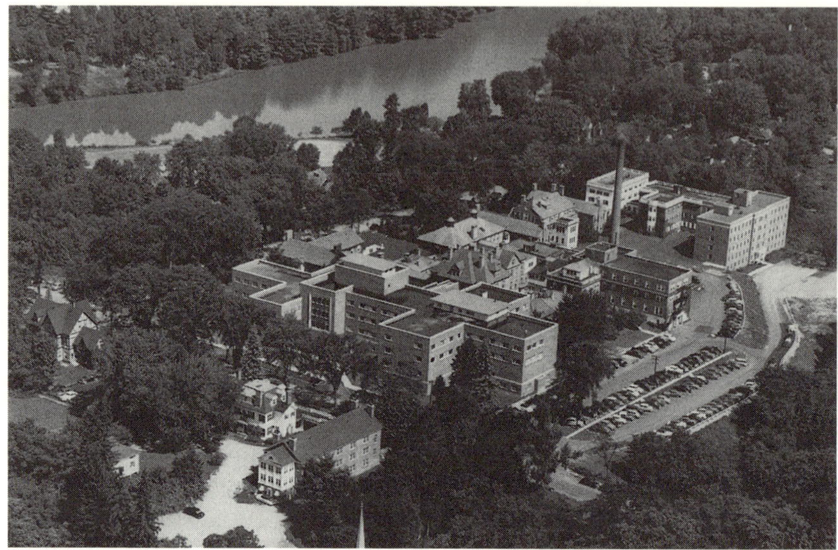

Dartmouth Medical School, Mary Hitchcock Memorial Hospital, and Hitchcock Clinic, early 1950s. Courtesy of Dartmouth Medical School.

Pharmacology—into one, Physiological Sciences." Such disagreements seem to have had no ill effect on Tenney's working relationship with Morrison, and a carefully reasoned letter from Tenney to Morrison in late November 1955 on the proposed "organizational set-up for a Physiological Sciences Department" demonstrated Tenney's effort to be fair to all parties.[20] In December, Tenney visited Hanover and made further specific proposals about laboratory space and ancillary facilities, having been given "a free hand to plan program and to begin a major recruiting effort."

In a November 25, 1955, memo headed "Study of Medical School Organization," the first item was: "Timing: After January 1 [1956]—when ad hoc committee will have determined its recommendations as to what kind of Medical School we should have."[21] This is fully in keeping with Tenney's recollection that by early 1956 it "was clear" that Dartmouth "was moving briskly to expedite matters." Among the indicators was that "President Dickey had written exploratory letters to the Rockefeller Foundation, the Commonwealth Fund, and the Ford Foundation saying that we would be submitting proposals within the next few months."[22]

All systems were being readied for the bright new world heralded by

Tenney's arrival in the autumn of 1956. He had, after all, been praised in Rochester as "one of the most generally promising young men that has come my way in a very long time. . . . With all his superiority as a laboratory man, he is also an excellent clinician. . . . [H]e is a prize winner."[23] But first there would be fireworks.

Confidential Probation

When a visit from the joint accreditation committee of the AMA's Committee on Medical Education and Hospitals (CME) and the Association of American Medical Colleges (AAMC) was announced for March 5–7, 1956, no one at Dartmouth appears to have been particularly concerned. The site visit was, after all, part of a regular and familiar pattern of visits by such joint inspection teams to medical schools. Furthermore, spirits were high because of the work that had already been done and the commitments to the future of the school that had been made in the TPC's memorandum to the trustees almost a year earlier (April 18, 1955).

This new-found optimism may help explain why no real preparations were made for the visit. Morrison had become exceedingly well informed on the subject of Dartmouth Medical School, but it appears—according to Tenney's later memoir—that "[Dean of the Medical School] Syvertsen had told [Morrison] almost nothing about the impending site visit and [the visitors'] expectations," even though these were explicit in the detailed form that the school had to fill out prior to the visit. "In fact," Tenney went on,

> most of the faculty, as well, were uninformed and were caught by surprise at the last minute when they were summoned to meet with the committee. Small wonder that the visitors were perplexed by the blank faces that confronted them in interviews. The language of the committee's report reveals an exasperation that was unleashed in intemperate expression. They probably couldn't believe that a formal site visit could be treated so casually unless it was designed to be a calculated rudeness, which it wasn't. It was just inept.[24]

Nor had the students been alerted that the visitors held the future of DMS in their hands. One student later recalled how Harry Savage, secretary of the Medical School, berated them afterwards for their behavior. When Savage took the visiting team to the Nathan Smith Laboratory, the students pitching pennies on the front steps (a frequent diversion during class breaks) blocked the entrance to an extent that Savage and his visitors had to shoulder their way through. Hardly the way to make a good impression on outsiders.

How much difference better behavior on the part of the students or better preparation on the part of the faculty and administration might have made is, of course, anyone's guess. In fact, numerous weaknesses still existed in the school. The grand plans for the future were themselves an admission that problems existed; there was indeed fault to find. Perhaps what Tenney called the "intemperate expression" in the final report would have been softened, but the conclusion probably would have been the same.

The members of the visitation team, Glen Shepherd and William Hubbard, wrote and dated their report in March, immediately following the visit. Three months passed, however, before official word on the outcome of the review came to Dartmouth, in the form of a joint letter (June 22, 1956) to President Dickey from Dean F. Smiley for the AAMC and Edward L. Turner of the CME:

> At the recent meetings of the Council on Medical Education and Hospitals of the [AMA], the Executive Council of the Association of American Medical Colleges, and the Liaison Committee representing these two Councils, full consideration was given to the report [of the Survey team] and to the recommendations made by the survey group. On the basis of these discussions and careful consideration both Councils and the Liaison Committee concurred in the recommendations of the Survey Team to the effect that Dartmouth Medical School be placed on confidential probation, subject to revisit within a period of two years prior to further reconsideration.[25]

With the wisdom of hindsight one is tempted to say that DMS should have expected something of the sort. Certainly the outraged reaction at Dartmouth seems out of proportion in the light of several factors that are often conveniently ignored. First of all, "confidential" meant just that; there was no report to the media, and knowledge of the whole matter was limited to members of the two councils, and the administration of the Medical School and its parent institution. Furthermore, Dartmouth Medical School would continue to be listed as approved and would maintain its membership in the AAMC. Thus the sky had not really fallen in, even if the initial reaction at Dartmouth was that being put on probation—even confidential probation—was "devastating," a "crippling blow," a "calamity."

Still, memories of Flexner and Weiskotten were bound to come rushing back. To some, this must have looked like one more instance of outsiders interfering in internal affairs of a venerable and valuable institution. And that wasn't all. Adding insult to injury, the "probation" label was slapped on DMS by *external* reviewers despite *internal* efforts underway to reevaluate and possibly reorganize the institution. The timing itself was an affront. Had the probationary status been announced two years earlier, before Dartmouth's Board of Trustees undertook to review their associated schools, it would have been less distressing. Coming when it did, however, it looked patently unfair. Couldn't the investigating team *see* that Dartmouth was hard at work? Couldn't they give credit where credit was due? Couldn't they have waited to see the outcome of the efforts in progress?

Yet honesty forces an admission that the accreditation team was not wholly wrong. "Some of the points raised," Tenney later wrote, were these:

> the medical school is essentially a department of the College (true); the Dean does not have the usual function and authority of that office (true); there is no Associate Professor rank and very few tenured positions (true);[26] the budget is barely adequate (true); the physical plant is inadequate (true). . . . The committee accurately, but with biting sarcasm, pointed out that absolutely nothing had changed at the School since the site review by Weiskotten and Rypins that had been made twenty-two years earlier.

The one criticism that could be challenged, Tenney said, was the claim that "there is no apparent planning to incorporate progressive development in medicine"; that, according to Tenney, utterly "failed to take account of the vigorous planning efforts underway."[27] The implied charge of current complacency at the Medical School was patently unfair, given what the College administration—under Donald Morrison's leadership—had started in mid-1956.

Still, the criticisms were so sweeping, and—alas—so true (as Tenney admitted) that the whole effort to rehabilitate Dartmouth Medical School could have come crashing to a halt on the spot. That it did not is, once again, largely to Morrison's credit. He did not cave in, though he was no doubt stung first by his realization that many (even most) of the criticisms were correct and second by the fact that he had not been prepared for them. Whether that was because the faculty had not kept him fully informed or for some other reason is unclear.

Morrison's Response

Morrison promptly went to Rochester to confer with Tenney. He also conferred (in mid-August) with Smiley and Turner, who invited him to present his view of the case for DMS to them. The resulting "Memorandum of Comments on the 1956 Report of the Survey Liaison Team on Dartmouth Medical School," dated September 7, 1956, is one of the great documents in DMS history, not least because it led directly to the "confidential probation" stigma being removed in short order. Morrison's detailed account of the ways in which the picture the two councils had received did not fairly represent the situation at Dartmouth is also a passionate review, a kind of manifesto, of where Dartmouth Medical School stood and where it was headed.

Part of Morrison's strategy was to note the points of agreement (some of those Tenney acknowledged to be "true" in his later account, such as the inadequacy of the physical facilities and understaffing). He then hammered away at the facts that the visiting team had either failed to note (the new administrative position to which Tenney had been appointed, the intensive examination of Dartmouth's role in medical education with outside advice—"notably" from Alan Gregg) or simply misunderstood.[28] It was, he wrote, "remarkable and disquieting" that the "careful review of our program should have failed to note and credit what is now being done; indeed, in these respects, things that have been studied and praised by students of the problem are casually treated in the report as weaknesses to be criticized and as grounds for probation." The survey team obviously did not have complete information on a number of points (admissions policies, faculty, faculty salaries, the department of physiological sciences, and so on). In particular, it did not seem to understand the curriculum and teaching methods at DMS. "The test," Morrison insisted, "should be whether the [DMS] students are adequately prepared in the basic medical sciences, not whether other methods might produce a better result."

In building to a climax, Morrison stressed what Gregg had also insisted upon—the high quality of Dartmouth Medical School's students and graduates. "Finally," Morrison wrote,

> it is not irrelevant to ask whether an enterprise that produces an admittedly superior product year in and year out under less than optimum conditions in respect to money and facilities and which on its own initiative is trying to get a few more of the better things in facilities and personnel should not receive commendation for a quality of resourcefulness and dedication which others tell us is exemplary in medical education and for which there is no substitute under even the most lush circumstances.

He concluded in a firm but conciliatory tone, making clear that Dartmouth had every intention of proceeding with its mission of reform—and that it wanted to be given a fair chance of carrying out that mission:

> We assume that a dispassionate review of this matter brings all of us out with a substantial feeling of inconclusiveness and dissatisfaction with the position in which both the Councils and we find ourselves. We cannot expect the Councils immediately to undertake another on the spot survey and we trust it is understandable to the Councils in the light of this memorandum why the "probation-

ary" judgment on this record cannot be regarded as merited, or helpful to our common objective.

May we suggest that, under the circumstances, the fairest and most practical approach at this juncture is to record a "suspended judgment" until a satisfactory resurvey can be scheduled and made in two years.

It was a masterpiece of diplomatic rebuttal. Morrison won as much as could have been hoped for, which was the promise of a new site visit in 1957.

A letter written by President Dickey a few days later made the seriousness of the ongoing discussions absolutely clear: "We recently concluded an extensive review of our premedical program here at Dartmouth and we are now in the middle of a terribly important and difficult decision as to whether we can see our way clear to finding the money to refound the Dartmouth Medical School in order to assure it a place in the future plans of the College."[29]

Tenney Arrives in Hanover

On October 25, 1956, a three-page memo that appears to be from Morrison to the TPC—"Status of Medical School Planning"—sketched rather grandly a major expansion at DMS in plant and personnel.[30] The following day, after reports on progress that had been made in persuading the Rockefeller and Ford foundations as well as the Commonwealth Fund to look more favorably on Dartmouth Medical School, the TPC voted affirmatively to hire an architect as the first step in preparing grant proposals for funding for a new medical school plant.[31] In the meantime, work had begun with a vengeance for Marsh Tenney, who had moved to Hanover with his family that same month. Morrison's "Memorandum" had staved off the immediate danger of disrupting the momentum toward rehabilitation of the school, but there remained much to do. For Tenney, the "opportunity:challenge ratio" to which Gregg had alluded "appeared strongly biased toward the latter. A time of total immersion had begun, and I couldn't see the end. There were many problems and they all merited high priority." Classes had started, which meant that "departmental concerns were pressing"—but "the need to quicken the pace of institutional planning and to formulate grant proposals, particularly to secure funding for building construction, was even more so."

In November 1956, a month after his arrival in Hanover, Tenney drafted a memorandum for the Board of Trustees stressing the benefits of Dartmouth's five-year approach to medical education so beloved by

Gregg (the old stratagem of collapsing the senior year of college and the first year of medical school into one), which helped fuse the liberal arts and medicine. He underscored this by emphasizing medicine as a branch of the life sciences, further appealing to the trustees' desire to build on the strengths of the undergraduate College. But ultimately the "most successful aspect" of the appeal on behalf of DMS, in Tenney's mind, was "the elaboration of an economic tactic." Insisting that Dartmouth's two-year transfer students could easily find places in four-year schools, where attrition always created vacancies, he painted a scene in which "the nation would benefit from an additional physician output without any significant extra cost" to the existing four-year schools. With Morrison increasingly tied up with other College matters, Tenney received valuable help in finishing "the basic presentation for the case of Dartmouth Medical School" from Robert Gosselin, one of the several Rochester faculty he had persuaded to join him in Hanover.[32]

The outcome was the "Dartmouth Medical School" report of March 5, 1957. The "Views of Dr. Alan Gregg on [DMS]" constituted Appendix A, just as it had for the April 18, 1955 report to the trustees. The refounding effort served as both the basis and the conclusion of the report. In the introduction, it was stated that "Dartmouth Medical School in the course of undergoing a virtual 'refounding' finds itself in an unusual position to re-examine its educational policies and formulate new concepts and teaching techniques if these seem advisable." After reviewing the proposed educational program (under the following subheads: "Premedical Education and Dartmouth College," "Convictions Concerning Modern Medical Education and the Role of Dartmouth Medical School," and "Medical School Curriculum Innovations"), the school's assets were listed. These included the quality of the students, the small size of the school, the close relationship between College and Medical School, the clinical facilities, and the presence of "teacher-investigators." Most striking—and a clear indication that things had changed since the days of the Flexner report—was the touting of the clinical opportunities as one of the strengths. The "Hitchcock Hospital and Clinic have grown in recent years to become a major center for upper New England. The strong clinical staff has been a major supplement to the [Medical School] faculty, and the wards of the hospital provide ample clinical material for teaching and for clinical research."

The special role that could be played by a two-year school was emphasized, using yet again one of Gregg's chief arguments (that DMS had an opportunity to be a national "prototype"). Dartmouth Medical School, it was said, "has demonstrated that the time required for the training of doctors can be shortened without loss of quality, and that a two-year medical school can contribute toward the fuller utilization of the clinical training facilities now available in the country." A reexamination of the school's needs, however, given the existing shortfalls in several areas, led the committee to the following position: "The conclusion is inescapable that a virtual refounding of the Dartmouth Medical School is required."[33] (The theme of the two-year school reappears in many forums. The November 1957 issue of the Maine Medical Association's journal, for instance, contained a guest editorial on the subject by John Bowler. The two-year school, he wrote, "Having existed as a neglected child for several decades, . . . can fill a large and important role in the immediate future."[34])

Other variously constituted committees and subcommittees met over the following months, and most of them issued reports and memoranda at one point or another. (Morrison, for instance, also chaired a "Committee to Study the Premedical Curriculum." That committee met for the last time in mid-1955 to discuss finalizing its report.[35]) Given the solidly grounded position in favor of continuing to support DMS that Tenney had argued for in the March 1957 "Dartmouth Medical School" report, one might have thought there was little more to discuss. Tenney's report notwithstanding, however, there was still a large question mark hanging over the TPC's deliberations. A confidential memo to Dickey and Morrison from Thomas E. O'Connell, executive director of the TPC, makes that clear. "I have been doing some thinking about the Medical School," O'Connell wrote. "Here are some of my second thoughts, for what they are worth, on the 'refound or close' assumption.'" He continued:

> [B]efore we take the courageous plunge to close our medical School [we should consider] this: What are the chances that five or six or ten years after the closing we would respond to pressures to open it up again? . . . Do we actually *have* to *refound* our [Medical School] right now? . . . Are we too far down the drain on our decision to refound or close . . . ? Have the Trustees themselves really faced up to closing and steeled themselves to going through with it?[36]

O'Connell seems clearly to have thought the answer to the latter two questions was negative. Yet the trustees and the TPC as a whole were equally clearly trying to keep an open mind and to review all the relevant arguments pro and con. On April 26, 1957 (after receiving Tenney's report), the trustees appointed a special ad hoc study committee of Harvey Hood (chair), Dudley Orr, and Ralph Hunter to make its own recommendations. The three relied heavily on the opinions and advice of the outside consultants in their recommendations to the full Board of

Trustees at the June 1957 meeting (as is evidenced by some of the supporting documents they attached to their report). But some of the sailing into that haven was done in rough seas.

Dudley Orr, for instance, still had considerable misgivings about the wisdom of the whole enterprise. His memo of May 6, 1957, provides evidence that the subcommittee was giving serious consideration to the drastic step of pulling back from all the grand refounding plans. "A decision to stop teaching professional medicine at Dartmouth obviously would be an important one," Orr wrote. "It should not be made without the careful study and deliberation which, I think, the problem has received already." He first reviewed the arguments in favor of continuing the Medical School: There was a national shortage of physicians[37]; DMS had a venerable history and had been successful by several measures; the Medical School helped attract doctors and teachers in life sciences to Hanover; and the very real needs of the School might be parlayed into an added appeal for the upcoming capital campaign.

He then proceeded to respond to each of these arguments: In fact, money was unlikely to be forthcoming; Dartmouth had long ago been affirmed as primarily an undergraduate college, and all available monies were needed to keep it in the front rank of colleges; it was the liberal arts that were central to American life; and the Hitchcock Clinic could do the job of serving as a "beacon" to attract physicians quite independent of the Medical School. Orr seemed to think these latter arguments were dispositive, though he implicitly acknowledged that "tradition" stood in the way. "We must frankly admit that in closing the Medical School, we will let an old tradition fail," he wrote,

> but we can continue [that tradition], to some degree, by a strong faculty and a strong curriculum in the life sciences. This development will also solve, to some extent, our commitment to medical school staff. It is an issue now of saving only a two-year medical school. Whatever Dr. Gregg or Dr. Wood or anyone else may say, we will be always on the defensive at this point. Dartmouth has the only privately supported two-year medical school in the country. If it was a mistake to abandon the four-year medical program 40 years ago, then it was a mistake that was made for good. . . .
>
> Confronted with a challenge, capable people often make the mistake of overestimating their own physical capacity. It is a wholly admirable characteristic of courageous men to make a last desperate effort to save a sinking ship. It seems to me clearly to be the duty of the Trustees to restrain our precious and irreplaceable administrative force from making this mistake. . . . Even if we found $5,000,000 for the Medical School, I would be apprehensive about the additional burdens thus placed on the shoulders of the President, The Treasurer, and the Provost.
>
> After ten years of remarkable accomplishment and achievement the trustees

may well want to consider the desirability of retrenchment and consolidation, particularly in the area of human resources.

Orr went so far as to propose what he thought was a suitable statement for the trustees to make following the vote they would take at their next meeting. It would, "in substance," read as follows: "'The Trustees of Dartmouth College voted on June 7 to discontinue offering medical school instruction in September 1959 unless before that time the College shall have received not less than five million dollars specifically for medical school purposes.' Then, of course," he continued, "the statement may be expanded to give a history of the efforts of the last three years, the reasons for the decision and the plans to fortify undergraduate instruction in the life sciences." Some of Orr's views can be read between the lines; others he stated outright. Further consultation "with men like Drs. Gregg, Wood and Loeb," he insisted, "would serve no purpose." He insisted that it was "hard to imagine what fresh knowledge or new ideas might be turned up by further consultation after all the effort and thought the President and Provost have put into this matter in the last three years."[38]

Despite Orr's strongly worded memorandum, the subcommittee in the end presented to the Board of Trustees a report that urged preparation of a statement that would "reaffirm the College's interest in continuing the Medical School." A draft of such a statement was included. The first of the seven conclusions reached by the subcommittee was that "The Dartmouth Medical School is making an important contribution to society, to the medical profession, and to the undergraduate college." (The influence of Alan Gregg is evident once more, and the memorandum of his views from January 1955 was yet again appended.) On the other hand, the subcommittee was suitably cautious about financial issues. The final item in the list of "Conclusions" read as follows: "The effort to secure the needed funds should be intensive and be completed within a period of three years. If the new capital and income are not available by that time, the Medical School should be discontinued and the College funds thereby released and devoted to the strengthening of the undergraduate pre-medical and science programs."

On June 7, 1957, the trustees received the report from the special study committee and voted to proceed as recommended therein. Thus this report and its supporting documents constitute the definitive basis on which the Board of Trustees decided to "refound" the Medical School—with the caveat concerning the clearly defined timetable having to do with money.[39]

Refounding Officially Begins

Two challenges in particular faced Tenney as he approached the end of his first year on the job. One had to do with the exceedingly awkward (perhaps even humiliating, Tenney later speculated) position in which Rolf Syvertsen had been placed. As Associate Dean, Tenney was nominally in a position to report to Syvertsen. Yet Dickey and Morrison had given Tenney "the full authority to run the Medical School and to implement the steps which would determine its future." Leaving Syvertsen to do what he had always done best "was all very satisfactory because it kept him fully and productively engaged," but the lines of authority and the chain of command confused the outside world; communication sometimes suffered. "Sy was never a willful obstructionist, and he never opposed me at any stage," Tenney wrote, "but his pride suffered."

The second major problem for Tenney concerned making overtures to foundations. The "failure to receive a clear, firm, unambiguous statement of commitment by the College Trustees to its Medical School" nagged. "Everything written was conditional on raising the necessary money, but for prospective major donors this appeared to be equivocating." A Rockefeller Foundation officer was openly hostile; Henry Heald, president of the Ford Foundation, succeeded in thoroughly flustering John Dickey by asking him point blank whether the Dartmouth Trustees really even wanted a medical school.[40]

Both of the issues troubling Tenney were resolved in the summer of 1957. On July 2, Dickey wrote the kind of affirmative letter to the Ford Foundation that Heald had said was essential; in that letter, among other things, Dickey announced that Marsh Tenney was being appointed "Director of Medical Sciences."[41] While this newly created position added confusion of its own, Dickey's internal memorandum on reorganization (of August 16, 1957) listed Tenney's responsibilities and made explicit that Rolf C. Syvertsen, Dean of the Medical School, was "Responsible to the Director of Medical Sciences for the operations of Dartmouth Medical School." Still awkward, but at least down in black and white.[42] At the same time, Henry L. Heyl—who had been Director of the Hitchcock Foundation—was made Assistant Director of Medical Sciences for Research and Planning. (The aim of this appointment was, among other things, to reduce the extent to which the Hitchcock Foundation and the Medical School were competing with each other for the same foundation grants.) In addition, Dickey announced the formation of a Policy Committee. The members were some of the same consultants who had earlier been asked for their advice—George Berry, Robert Loeb, and Barry

Wood—plus Waltman Walters of the Mayo Clinic and John Bowler (both DMS alumni).[43] It was a powerful group of individuals, whose influence, Tenney later wrote, "cannot be overemphasized." Not that they were always in full agreement. "There were often fundamental differences in point of view regarding where emphasis should be placed," Tenney went on,

> primarily in faculty recruitment and educational program, but the three academicians on the committee [as opposed to the two DMS graduates, both practicing physicians] always came down strongly on my side. The support that they gave me, without fail, over the entire life span of the committee, certainly helped to alleviate my occasional waves of insecurity, but the committee's division into 3:2 opinion on some issues was unfortunate.[44]

In September 1957, Tenney submitted the first of his three progress reports to the trustees. He skillfully wove together what had been done and what was going to be needed: The president and trustees had "reaffirmed their belief that medical education is an important part of Dartmouth's over-all educational opportunity and responsibility." They had also recognized the need for "sweeping improvements"; they had endorsed a program for reorganization, an enlarged basic science faculty, and the construction of a new medical science building. It was understood that there needed to be greater financial assistance from the College and that a $10 million fundraising effort for the Medical School would be undertaken. Tenney also reported the changes in administrative titles (and responsibilities) and the formation of the Policy Committee.

Of some interest is his statement that the rationale for the new program was that the "national need for medical teachers and investigators is fully as great as that for practitioners." To the extent that this was to become a central theme in the plans for the future, it could have been argued that it was something of a move away from the founding mission of Nathan Smith—to train practicing physicians—and of most of the years between his day and the late 1950s. When Tenney went on to say that the object of the educational program would continue to be "to provide the best possible grounding in the basic medical sciences" and that "a distinctive feature . . . will be an experiment in medical education providing six months of elective research experience during the first two years of medical school," one could perhaps also read into this the beginnings of tensions that would arise in the decade ahead, as misunderstandings developed concerning the Medical School's primary purpose.

The most impressive sign of change recorded in the report had to do with the growth of the full-time faculty. With Tenney's arrival it had gone from six to seven. One year later, by the autumn of 1957, it had exploded to twenty. There was a "completely new faculty in . . . Physiology, Biochemistry, and Pharmacology."[45] (In fact, though Tenney did not mention it, much of the growth had been at the expense of his former employer; Rochester had been absolutely robbed. Of six new people in physiology, all had Rochester connections—and all but one had come directly from Rochester.) One of the two new people in pharmacology also came from Rochester; Robert Gosselin had been appointed Professor and Chairman of Pharmacology already in 1956. (Tenney essentially brought Gosselin with him.) In 1957 Manuel F. Morales came from the Naval Institute in Bethesda, bringing some faculty with him. He was made Professor and Chairman of Biochemistry, thus completing the process of dividing up the old conglomerate "Department of Physiological Sciences" into its more logical disciplinary components: physiology, pharmacology, and biochemistry.[46]

Probation Comes to an End

A month after this first progress report, the promised revisit by the AMA/AAMC Accreditation Committee took place. Tenney in his "Memoir" gives such a brisk and concise account of this significant event that its importance might almost be missed. "This time it was a large group," he wrote (naming the five members of the team):

> These were senior, respected leaders in medical education (the AMA/AAMC was now defensive about the previous site visit) and they rendered a strong endorsement of our program and of our progress. Full accreditation was granted. The blemish of "confidential probation" was now erased, and we were no longer burdened with that handicap in fund raising. Further, Ward Darley [on the visiting team] who was Executive Director of the Association of American Medical Colleges became our strong advocate after his visit here. Foundations frequently sought his judgment about Dartmouth Medical School and he unfailingly gave us his strong endorsement.[47]

The next two years were filled with a great rush of satisfying achievements. All major foundation grants were awarded. Building plans were approved; the contract was let. (The idea was to double enrollment to forty-eight per class when the new science building was finished.) The first appointments to full-time positions of women faculty—Jean Botts and Jane Sands Robb—were made. By 1959, Frances McCann and Lucile Smith had also joined the faculty. In fact, by the time Tenney issued his "Second Progress Report" in December 1959 the teaching staff had again grown significantly; there were by then thirty-eight full-time faculty in the basic science departments.[48] Furthermore, five faculty members had been made Senior Research Fellows by the U.S. Public Health Service, two had "Established Investigator" awards from the American Heart Association, and Tenney himself had been made a Markle Foundation Scholar in the Medical Sciences.

Near the end of his report, Tenney took pains to underscore how DMS was an asset to the College as a whole. Research collaboration was under way, some crossover teaching was taking place, and joint appointments had been made. "Past experience at Dartmouth has shown that a basic science medical school and a liberal arts college can draw on each other's strength to mutual advantage," he insisted. His summary was full of optimism: "Dartmouth Medical School looks forward with increased vigor and enthusiasm to the further steps which will be necessary, firmly convinced that the 'experiment' it is engaged in is important to the solution of a national need for new and imaginative approaches to medical education."[49]

"Medical Metamorphosis"

It was too much to hope, perhaps, that everything would go as planned. Death cast a pall over the Dartmouth community in 1959 and then again in early 1960. Long-time and much-loved faculty member Ralph Miller and his young colleague Robert Quinn died following the crash of Miller's plane in February 1959; almost exactly a year later, Rolf Syvertsen was killed in an automobile accident. In between, equally shocking and tragic for the medical school, Provost Donald Morrison died of a heart attack at forty-four. John Masland was appointed Provost to succeed him. That so much positive happened during this period is a tribute to the commitment that College and Medical School administration alike had by this time made to putting DMS on solid ground again. Several additional stellar appointments were made: Shinya Inoué (another Rochester connection, a distinguished and well-established researcher) was brought in as Professor and Chairman of Anatomy-Cytology. Robert Weiss was appointed Professor and Chairman of Psychiatry, and Allan Tisdale came from Yale to coordinate clinical teaching in the second year; these were the first *clinical* appointments. Another fine appointment was made when Kurt Benirschke became Professor and Chairman of Pathology (replacing Ralph Miller). And then Dartmouth Medical School—having already added women to its faculty—took another dramatic step into the future by admitting its first female student, Valerie Leval, in 1960.

In the aftermath of Syvertsen's death, Marsh Tenney was appointed

Dean, and the "Director of Medical Sciences" position was eliminated. Henry Heyl's title was changed to Assistant Dean; Philip Nice became Assistant Dean for Student Affairs. Harry Savage remained in charge of Admissions. Also at this time, R. Clinton Fuller came from Oxford (where he had been on a Fellowship in the Department of Microbiology) to become Professor and Chairman of Microbiology, and—when Manuel Morales was awarded a prestigious Career Award by the American Heart Association and left for San Francisco—Lafayette Noda was appointed Chairman of Biochemistry.

The future looked bright. Tensions between the College's Development Office and efforts by the Medical School to raise its own money other than from the "big four" foundations primarily concerned with medical education eased considerably once the College closed its bicentennial capital campaign. In December 1959, the *Dartmouth Alumni Magazine* published an article aptly titled "Dartmouth's Medical Metamorphosis," which outlined the "amazing progress in the recent past." The article ended with reference to the $10,000,000 capital campaign that DMS was then about to undertake.[50]

Yet another site visit and review by the AMA/AAMC Liaison Committee on Medical Education resulted in a recommendation to continue full accreditation. Particularly gratifying, according to Tenney, was the CME's acknowledgment of all the progress that had been taking place."[51] The new medical science building, Remsen, was ready to be dedicated in the autumn of 1960 (a year later money was in hand or committed for three more buildings—the Kellogg Auditorium, the Strasenburgh Dormitory, and the Dana Biomedical Library). The dedication was scheduled in conjunction with a major symposium on "Great Issues of Conscience in Modern Medicine," held in September 1960. Ward Darley of the AAMC thrilled his audience when he said at that occasion, "I do not think I exaggerate when I compare the importance of Dartmouth's opportunity in 1960 with that which confronted Johns Hopkins in 1893."[52] This was high praise, indeed. The convocation itself, chaired by microbiologist René Dubos from the Rockefeller Institute, was a splendid affair. The panel discussions and assemblies featured author Aldous Huxley; writer and scientist C. P. Snow; George B. Kistiakowsky, physical chemist and special assistant to President Eisenhower for science and technology; Hermann J. Muller, professor of zoology at Indiana University and winner of the 1946 Nobel Prize in physiology or medicine; Sir George Pickering, Regius Professor of Medicine at Oxford; and another half dozen speakers of similar distinction. Attendance exceeded all expectations.

Though in a very real sense it could be said that the refounding of

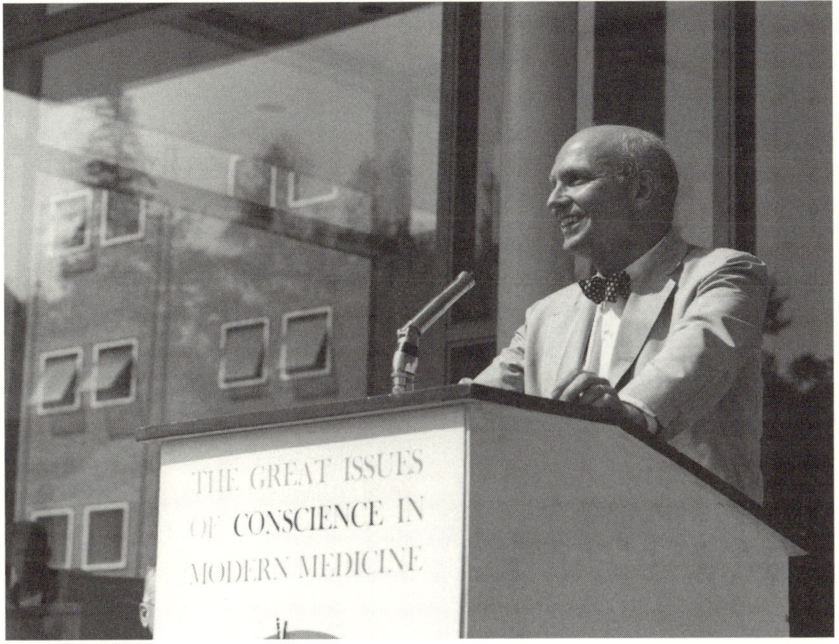

Stephen Marsh Tenney at the Great Issues Convocation held at DMS, 1960. Courtesy of Dartmouth College Library.

DMS had been accomplished by the time of the convocation (as Tenney stated in his third progress report, in February 1962), it would turn out that some local issues had not yet been fully resolved.[53] Still, the phase of rapid growth had clearly come to an end, and implementation of plans for further expansion and development seemed under control. In October 1961, Tenney submitted his resignation as dean, to take effect the following September. He was eager to be relieved of the administrative work—much though he had relished the initial "challenge of developing a first-rate institution." His relationship with the new provost, Masland, had proved somewhat less congenial and was therefore perhaps also less effective than his partnership with Morrison had been. Masland's view of the Provost's administrative function was not the same as Tenney's, and Tenney wanted in any case to return to teaching and to his own research.[54]

Whether Tenney had any idea just how big the institution's next challenge would be—and of the extent to which he would become once again (or remain) a key figure—is anyone's guess. He almost certainly did not imagine that he would return as acting dean not once, but twice in the years ahead. Once Gilbert H. Mudge came on board as the new dean, Tenney was able (for the nonce) to return to physiology full time. The Medical School was not, however, on quite such a firm footing as he may have thought. To be sure: DMS was definitely back on the map, clearly having been successfully refounded, and great talent was being drawn to Hanover. There was much reason for optimism. Ironically, however, it was the very success DMS had had in bringing outstanding scientists and researchers to the school that laid the basis for what happened next.

CHAPTER TEN

A Question of Balance

. . . forsan et haec olim meminisse juvabit.

[Some day, perhaps, remembering even this will be a pleasure.]
—VIRGIL[1]

The Context of Controversy

On March 20, 1961, John W. Masland—Provost of Dartmouth College since Morrison's death—sent a memo to President John Sloan Dickey. The topic was a new "Medical Science Graduate Program"; the purpose of the memo was to put into President Dickey's hands a resolution voted by the chairmen of the Medical School departments two weeks earlier (March 6, 1961). "Be it Resolved," the memo read:

> That, graduate education leading to the Ph.D. degree within the Dartmouth Medical School should take form as interdisciplinary programs under the broadest categories of major faculty research interest and capability. These categories are:
>
> a) Molecular biology
>
> b) Physiological mechanisms in Health and Disease.
>
> That, although these programs will have their roots in the basic educational and research opportunities provided by the Medical School, there will be important participation by members of the Science Division of the College.
>
> That, although interdisciplinary in concept and operation the training will have a specific departmental focus for each graduate student.

This brave new start to building serious graduate programs in the medical sciences, quite apart from guiding prospective medical doctors through the first two years of their training, sounds simple enough. But even getting to this point had taken some time. Two years earlier, a report "On Graduate Study at Dartmouth Medical School" had been generated by a committee comprising Manual Morales (as chairman),

Shinya Inoué, and Jane Sands Robb.[2] A few months after that, Tenney had met with Masland and the deputy provost, Leonard Rieser, to brief them on plans for Ph.D. programs at DMS. This was, Tenney said, a venture "supported by a unanimous resolution of his entire faculty." One of the major questions the three colleagues discussed was how the relevant science departments in the College were likely to respond to DMS-sponsored Ph.D. programs in what the undergraduate faculty considered "their" fields.[3]

Tenney had come from a medical school faculty meeting just two days earlier where considerable enthusiasm for introducing a Ph.D. program had been expressed. Somewhat later (in May 1961), shortly after Clinton Fuller was hired as Professor and Chairman of Microbiology, Tenney appointed him chairman of a new Molecular Biology Graduate Committee.[4] Not until January 1962 was it appropriate for the *Dartmouth Alumni Magazine* to announce (with the appointment of Gilbert Mudge as dean) that the medical school was "joining with the Science Division of the College to offer a new Ph.D. program in molecular biology, a step in the development of graduate education that was inherent in the growth of the School and the type of faculty and research now flourishing there."[5] Long before the pieces neatly fell into place, tensions over Ph.D. programs in medical science at Dartmouth began to arise and then fester. Those surrounding molecular biology in particular shape all memories of DMS in the 1960s; the disagreements and the resulting changes in direction defined the immediate future of DMS in unanticipated ways.

With the stigma of probation removed, new financing was being pursued and obtained; an ambitious building program was under way, as was the development of programs that would lead to Ph.D. and M.D. degrees. Furthermore, by the early 1960s, there were signs that DMS was neither so provincial nor so small as it had been. The entering class in 1962 was twice as large as the class that had entered five years earlier, and fully half those students came from undergraduate institutions other than Dartmouth.

No one, however, seems to have expected that these dramatic innovations would soon lead to dissension. What was meant to be the crowning touch in the refounded medical school—some kind of a "cross-field" program that would put DMS on the map with a unique program in the basic biomedical sciences—all too soon looked like gold turned to dross. That a Ph.D. in molecular biology should have been the first to be proposed has as much to do with who the first faculty recruits were as with any deliberate determination on Tenney's part that this was the best place to start. On the other hand, it *was* theoretically a good place to start; the "alignment of genetics and physics and chemistry to focus on the relation of information to molecular structure was the intellectual force that brought the term *molecular biology* into vogue in the 1950s."[6] And here was DMS, in the early 1960s, trying to do something important and impressive. Difficulties began to emerge as early as 1963, however, and by 1966 they were visible to all. Uncovering the full story is not easy, though it is a matter of verifiable record that a significant number of faculty members (including some of the very recently arrived) left DMS—most of them sad or disappointed or angry or bitter. Some were all of the above. A similarly wide range of emotions was shared by many of those who stayed, with a sense of relief or triumph or vindication for a few, but a deep sense of loss for many others.

Getting at the core of the problem is no easier than uncovering the full story. Even at the time, disagreement existed over what the issues were; in hindsight one can see more than one possible interpretation of the central concerns. Carleton Chapman, writing in 1972 (thus not long after the faculty exodus), insisted that "the elements of the controversy included problems that were—and still are—deeply ingrained in American medical education and in general academic philosophy."[7] For medical schools today the basic question remains: Should medical schools be training doctors or educating scientists? Yet the view that tensions at Dartmouth Medical School in the 1960s arose primarily as a result of seemingly inherent conflicts between Ph.D.s and M.D.s, between the desire of medical departments to have a full-fledged medical school and science departments eager for a research institute, is not shared by everyone. Some, to be sure, did believe that the next logical step for DMS—once it had been liberated from its probationary status and was being acclaimed as successfully "refounded"—was a return to its M.D.-degree-granting status. Yet "research institute or full medical school" was not generally viewed as an either/or question in the sense that a choice would have to be made between a Ph.D. program and an M.D. program. The issue was rather whether an entity with the characteristics of a research institute was compatible with a traditional medical school program—which at that point really still meant the first two years of medical school.

Others saw the disagreements at DMS as being based to a far greater extent on differences between the faculty and the administration over governance. The administration for the most part tried to downplay the formal *institutional* nature of the problem by insisting that the difficulties lay within the faculty itself, between one faction of the faculty and another. But any attempt to say "the problem was *X*" or "the problem was *Y*" is bound to be an oversimplification; it assumes that the controversy can be brought into sharper focus retrospectively than it ever had in the first place. There was more than one source of irritation, and that many members of the faculty did not trust each other (and in some cases actively disliked each other) is all too evident, even decades later.

Yet another view often expressed is that the real underlying issue was the classic Dartmouth ambivalence about anything that might turn the cherished "small college" into a university. In the mid-1960s, the rise and fall of the Dartmouth Eye Institute was recent history; the possible implications of that story for the future of Dartmouth Medical School cannot have escaped notice altogether. Other issues would also arise (or resurface) in the aftermath of the refounding. The planned expansion of the physical plant went well beyond dedicating the first new building. Money continued to be a concern. Territorial questions abounded, such as whether the College or the Medical School was to be responsible for fund raising. Discussions started all over again within the Board of Trustees about whether Dartmouth should be in the business of medical education at all. But the topic that consumed the most time and energy in the 1960s was the fate of the new molecular biology graduate program.

Molecular Biology at DMS

Granting some ambiguity about when this particular story begins, one might point to the recruitment of Manual Morales in 1957 to head the Biochemistry Department. Critical to Tenney's vision was that the science being taught at DMS should be strengthened, yet in retrospect it is not clear that even he recognized quite how great the culture shock would be once the faculty had a significant number of members on board who were themselves products of Ph.D. programs and who were interested in making their teaching of medical students as scientific as possible. Their focus was somewhat different from that of their colleagues who had come out of M.D. programs.[8] Serious scientist though Tenney was, he was committed to the DMS he knew and loved (and had known and loved as a student) and endorsed its orientation toward medicine. When Shinya Inoué was hired (in 1959) as Professor and Chairman of Anatomy-Cytology and began to build that department, the earliest signs of a serious mismatch could probably already have been seen by anyone alert to them. Inoué was thoroughly wedded to the idea of continuing to do the kind of serious scientific research he was known for; that he was to be attached to a *medical* school was probably less of the attraction for him at DMS than the fact that he and other up-and-coming research stars had been vigorously recruited. The mood at Dartmouth seemed upbeat; the future there looked very promising.

Clinton Fuller, as mentioned, had been appointed Professor and Chairman of Microbiology. Meanwhile Morales, for personal reasons and because he was offered an endowed professorship elsewhere—something DMS was not yet in a position to match—left in 1961; the chairmanship of Biochemistry fell to Lafayette Noda (already a member of the department). In addition, three members of the biochemistry department (including Jean Botts, one of the first women faculty members at DMS) left with Morales, followed by another three the next year. These departures probably contributed to a sense of instability or even confusion about the direction scientific research was going to take at Dartmouth. Those who remained, however—Noda, Lucile Smith, Peter von Hippel—were certainly strong contributors to the new work being done. Furthermore, it was a wide-open and innovative era in the biological sciences, so that turnover, even at a place like Dartmouth that seemed to be offering such promise of great things to come, was not shocking in itself. The decade of the 1960s generally was the period of the greatest academic mobility during the twentieth century.

Nonetheless, as some of the first recruits left, the character of their departments changed. As other new faculty members moved forward with their work convinced that they knew better than those who had recruited them what was important, the unified front that had been so typical of Dartmouth Medical School for most of its history began to show cracks. Yet in 1961 and 1962, no one could have imagined how embattled some members of the biochemistry, microbiology, and anatomy-cytology departments would soon feel. No one would have been able to predict that the chairmen of those three departments—Noda, Fuller, and Inoué, respectively—would soon find themselves caught in a vortex not altogether of their own creation.

On January 1, 1958, the Policy Committee for the Medical School that President Dickey had formed in mid-1957 issued a detailed statement on "The Potential Role of Dartmouth's Two-Year Medical School." The several paragraphs on curriculum began thus:

> The object of the program should continue to be to provide a thorough and stimulating education in the basic medical sciences. We see at Dartmouth the opportunity to teach these sciences as part of the broad discipline of biology.
>
> One feature of the new curriculum will be an experiment in medical education providing six months of guided elective research experience during the first two years of medical school.[9]

As for the faculty, the statement said that any "additions should be chosen with a keen eye to their ability to contribute to the spirit as well as content of the proposed curriculum. The new faculty will, as an aggregate, combine investigative distinction with inspiring tutorial teaching." Thus it should have been clear that all faculty members were expected to engage in both research and teaching. While Tenney's most admiring colleagues were caught up by his qualities of brilliance, vision, and charisma (he had a "scintillating" intelligence, "he excelled in everything," it was he who "held things together"), others began to wonder whether Tenney was wholly sympathetic to their aspirations. If he in turn—with a self-confident proprietary attitude toward the school he had played an instrumental role in rescuing—sensed that a degree of hostility was growing, it would be understandable if in subtle (perhaps subconscious) ways he did begin to block some of what the most ardent researchers among the biologists sought. (Much, much later it would come out that there had been something like unanimous distrust of—"lack of confidence" in—Tenney among the "dissident" faculty members.[10]) It is not clear that Tenney ever appreciated quite how deep the antagonism and distress ran.

Anyone asked today to recount what transpired, or to identify the underlying causes of the disagreements that reached the fever pitch of "mass resignations" in April of 1966, resorts very quickly to describing the personalities of one or more of the faculty members involved. What is really striking is how differently the same person is described by different individuals. Nor is the language used always temperate. One and the same person has been labeled as an "ogre" and as a "very likeable person"; another individual was both "a sweet guy," "one who "behaved well"—and "absolutely hostile to all scientists." A colleague could be described as an excellent scientist in one breath and dismissed as isolated and selfish, even "despised," in another. Someone could be identified by one person as "fair" and by another as having "absolute integrity"—and yet have a third individual describe him as "devious," and as someone who "handled truth with a certain slippery hand." Words like "ineffective," "inept," and "stubborn," and phrases like "harsh, powerful, and proud of it" or "heavy, stubborn, rigid" have been bandied about to describe one or another of their colleagues by those then at DMS. One "very wise man" was also identified as "arrogant"; someone who "deserves lots of credit for progress made" was said by others to be "guilty of subterfuge" when it suited his purposes. Another was said to "understand well how medical schools work" but (by someone else) to have "no deep understanding of graduate programs," thus drawing a distinction that not everyone wanted to accept.[11] According to one participant, "the controversies appear to have been blown out of proportion and in some instances are unintelligible." Left dangling is the wistful remark, "If we hadn't been so young, if we had all been a little smarter. . . ."

They *were* smart. Yet most were also pretty young, as well as ambitious and fully committed to their own visions of what Dartmouth Medical School should be and could mean to each of them and their work. Furthermore, they may not all have fully understood the route Tenney was following. Like John Sloan Dickey, Tenney wanted to build bridges between the College and the Medical School; he saw biology as the area in which that could most easily and effectively be done. In his "Second Progress Report" (1959), he wrote that the "graduate program leading to a doctorate in the basic medical sciences is considered an important component in bringing the Medical School's educational responsibility to full maturity. . . . It is likely that a 'cross-field' program will emerge—'molecular biology,' for example—which will utilize the combined resources of the Medical School and liberal arts faculties of Dartmouth College." The aim, he went on, was to provide "local opportunity" for medical students whose interest in basic science "has been sharpened by the Medical School curriculum" to stay for a Ph.D. (they would still have to go elsewhere for the M.D.).[12] And sure enough: In Tenney's "Third Progress Report" (1961) he was able not only to claim that "the major objectives for this School as outlined five years ago" had been accomplished, but to announce that the anticipated cross-field program in molecular biology, the first graduate program leading to the Ph.D., would "be offered through a joint effort of all the basic science departments of the [Medical School] and certain departments of the Division of Science in the College."[13] The refounding had effectively been accomplished; partial evidence lay in the considerable expansion of the Medical School's program that had already been achieved.

The new Medical Science Building was occupied in 1961, and all the old buildings were vacated. The search for a new dean had culminated with an offer to Gilbert H. Mudge, Chairman of the Department of Pharmacology and Associate Dean at Johns Hopkins University School of Medicine. Though there might have been some reason to be concerned about whether the new dean (Mudge) could work effectively with a former dean (Tenney) still on the faculty and actively engaged in all aspects of the school's welfare, a letter from Mudge to Tenney on December 8, 1961, shows no hint of any such problem. Mudge expressed his gratitude for being brought up to date; he also took the opportunity to claim neutrality on the issue of whether DMS should remain a two-year school or move toward becoming a four-year institution again. He did, however, stress his conviction that the clinical facilities of the VA Hospital would be essential if DMS were to add the clinical years, thus going on record as very much hoping the VA would not move the hospital, so that all options for DMS would remain open.[14] There seemed to be agreement all around on this point. In a confidential memo to John Meck (college treasurer) and Masland written a month later, President Dickey reported Tenney's "reiterated insistence" that the Veterans' Hospital was of vital significance to the Medical School. The increase in the size of the Medical School to forty-eight students per class was predicated on the availability of the teaching beds in the Veterans' Hospital for second-year students.[15]

Meanwhile, Fuller, in his role as chairman of the Molecular Biology Graduate Committee, wrote to President Dickey announcing that implementation of the program was ready and spelling out how the conditions laid down by the Board of Trustees were to be met.[16] A short letter from Fuller to Mudge welcomed the latter eagerly, saying how much all at DMS were looking forward "to continuing with you, the magnificent effort that Marsh has started." A new era was about to begin, and spirits were high.[17]

A New Dean Begins His Work

Mudge (like Tenney before him) did not wait to arrive at Dartmouth before putting his oars in the water. In May 1962, he wrote to Allan Tisdale expressing his concern about the lack of clear definition of "clinical investigation" at Dartmouth, while also insisting he had "tried not to have too many pre-conceived notions." His letter sounded a word of caution: "There are a large number of very closely inter-related problems, and it will be better in the long run to go slowly rather than in the wrong direction."[18] Certainly the attempt to get on the same page with Tisdale was a good idea. Tenney had identified Tisdale's appointment to a full-time position on the clinical faculty as a "step of signal importance in the fulfillment of [DMS's] education program." His responsibilities, Tenney had continued,

> include the supervision of all clinical instruction in the [medical school], not only in the first two years of medicine, but in the internship and residency programs as well. . . . At Dartmouth, the large and very active clinical group is a magnificent asset, but without someone who is full-time and able therefore to administer and coordinate the clinical courses, it is difficult to maintain essential continuity and perspective. Dr. Tisdale has brought this kind of leadership to our clinical programs.[19]

Nor was Tenney alone in his assessment of Tisdale's importance to the whole enterprise. Another former member of the faculty once said that, as a "transition figure," Allan Tisdale was a "gift of God"; it was he who, among other things, helped establish a workable departmental structure.

Marsh Tenney, reflecting on his decanal experience during his final year as dean, later wrote that he had been "presented, on several occasions, with arguments over familiar subjects of concern in any faculty group: governance; tenure; finances; space. These matters grew in importance subsequently," he continued, and "new ones were added." But by that time Mudge was dean; Tenney could stand back and observe. "Not much time had passed before the faculty of the school was divided over a number of contentious issues," Tenney went on, "and Mudge found himself fully occupied with a turbulent storm that was not of his making."[20]

The worst of that storm still lay some distance in the future, though Mudge had no way of knowing this. Things looked bad enough to him already in his first meetings with members of the medical school faculty and with the Advisory Board (essentially the renamed "Policy Committee," which included department chairmen and college administrators but not other members of the medical school faculty).[21] At least that is the impression one gets from the extensive notes he wrote to himself. Indeed, Mudge seems to have come away from the initial encounters with his faculty surprised and distressed at how close to the surface underlying tensions were.

Years later he said that, having been apprised by Tenney when he was recruited for the job, he was "fully aware of a divided point of view within the School." Yet he seems to have been unprepared for the extent to which the rapid growth of the faculty had produced a group that lacked collegial experience. The picture emerges of a dean who was somewhat conflicted. On the one hand, he wanted department chairmen to play a major role in the running of the school, but he also seems to have wanted them simply to accept the wisdom of his views. Again and again, in memos to the file and to others, Mudge wrote of the need for department chairmen in particular to "accept responsibility in a mature way." He was from the outset of his deanship frustrated and disappointed by what he deemed unreasonable and uncooperative responses from the faculty.

At the Advisory Board meeting on October 1, 1962, Mudge announced that it was not the plan "to set up separate research institutes here and . . . we are not going to want to have a postgraduate faculty." He also said that "all individuals should be appointed for their ability to both teach and perform research."[22] It is easy to see how some of those hired to establish an exciting and innovative cross-field research program in molecular biology might have taken umbrage at these words.

The handwritten notes on which Mudge based his remarks at a special meeting of the Advisory Board on November 19, 1962—some three weeks after the most recent faculty meeting—indicate that he was by that time aware of the nature and seriousness of the situation. He knew for sure after receiving a detailed response the next day. In a nine-page confidential memo, one department chairman responded item by item to Mudge's fourteen enumerated points. Occasional conciliatory remarks—"I cannot agree with you more," "That is certainly true," "I concur with your wisdom in not attempting . . . a rash decision"—were for the most part followed by "but" clauses. Overall, the memo was characterized far more by correction and amendment than by agreement. What the dean presumably still did not know is whether the memo reflected the views only of the memo's author or of the entire "dissenting minority" (whose size and significance Mudge acknowledged he did not yet know). Looking back, it is difficult to tell how much the increasingly uncomfortable position in which Mudge found himself was caused by his own heavy-handed and too-authoritarian management style. Equally possibly among the causes of the difficulties Mudge faced was a combination of poor information and communication in the first place and bad luck or bad timing in the second.

Faculty Governance Becomes an Issue

A further blow, and an explicit statement of the nature and source of at least some of the problems that were surfacing, came in a post-Christmas letter to the dean from Clinton Fuller. A mere six weeks after having written to President Dickey that implementation of the program was ready, Fuller found himself explaining to Dean Mudge why he had felt compelled to resign as Chairman of the Molecular Biology Graduate Committee. The letter is an important one, for it shows very clearly what at least one critical faculty member believed to be the focal point of the differences between the dean and the faculty. Certainly "faculty organization" was the overall theme of the letter. More specifically, the issue as Fuller saw it was the existence of a fundamental difference between how Mudge thought the medical school should be organized and how Fuller (and, presumably, others) thought a "special kind of graduate program" should be organized. "I am sorry," he wrote, "that graduate education was the victim of faculty organization problems in the medical school—but by the very nature of your ideas of the organization and operation of a classical medical school and my ideas on the organization and operation of a hopefully special kind of graduate program, this clash was inevitable." The crux of the matter, according to Fuller, was Mudge's conviction that the medical school had to have a "highly departmentalized structure with permanent, strong department chairmen," whereas the graduate program in molecular biology was by definition a "*non-departmental* and *non-school* oriented program," one designed to run under the aegis of the Graduate Council in any case rather than the medical school as such.[23]

Six days later (on January 3, 1963) Mudge distributed to his faculty a document on "The Organization and Responsibilities of the Faculty," to which he added a request (on January 9) that responses be made in writing. Fuller, Inoué, and Noda each replied, offering a variety of suggestions for changes and making clear that alterations in the dean's proposal were essential. Noda's letter, for example, ended with a firm indication that the issues at hand were not trivial: "I believe," he concluded, "that the times ahead are very important as Dartmouth Medical School comes of age as a leading two-year school and that the tasks are large, falling on the shoulders of the new Dean as upon each of us, for we all have invested tremendously in a new and inspiring enterprise."[24] And Fuller, insisting that he had proposed "only *one* basic change," pleaded, "I really feel you will have your faculty behind you if you can by this gesture show them you are willing to let *them* participate in the overall operation of this School directly."[25]

The extent to which the distress expressed by the three department chairmen was shared by members of their respective departments is unclear. Tenney, in his "Memoir," giving what he called "my version" of the whole "developing storm," treats them as a unit. "The dissident group," he wrote,

> were members of the Departments of Biochemistry, Cytology and Microbiology. They had all come to the Dartmouth Medical Faculty from positions in university or institute departments. None had had a medical school experience. Therefore, it was natural that their orientation was different in many regards from that which is traditional in a medical faculty. Faculties in the liberal arts have a greater concern for academic government as a participatory democracy; medical faculties are more inclined to accept a good deal of authoritarian management.[26]

This analysis could help explain why Mudge—with his considerable medical school experience—so quickly came into conflict with faculty members used to faculty self-governance.

Bit by bit, the three central departments of the "exciting" cross-field program in molecular biology were beginning to be viewed by the administration—starting with Mudge but by no means ending with him—as problematic. Or, to be more precise, the three chairmen were seen as difficult to work with. Mudge came to see Inoué and Noda especially as contrarians, "dissidents," perhaps even as leaders of a genuine faction. President Dickey perceived the disagreements between Mudge and the three department chairmen as serious. Anticipating that changes in the department chairmanships might need to be made, the president—in a startlingly candid memo to Mudge—expressed the hope that Fuller could be "saved" as a department chairman even if Inoué and Noda could not be.[27] Among the reasons was that this would be a means of further isolating "the dissident two" and clearing the way for the Advisory Board to become a more cohesive working unit, one that would experience a "growing sense of solidarity for the future in their collective action *with the Dean.*" The memo in which these observations appear was written by Dickey while he was en route to Florida, on February 28, 1963. Addressed to Masland and Mudge, it was obviously meant to propose ways of smothering the flames of mutual distrust and antagonism that had flared in the aftermath of a contentious faculty meeting three days earlier. The effort failed in the short term.[28]

The College Administration Takes Action

On April 26, 1963, President Dickey sent a memo to "The Dean and Faculty of the Dartmouth Medical School." The memo's key feature was the president's announced intention to have the Trustees Planning Committee form a new planning group "made up mainly of Medical School faculty members," which would "undertake a thorough review of the professional aims, principles and policies governing all teaching and research activities of the School." In addition, he said, as "a parallel but independent undertaking I propose to appoint an *ad hoc* committee to examine the organizational structure and the current administrative problems of the school."[29] Dickey was extremely concerned about what looked like major breakdown in communication within the medical school. The TPC gave unanimous approval to the idea of a subcommittee on the medical school on May 10, 1963.

Establishing a committee is one thing, however; achieving the desired results is another. Less than two months later, in a formal letter to the dean of the medical school, Dickey reported on the work of the first committee: "Manifestly neither the Ad Hoc Committee nor any other individual or group has been able to suggest a comprehensive course of action which is wholly wise and feasible in all eyes."[30] The very next day, a personal letter ("Dear Bert") followed, sent to Mudge's home. "I think the most basic thing for you and me to be clear about is that we are at a point in the affairs of the Medical School where the deanship must be able to contribute positively to the unity of both the School and the larger bio-medical community." He left it for Mudge to decide whether he felt he could be an effective dean and keep the deanship from being "a prisoner of either that [unhappy] past or of a present that gives any indication of being a repetition of that past."[31] Mudge stayed on as dean.

The Medical School's "Primary Purpose"

Roughly a year after all the discussion about whether an irreparable split was forming between the research scientists and the people teaching medicine, a new but closely related issue began to emerge. A proposal to establish two new clinical departments—in medicine and in surgery—when coupled with the increased needs of the molecular and cellular biology team for space and faculty support highlighted the differences in agenda among members of the faculty. A simple statement on what the primary purpose of Dartmouth Medical School was set off fireworks of its own when the report of the TPC subcommittee (two years in preparation) came out in May 1965. Leading up to that was another furious round of lengthy memos, letters, and reports in the early months of 1964. At the beginning of March a document being prepared for the Advisory Board, on the proposal to establish departments of medicine and surgery, was circulated. Shinya Inoué distributed a copy of it in the cytology department. One reaction is preserved in an unsigned memo back to Inoué with twenty-one pointed and sometimes sarcastic questions about the implications of the proposal. The undercurrent of anxiety over what role Mudge had played in putting the plan together and whether Tenney was actually the main force behind it (both Mudge and Tenney were on the committee that had prepared the proposal) gives full evidence that disaffection and distrust were by no means a thing of the past.[32] At the end of March 1964, a memo from Inoué to Leonard Rieser (in the latter's capacity as Director of Graduate Study) outlined the "Space Needs and Faculty Support for Graduate and Research Training in Molecular and Cellular Biology." The real point of the memorandum was to press the case for Dartmouth to take advantage of the National Science Foundation's new grants to support "Centers of Excellence." A response from Mudge, who—along with several others—had been sent a copy, shows cautious support in principle while raising the issue of where the necessary additional money would come from.[33]

Mudge's "Report on the Dartmouth Medical School to the Trustees of Dartmouth College," covering roughly the first eighteen months of his deanship, appeared in April 1964. References to the Ph.D. program in molecular biology (then in its second year) were matter-of-fact; Mudge stressed that this was "a joint program between the Medical School and several departments in the College." In a much fuller way, he devoted a whole section to "The Role of Academic Clinical Medicine in the Two-Year Medical School" and another (even longer) section to "Research." More than once, he reiterated the necessity of research and education going hand in hand. "Indeed," he wrote in one place, "the refounding of the Dartmouth Medical School was undertaken with the conviction that research and education were opportunities of equal importance." And elsewhere: "research and education can *not* be separated."[34] Mudge was clearly walking in step with his predecessor Tenney.

On April 6, 1964, Mudge sent Dickey the proposal concerning new departments of medicine and surgery, which had been unanimously endorsed by the Advisory Board. The next step was for the Board of Trustees to approve it. As Mudge said in a letter to Dickey some five months later, establishing these two departments was "tangible evidence that the Hitchcock (either Clinic or Hospital) and the School will in the future be collaborating towards a common goal." He rightly pointed out that this was by no means something that could be taken for granted during the initial phases of the refounding.[35]

Mudge then turned his attention back to the issue raised by Inoué's proposal that Dartmouth should apply to be one of the "Centers of Excellence" being funded by the National Science Foundation (NSF). In a long memo to Rieser, Mudge spelled out the well-established reasons that the Dartmouth Medical School should not undertake to support graduate education as such—since it had been agreed that was to be "under College-wide sponsorship." Medical school faculty should have the opportunity to participate in Ph.D. programs, with no requirement that they do so. It followed from this, in Mudge's view, that building the molecular biology program in a way that would require greater commitments of time, money, and personnel from DMS was not advisable. "To recapitulate," he wrote, "the Medical School has Medical Education as its mission," not "Graduate Education (Ph.D.)." He did not explicitly say that he was opposed to having the faculty in the molecular biology program turn it into one of the "Centers of Excellence," but he certainly laid the basis for not supporting their application to the NSF.[36]

The Beginning of the End

The lines were being drawn once again. Three weeks later, Fuller, Inoué, Noda, and John Copenhaver (of the College biology department) submitted to Rieser their proposal for an application to the NSF. Their covering memorandum indicated an understanding of the situation very different from Mudge's. They included in their plea and defense a statement obviously intended to show they were in full support of what else was going on in the medical school: "Concurrent with the strengthening of clinical medicine, the improvement of the medical curriculum and research efforts, the time has then come when graduate education in the basic science departments needs to be placed on a sounder financial basis and to be provided with necessary space and facilities to fulfill this aspect of our academic mission in medicine and science."[37]

They were not to get their wish. The administration at Dartmouth concluded it was too risky to become involved in a program that would require the College to pick up the tab after the initial funding ran out. (Marsh Tenney's summary of this episode was that although "this was a possible development with considerable merit," guaranteeing its "future financing was a problem. . . . The School was also dubious about fitting an institute into its structure, and eventually a question of 'balance' among the programs of the school was raised." By his own admission, when after "prolonged discussions the NSF overture was rejected, . . . a storm of protest followed."[38])

That was not the only crushing blow to the molecularists. Around the same time, the National Institute of General Medical Sciences at the National Institutes of Health (NIH) had established a new interdisciplinary program in "Molecular and Cellular Biology." The group at Dartmouth jumped at the opportunity to submit one of the first grant proposals. To their delight, the funding they sought for a tenured position was approved in principle—though not for the full amount—by the reviewers and by the Council of the NIH. A revised budget was requested. At that point, the group hit an unexpected wall. Once again, the College administration balked at the requirement that it take on the financial responsibility for a tenured position after the five-year grant ran out; this meant that submitting a revised application was a waste of time.

Despite these terribly disappointing setbacks, the success of the new program was on display for all to see when the first Ph.D. in molecular biology was awarded in June 1964. And the College clearly had not decided altogether to block new initiatives in graduate education at the medical school, for a second Ph.D. program—in physiology and pharmacology—was also announced.[39] This made the denial of approval for the grand plans in molecular biology all the more shattering. The affected faculty members were angry and frustrated.

Things came dramatically to a head early in March 1965. Mudge became convinced that opposition from Inoué and Noda in particular was putting wholly out of reach any progress on the issue of governance, which he believed was of paramount importance. He demanded that the two scientists resign their respective department chairmanships; then, on the heels of that meeting, he met with Fuller and earnestly requested him to remain as the microbiology chairman. By his own account, Fuller was both astonished and outraged. He promptly announced that he, too, would resign his chairmanship. The same day, Mudge sent Dickey a memo "to report on policy matters relating to the development of the Medical School." The content of that memo (which Mudge hoped to discuss with Dickey) becomes an insignificant footnote to history in comparison to a revealing document full of personal notes that Mudge made in the days following the resignations. As he met with some faculty members, or tried without success to meet with others (who said they would be working at home but did not answer phone calls to their houses), the dean filled several pages with handwritten fragments of what he heard and his own commentary. What emerges most clearly is that virtually everyone on the DMS faculty seems to have been distrusted at one time or another by at least one other person or group. Accusations were made that actions had been carried out in secrecy or with devious intent, and just about everyone charged that someone else was overly emotional.

For nearly two weeks, Mudge looked for solid ground on which to stand. None came into view. Finally, after writing personal notes (on March 23 and 24) explaining his plan of action to the members of the Policy Group, Mudge sent a letter of his own to the president, announcing that he would resign his position as dean effective September 1, 1965.[40] He stressed in those personal letters how "infinitely complex" the "academic squabble" had become. He also made it clear that he had decided to step down only after having been blocked on two of the three distinct goals he had set for himself (he did not explain what they were). In these letters as well as in his formal letter of resignation addressed to President Dickey, he emphasized that he believed he was acting in the best interest of the institution. He elected to stay on at DMS as a member of the faculty and later as chair of the Department of Medicine (he was appointed by Tenney, during the latter's early 1966 acting deanship), testimony to his intense loyalty to the school and the importance to him of the reforms he had tried to put in place. He must, however, have been

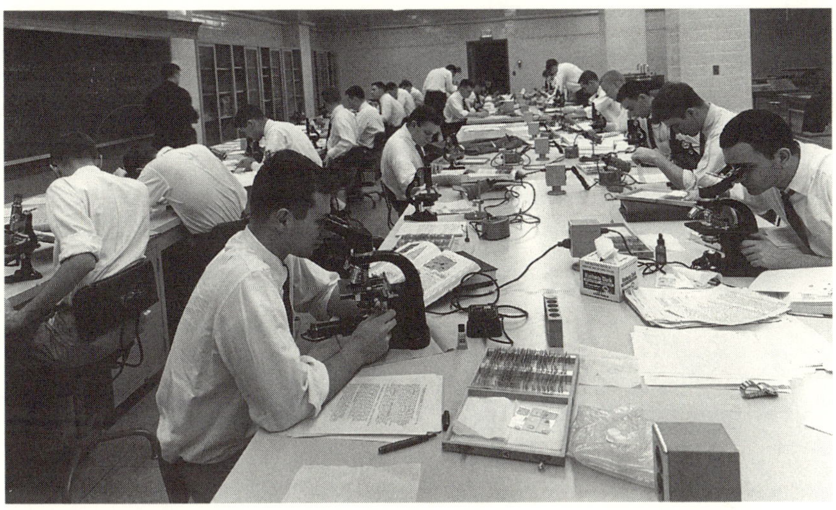

Medical students in the microscopy laboratory, early 1960s. Courtesy of Dartmouth Medical School.

monumentally disappointed and frustrated at the way things had worked out.

Further Grounds for Distress

The long-awaited Report of the Subcommittee on the Medical School was submitted to the TPC on May 15, 1965. A covering letter clarified the significance of the dissenting views attached in a minority report and explained how the subcommittee had "attempted to evaluate objectively the needs of the Medical School now and in the near future *without restriction*." They had been at work for nearly two years.[41] The report was a model of careful and thorough work, with a clear opening statement in the main section on "The Principle of Balance." (Precisely this would turn out to be first the sticking point and, eventually, the breaking point.) As soon as the subcommittee began its work, Marsh Tenney recollected in his "Memoir," it was "apparent that trouble lay ahead. The very first item on the agenda was introduced in complete innocence: it was a simple statement that the primary purpose of the Medical School was to educate medical students. This provoked an immediate objection by [Peter] von Hippel and [Andrew] Szent-Györgyi that the word 'primary' was unacceptable, that graduate education and research were of equal importance to medical education."[42] As early as August 1964 (roughly halfway through the period in which the subcommittee had worked), Tenney had written to Dickey expressing his concern over the continuing differences of opinion on these critical matters:

I think (unhappily) that the woes of [DMS] are not yet past history. . . . I think the most important aspect of the problem derives from our still unsatisfactory incorporation of graduate education *into the concept and operation* of a basic science medical school; and now even more significantly, into the biomedical center. However the divided ranks in controversy have been labelled, . . . *the issue* has always been graduate study (excluding of course, personnel problems).[43]

Yet the minutes of a September 1964 Advisory Board meeting stated that "it was nevertheless generally agreed that the primary mission of this Medical School is medical education" and that "the trend of thought seemed to be that whereas the primary mission of DMS and each of its departments is medical education, the specific role of individual faculty members may be variable." These remarks might have led one to think that all parties had agreed on how to proceed and that the school's "primary mission" was not something still under discussion.[44] Not so, as the "added comments" appended to the subcommittee's report by von Hippel and Szent-Györgyi tell us. Stressing first that complete agreement did exist on the critical importance of a medical school having medical students *and* "active research programs, graduate students, post-doctoral fellows, etc.," the dissenters nonetheless wanted to "enter a philosophical objection" to labeling any one part of the medical school's mission as "primary." The point of view represented by von Hippel and Szent-Györgyi was that the principle of "balance" made it imperative for no part of the equation to be labeled "primary."[45]

Tenney, however, clearly saw no inconsistency in talking about a "primary purpose" of the medical school while insisting that the faculty engage in both research and teaching. A decade earlier, in July 1955, he had written to Donald Morrison:

Why can't a faculty be created which is interested in teaching and research? Many of the qualities of a good research worker are just those things that make him a stimulating as well as a critical teacher. Conversely, investigation can easily wither in the absence of teaching—the plague of research institutes. I am fundamentally opposed to faculty appointments of the either-or choice, teacher or researcher. The superior faculty will contain qualities of each in the individual, though it will rarely be 50:50 or whatever balance is deemed "best." I don't see how a small school can afford to make any appointment in which the individual concerned has "little personal interest in research."[46]

Given that Tenney was already taking this strong line when he was still being recruited to rescue (refound) the medical school, it is understandable that he was troubled when others did not see things his way.

A five-page summary of Provost John Masland's remarks to the medical school faculty at a meeting on May 21, 1965, focuses almost entirely on the need to begin the search for a new dean and the challenge of finding new acting chairmen for the departments of biochemistry and anatomy-cytology. Nothing appears to have been said about the subcommittee report, as such, nor does there appear to have been any discussion of it. The chairmanship vacancy in microbiology was filled when Clarke Gray agreed to serve. A clinical microbiologist, he had—with the subsequently hired Lawrence Kilham—helped give that department a more balanced clinical/basic-science presence than either biochemistry or anatomy-cytology. But Gray's action surprised and disturbed his colleagues, since he had not discussed the matter with any of them. Up to that point the faculty in the three departments had all loyally supported their resigned chairmen by refusing to replace them even as acting chairmen. Gray's acceptance may have made Masland's evident frustration at the stance taken by members of the other two departments all the greater. Peter von Hippel rejected an explicit offer to head the biochemistry department, and no one in anatomy-cytology was willing to step forward.[47]

Searching for "Balance"

Many of those reminiscing more than three decades later about the tensions of the time say the real problem was fear among those *not* in the molecular biology program that it was growing disproportionately with respect to other departments and initiatives within the school, and so would inevitably detract from the College. Clearly this was a subjective matter. One faculty member who left remarked later, sadly, that despite all the "wonderful" things about DMS in the 1960s, "to create a really first rate investigative academic environment [there] was hard." Another faculty member, among the "dissidents" who stayed, admitted that they had paid little attention to the rest of the medical school and didn't realize how grandiose, ambitious, and self-aggrandizing their plans looked to others. Still another acknowledged that there came a point when people were nervous about the attention the molecular biology group seemed to be receiving; "the department grew out of any proportion to its teaching responsibilities." One commentator close to the matter later wrote that the molecular biology program, "desired by most of the basic-science faculty, was opposed by others who saw the program as the tail of avant-garde research wagging the dog of medical tradition."[48]

In a May 26 memo to Dickey, Masland reported that the issues of the "primary purpose of the Medical School" and of "balance" had come up again. The molecular biology group still troubled him most. "There will never be enough time," he despaired,

> to tell you in any kind of detail about the protracted conversations with these people [Inoué, Wayne Thornburg] and their associates, particularly the biochemists. . . . Basically, they kept coming back to a central theme, to the effect that the school has been "stacked" against the molecularists. Thus they once more argued that some kind of reorganization at this time was called for. They seemed to feel that this was even more important than the appointment of a new dean.[49]

Mudge (with only a few months remaining before his resignation as dean would take effect) thought Masland was making matters worse. Masland had, he noted, on May 29, "attempted a greater degree of reorganization than ever previously proposed by anyone . . . and this without consultation with the Dean, either present or Dean to be appointed." Mudge's anger led him to prepare "A Chronology of Recent events relating to Dartmouth Medical School, with a few comments" (it is not clear to whom—if anyone—he sent, or intended to send, this memorandum), in which he attacked the provost directly for the "charge" he had issued on May 29; that charge by the provost, he declared, "has been arrived at in such a manner as to virtually guarantee failure."[50]

Mudge's remarks at an Advisory Board meeting a week later were even stronger. To say that an appointment had been blocked "by labor-union tactics, by the creation of an 'academic Junta,'" to refer to "a lone Ph.D. amidst a sea of snarling wolves," to remark that "it would be imbicilic to assert that tranquility is the order of the day"—observations typical of most of the seven pages (single-spaced) of his remarks—was to risk having the whole presentation seem nothing more than an angry rant. Some sensible observations got thoroughly buried under the rhetorical excesses, so that the lasting impression is one of overblown melodrama: "The affairs of the School are now in a state which can not become worse, for indeed if they do worsen there will in fact no longer be a Dartmouth Medical School and the matter will have been resolved," he intoned at one point. He would be proved wrong the following April—when things *did* get worse without the medical school collapsing.[51]

A calming and stabilizing influence came with the appointment of

Ralph W. Hunter as acting dean, beginning September 1, 1965. No one could doubt his loyalty to the institution; he also knew the ins and outs of academic medicine. As one of the "dissidents" later remarked, it was Hunter who saved the moment and really held the place together with his "enlightened leadership." And in October of 1965, the Trustees passed three resolutions based on the TPC subcommittee's report, having to do with "Purpose" and "Future Expansion," as well as with the "Possibility for a Tutorial M.D. Program."[52] When Hunter decided four months of leadership was enough, Marsh Tenney was once more asked to step into the breach beginning January 1, 1966. Thus it was he who was dean at the time of the dramatic dénouement to the "molecular biology blowup" (as Tenney said it came to be called), in April 1966.[53]

Enter the AAUP

The drama that ensued had two dimensions, one very public (and often recounted, if in fragmentary fashion) and one mostly private (and poorly understood). The public part concerns the oft-mentioned "mass resignations" of faculty from the molecular biology group in April 1966—dramatic, but hardly unexpected. A December 1965 article in *The Dartmouth* announced Tenney's appointment as acting dean. The same article reported that Mudge's resignation earlier in the year had come "amidst speculation that several other professors were planning to resign in a high-level shake-up at the school. Subsequent action has not borne this out, however."[54] Yet at the very time that article was being written, the rumblings that would indeed lead to a "high-level shakeup" were gaining momentum.

The first formal communication to the national office of the American Association of University Professors (AAUP)—many would follow—was sent on December 16, 1965, over the signatures of fourteen members of the departments of biochemistry, cytology, and microbiology, including the three resigned chairmen and all the tenured members of those departments (five of them with professorial rank).[55] The request for "assistance" from the AAUP looked to some like a gauntlet thrown. Letters flew back and forth, from one faculty member or another to others on the faculty (as upset as anyone was the former dean, Gilbert Mudge; the correspondence between him and Shinya Inoué became increasingly testy) and from various faculty members to one or another of the AAUP staff in Washington, D.C., demanding to be informed of exactly what the nature of the complaint to the AAUP was. Charges and countercharges were leveled. Henry Payson (an assistant professor in the psychiatry department) also wrote to the AAUP, demanding to know the "specifics of this complaint"—to which he felt he was entitled as a fellow member of the Dartmouth chapter of the AAUP. He also wanted to register his belief that "the conflict really exists between a faction of the faculty represented by Professor Inoué and a majority of the faculty . . . not between this faction and the Administration of the Medical school or College."[56]

Fortunately, there was a voice of reason in all of this. AAUP Staff Associate Philip Denenfeld's responses to the sometimes "demanding" letters were models of patient explanation. "First," he informed them, "no formal 'investigation' of Dartmouth Medical School has been requested, and none is presently contemplated." Only after attempting to understand the situation, deciding whether "the allegations are accurate, and reflect serious departures from our recommended standards," would advice be offered.[57] (This is a critical point. Having someone from the AAUP look into these matters is by no means the same thing as conducting a formal investigation.) Denenfeld then dealt firmly with what amounted to a demand to breach confidentiality (several at DMS wanted to know exactly who had said what to the AAUP). "I do believe," he wrote, "that our record of a half century warrants the assurance that we do not abuse information submitted to us." On April 8, 1966, both *The Dartmouth* and the region's local paper, the *Valley News*, trumpeted headlines that made internal affairs suddenly very public indeed: "Eleven Professors Quit Posts In Med School Controversy" (*The Dartmouth*), and "11 Med School Profs Resign: Doctors Quit In A Hassle Over Complex Policies At Dartmouth" (*Valley News*). The *Valley News* ran another page-one story the next day ("Resigned Profs Explain Position"), and other papers soon picked it up.[58] The *Boston Globe* put it on page one on April 9, and the *New Hampshire Sunday News* carried it on April 10.[59] Predictably, no two versions of the story in the media completely agreed. The number of faculty members resigning, their reasons, and what it all signified were variously reported. Particularly bad from a public relations point of view was the *New York Times* story of April 15. Yet that story (buried on page 41) had perhaps the best concise statement of the views of those who had decided to leave. Andrew Szent-Györgyi was reported to have said that "Dartmouth 'has done the impossible' by recruiting a strong faculty and rebuilding a medical school 'but it has failed to do the possible—keep it together.' "[60]

Former Dean Gilbert Mudge was among those who held Inoué chiefly responsible. And in a long letter to the provost, reviewing in detail the complexity of the circumstances that had built to this public crescendo (and his own attempts to "keep the Medical School situation out of the press"), the former dean referred to "Professor Inoué's epidemic of press conferences."[61] Mudge's concern was first and foremost to assist Masland in the damage control he assumed would be necessary. "At the present time it would be absurd to deny that the nationwide publicity has been harmful to the School." Mudge distributed the letter to several administrators at Dartmouth, the president of the DMS Alumni Association, the president of the AAMC, and the full membership of the medical school's Policy Group (most of them not at Dartmouth). Several of the latter replied. Barry Wood (from Johns Hopkins) praised Mudge's "excellent statement" but added that he was "sure that the long-range reputation of the medical school will not be injured by the flurry of public complaints." DeWitt Stetten (at Rutgers) found it "an entirely satisfactory defense of your position and an explanation of your deanship." Robert Loeb (writing from Columbia) called it "an absolute masterpiece." Francis Dieuaide (retired from the Columbia medical faculty), agreed: "I can't believe the recent publicity and the departure of your late colleagues will really injure the School or anyone there."[62]

Mudge's statement provides a reasonably balanced and detailed account of the situation at DMS at the time along with a review of the precipitating factors. But the sharp tone that is characteristic of so many of his memos and letters is still present: "To the extent that this statement is based on the facts . . . I find the newspaper release incredible," he wrote in one place; in another, he stated baldly, "The allegation is fatuous." Thus the "detailed statement of fact" must still be read as one from Mudge's point of view.[63]

A much briefer review of the medical school's affairs appeared in the May 1966 issue of the *Dartmouth Alumni Magazine*; this is helpful to anyone who wishes a quick summary of what transpired. None of the "dissidents" was interviewed, however, and—not surprisingly, given where the piece appeared—the article presented what was essentially the "company line."[64] Readers were obviously meant to take away the message "All's well that ends well, and this is going to end well."

In early May, Philip Denenfeld informed President Dickey officially that the AAUP had received communications several months earlier from "a number of faculty members of the Dartmouth Medical School" seeking "the advice and assistance of this Association." Dickey responded a few days later, saying (in effect), "Thanks for informing us; we don't think we need a consultant—but tell us more about what a visit would achieve and we'll consider it."[65] Despite that brush-off, by June it was clear that Denenfeld's calming voice was still needed. Mudge wrote him again, once more agitating for "clarification of the status of Dr. Inoué's charges"—which, Mudge said, Inoué "has refused to disclose."[66] Denenfeld brought Mudge up to date, informing him that the allegations were part of an "open file" at the AAUP (in other words, their seriousness was still being considered); he would not, naturally, reveal any of the substance of the complaints.[67] Mudge, having failed to get the answers he wanted from the AAUP, wrote to both Inoué and Noda in June, urging them to make public the particulars of the complaints. It does not appear that either responded to him.[68]

Meanwhile, on a happier note (though with a passing reference to Dartmouth as a "scene of unrest"), the *New York Times* on May 19, 1966, announced the choice of Carleton B. Chapman, a former president of the American Heart Association then at Southwestern Medical School of the University of Texas at Dallas, to take over from Acting Dean Tenney in the autumn. A telling point in his appointment, the article implied, was that Chapman was "well known for his concern over problems of medical education and research."[69] Without question, Chapman came highly recommended, and several members of the Policy Group expressed their relief and pleasure at his appointment.

Yet the appeal to the AAUP continued to rankle. In late July, Kenneth W. Cooper (who had taken over as spokesperson for the dissident group after Inoué's departure), Noda, and Fuller wrote another letter to Denenfeld. Reviewing the fact that "forty-four [Dartmouth] faculty members submitted a petition to your office appealing for an investigation by Committee T," they begged him to take action on the grounds that the Dartmouth administration's refusal to accept the offer of mediation proved just how serious the problem of intra-institutional politics had become. (A Committee T investigation is authorized by the AAUP's General Secretary only in selected cases presenting major unresolved issues of academic governance.) The authors of this letter followed it with another the next day, in which they enclosed (among other documents) a seven-page statement describing "The means for participation of faculty in the affairs of the Dartmouth Medical School." Again they pleaded for a Committee T hearing.[70]

Numbers played an important role in the statement on faculty participation in the affairs of the school. Citing the 1965–1966 DMS catalogue, Cooper, Noda, and Fuller wrote that the full-time faculty—those "who have invested their total activity in teaching and allied scholarly pursuits in the Medical School's academic program administrative officers included"—numbered 52. By this count, the 14 resignations up to date represented 27 percent of the faculty. In sharp contrast, Acting Dean Tenney and Associate Dean Philip Nice had repeatedly stated when interviewed by the news media that DMS had an "instructional staff" of 135, of which 14 is obviously a much smaller percentage and thus, by implication, less significant.[71] But to reach that number, Tenney and Nice had to count all the part-time faculty, the staff members of the Hitchcock Clinic who had been given faculty status as part of the effort to create a true "medical center" in Hanover. At least some of the basic science faculty believed that this award of status was the result of administrative fiat, a maneuver calculated to ensure that clinical ("medical") faculty would outnumber research ("science") faculty.

President Dickey, when he turned down the offer of an AAUP consultant, had made clear to Denenfeld that Masland would be his intermediary in any discussions of medical school matters. On August 19, 1966, Masland met Denenfeld in Washington, D.C., for a discussion that lasted more than four hours. Four days later, Denenfeld wrote a seven-page confidential memorandum to a Committee T File and sent a copy to Masland. The provost wrote back immediately, indicating that he did not think the AAUP officer had accurately represented their discussion at all points, though he did acknowledge he found "that in general you have recorded the principal elements of our discussion."[72]

In October, Cooper—who had been in touch with Denenfeld since late June—went to Washington for a personal meeting. Again, Denenfeld wrote a long memo to the file (again marked "Confidential") and sent a copy to his discussion partner. Like Masland before him, Cooper expressed gratitude for the opportunity to pursue the matter—and proceeded then to respond to several of the points Denenfeld had made. In particular, he contested the recurrent canard (as he saw it) that those who had left or were about to did not really understand medical schools and were (therefore?) all going to university rather than medical school posts. He gave evidence that this was false ("8 of 16 *are* continuing in medical education," he wrote, naming the individuals and the institutions to which they were moving). "I don't believe it can seriously be held that we came here with unrealistic views of medical education," he continued with obvious sadness. "We came [to DMS] not because of salary . . . but because of ideals, the pleasure of participation in a new venture in medical education. . . . Needless to say, we and our families have been demoralized by the . . . strongly biased treatment we have received."[73]

Moving On

At the end of September 1966, Marsh Tenney relinquished his temporary decanal responsibilities on the arrival of the new dean, Carleton Chapman. A few weeks later, Chapman detailed for the DMS faculty some of his hopes and dreams for the school. He spoke of the "singular advantages of Dartmouth" and expressed his belief that Dartmouth was "uniquely equipped to bring the more academic aspects of education for medicine in line with the emerging needs of the last quarter of the twentieth century." Sounding excited, enthusiastic, and engaged, he used good judgment in not dwelling on the recent tensions except "to conclude by reminding you that the gaze of the academic world has been attracted to this school and that our academic colleagues over the country consider us on trial in a very real way." His optimism was explicit: "The recognition of the unique opportunities at Dartmouth is very widely shared indeed. . . . The job [of reconstructing the nation's system of medical education] requires talent, it requires courage, and above all, generosity. We have them all here and it's time now to get moving again."[74]

In Washington, on December 14, 1966, Philip Denenfeld wrote a memorandum on the situation at Dartmouth (with copies of various documents attached) for the AAUP staff to consider "as carefully as you can" prior to the next staff meeting. The issue to be discussed was "whether this case should be referred to Committee T with a recommendation for formal investigation." He apologized for confronting the staff with an "unusually large" briefing ("I found the file difficult to summarize briefly without sacrifice"), but his ability to clarify an admittedly complicated and protracted case is much in evidence. The four-point summary of the "current situation" on the final page is a masterpiece.[75] In January, Denenfeld wrote to Dean Chapman to say that as far as the AAUP was concerned, the Dartmouth matter was temporarily tabled to give the new administration—Chapman's—time to try its hand at resolving the issue. Denenfeld expressed a desire for a meeting as soon as possible "since we do not feel we should delay much longer in determining our position."[76] Chapman agreed that a meeting in the near future was a good idea.[77]

A powerful corroboration of the view that morale had improved with Chapman's arrival is found in a long letter from Kenneth Cooper (endorsed and signed by Lafayette Noda as well) to Philip Denenfeld, written in mid-February 1967. By then Chapman had been in Hanover a little more than four months. Cooper's letter is written with controlled enthusiasm; it is also full of optimism: Chapman has acted with "graciousness . . . that kindles cooperative desire"; he "could not . . . have improved his handling of [the first real faculty] meeting"; and "what is especially important is that our Dean, for the first time in my eight years here, has asked the faculty to discuss and to decide an issue very important to it. . . . [T]he prospect of such faculty action has more of the staff talking to one another, and in reasonably good spirits, about their school's future." As a result, "morale is growing, and the faculty is gaining self respect."[78] Denenfeld, in response, called the letter "a joyous document" (despite Cooper having ended by repeating his insistence that "investigation by Committee T is still greatly to be desired").[79] Further correspondence between the two during March made it clear on the one hand that the AAUP would continue to monitor the situation at Dartmouth, but that on the other hand there was no plan to make any public statement at the time "since it might well jeopardize some promising beginnings," according to Denenfeld.[80] In May, Cooper and Noda had a lengthy phone conversation with Denenfeld, during which—among other things—Cooper's repeated use of the word "surveillance" to describe what the AAUP was engaged in with respect to Dartmouth came up. Although Denenfeld acknowledged that the word was accurate, he also reported that Dean Chapman in discussion with him had strongly objected to it. True to his manner throughout the whole Dartmouth case, Denenfeld urged caution and suggested giving way on the point—he suggested alternative words—to avoid roiling the waters with Chapman just when things looked so promising.[81]

Finally, after months of discussion, memoranda, and letters, the whole molecular biology upheaval at Dartmouth came to an end—at least as far as AAUP involvement was concerned—not with a bang, but with something closer to a whimper. Denenfeld effectively signed off on the case (while saying that the AAUP would of course stay interested in the further improvements that were still needed at Dartmouth) in a letter to Dean Chapman with the observation that it seemed to him "that in your relatively brief tenure as Dean you have made remarkable progress away from a grave situation, and have achieved a sound basis on which to build cooperatively." Chapman responded a week later saying simply that he thought the AAUP had been "very fair indeed."[82] Nothing had happened, in the judgment of the AAUP officers, to warrant an alteration in their conclusion in January that they should take "no definitive action" in light of the way issues of governance seemed to be approaching resolution under Chapman.[83] Once the AAUP was no longer receiving complaints from members of the faculty, the file was closed. Denenfeld had engaged in a lot of hand holding and sympathetic consulting, but DMS was never formally investigated, censured, or put on probation.

Looking Back—What Difference Did It Make?

When all is said and done, especially after so many years have elapsed, it is difficult to know whether the sharp reactions by those who believed their legitimate paths were being blocked were either necessary or appropriate. The decade of the 1960s was a period of enormous ferment in the biological sciences in particular. What most sharply defined the period for many scientists was "the rise of molecular biology—that burst of discovery between the mid-1940s and the early 1960s that revealed the nature of the gene and its mode of expression."[84]

The memo from Masland to Dickey naming molecular biology as the first area in which DMS would establish a graduate program had been bold and made sense; molecular biology was preeminent as one of the "broadest categories" (as Masland's memo had it) of scientific disciplines. That notwithstanding, non–molecular biologists for the most part had no understanding of the extent to which molecularists during the 1950s "looked down upon the traditional biochemists." Furthermore, "the latter were smugly ignorant of the powerful forces the devotees of the new approach were mobilizing to change the way biological problems would be thought about and tackled in the coming decades."[85]

Given the way things played out at Dartmouth, it seems unlikely that these tensions were apparent to those in charge at DMS. Dean Marsh Tenney, in his "Third Progress Report" (covering the period 1959–1961), stated what had resulted from the resolution reported in Masland's memo to Dickey of March 20, 1961. "Dartmouth's first graduate program leading to the Ph.D. degree," Tenney wrote,

> will be offered through a joint effort of all the basic science departments of the Medical School and certain departments of the Division of Science in the College. This cross-field program in Molecular Biology seeks to examine the phenomena of living systems at the molecular level. It is expected that the first group of candidates will be enrolled in the Fall of 1962. The Ph.D. candidate will have an opportunity to do his thesis research in any of a number of areas.

Tenney went on to list an impressive array of the "current research interests of the Molecular Biology faculty."[86] No one would have imagined, reading that matter-of-fact account, that only a few years later that selfsame molecular biology program would engender such controversy. And yet, as we have seen, it became the centerpiece in what has been variously described as a "grievous burden," a "turbulent storm," an "unfolding disaster," a "brouhaha," a "crisis," a "rocket that blew," a "devastating controversy," a "horrible business," "an unfortunate incident," "a nasty academic imbroglio," and—purely and simply—"anarchy." Others have insisted, however, that the situation was by no means so chaotic as it seems in retrospect. On what he described as a "social visit" in the midst of the "revolution," one former member of the molecular biology faculty at DMS said he came to the conclusion that there actually *were* no issues, "just slogans, such as 'medicine vs. biology,' in a struggle for resources." Others have said that the whole thing was "dumb," and that the "Dartmouth thing was silly."

Leaving aside the problems caused by large egos—Dartmouth had its share—coupled with an unwillingness or inability to back down or compromise, there are reasons for viewing the debates and tensions at Dartmouth during this period as different from comparable ones elsewhere. The issues loomed particularly large at DMS for three reasons.

First, the excitement that resulted from the successful refounding of the medical school was enormous. Students and faculty were eager to be recruited to Dartmouth Medical School as its new life was beginning. And once the humiliating "confidential probation" tag had been removed, the future looked very bright. This was in no small part due to Marsh Tenney's charisma, as numerous people have attested. He was "energetic, modern, enthusiastic"—and he had "great vision," according to one former faculty member. This is only one of many accolades routinely heaped upon Tenney from many directions.

Second, DMS's parent institution was not a university, but rather a liberal arts *college* that took great pride in being just that. This meant there had always been a certain dis-ease (administratively speaking) about the very existence of the Medical School. Except for brief embarrassment at having its medical school not listed among the Class A schools, having DMS reduced to a two-year "incomplete" feeder school for other full-fledged medical schools at major universities was apparently acceptable to the administration; the College could still lay claim to being home to the fourth-oldest medical school in the country. The anomalous position of Dartmouth's medical school gave discussions about the "primary purpose" of a medical school—of this medical school in particular—a larger significance than they did elsewhere. Decisions about the "balance" between teaching and scientific research really mattered for the future of the institution.

Third, in the early years after the refounding of DMS, the available resources for assuring the school's future were manifestly inadequate. Every school and college has, during at least some periods, the problem of resources falling woefully short of what is needed; buildings, lab and office space, money for faculty and staff salaries, and even parking places are commodities typically in short supply. But at Dartmouth Medical School, which in the 1950s was starting very nearly from scratch, there was a special urgency about the inadequate resources. Simply put, it was not going to be possible in those early years simultaneously to build powerful graduate programs in science as an adjunct to a premier two-year medical school and to move toward a restoration of a full curriculum leading to the M.D. degree.

This, finally, is what made the arguments over the molecular biology program so important. Today it is clear (as it has been for some time) that it *is* possible to have both M.D. and Ph.D. programs—at Dartmouth as at many other institutions. The record is unimpeachable. We also now know how relevant and important a molecular basis is for an understanding of medical science. But in the 1960s, as one of the faculty members who left has said, it was "more an article of faith with all of us." It just wasn't a time when the risk of having graduate research programs overwhelm the historic and "primary" purpose of the school, the training of doctors, seemed acceptable to enough of the key people.

And so the die was cast. A further push in the direction of establishing a research institute, which some of the molecular biology faculty (perhaps predominantly Shinya Inoué) wanted, would have taken a major commitment of resources of all sorts. Almost certainly, it would have been impossible a few years later (beginning roughly at the time Chapman became dean) to make the move that many in the *medical* departments wanted, namely, for Dartmouth to return to the business of training medical doctors through four years of medical school. In other words, it seems likely that resisting the temptation to commit large and uncertain sums of money to the ambitious dreams of the molecular biologists was a critical piece of being able to reinstitute clinical education at Dartmouth Medical School sooner rather than later. And that was essential if DMS was again to become a medical school from which it would be possible to graduate with an M.D. degree. As scientists who stayed at Dartmouth and scientists who left have remarked, in the aftermath of the "blow-up" the balance at DMS did—unquestionably—tip toward the more *medical*, but it did so without halting significant research in the basic sciences. This in turn enabled DMS to develop and expand connections with the Hitchcock Hospital and the Clinic. And *that* in turn is what made possible the transformation of the medical world of northern New England into what is is today. If the fallout in the 1960s had not landed where it did, it is plausible to think there would be no Dartmouth-Hitchcock Medical Center today.

If this assessment is correct, the "molecular biology brouhaha" was one of the most important events in the history of Dartmouth Medical School. As to how much it hurt Dartmouth to lose so many faculty members from the molecular biology program in such a relatively short period, there is still disagreement. A core group stayed, so it was not a total loss even then. But when a Harvard review committee was brought in after the mass resignations and recommended that the school start—of all things—a molecular biology program, one former member of the faculty says that "people were clutching their heads and saying, 'Not again!'" Today, DMS clearly has recovered, even if slowly (in the minds of at least some commentators once on the inside at DMS). And despite the "travails," one person said, DMS "has turned into a good school.

What is bothersome is that . . . it should have turned into a great school."

The fraction of the faculty that left may have had to leave, according to one of those who did so. But what makes many people sad is the sense that, although DMS ended up all right, it took years longer than necessary. The molecular biology group of the 1960s was an important part of the evolution of DMS. In the 1960s, DMS could have been a major leader in genetics; instead, it seeded a lot of places that saw a good opportunity and took it, according to one of those who did some of that seeding. And one who stayed says that a beautiful cell-biology department, which was definitely in the making in the 1960s, would have put DMS on the map in an important way. ("It was," says a cell biologist who left, "one of the first" such programs. The "whole place was very exciting"—there's that word again.) Instead, although there is a second renaissance today, some of the ashes of the explosion caused by the multiple departures are still in the air forty years later.[87]

CHAPTER ELEVEN

Tradition and Innovation

We must have been walking through it all our lives.
—GALWAY KINNELL[1]

Building on the Past

HAVING MARSH TENNEY back in the dean's office during the most public phases of the molecular biology controversy had had its advantages; he was, after all, the architect of the partially rebuilt school. And having him continue to serve into the autumn of 1966, to accommodate the schedule of the dean whose appointment had been announced in May—Carleton B. Chapman—was, for many, a reassuring sign. For others, however, early 1966 was an awkward time. Some were frankly uneasy, seeing Tenney's willingness to accept the role of acting dean (later he would do so again[2]) as an indication that he had never really wanted to give up the authority and power that came with the office. More than one individual among those who had stayed at DMS was convinced that Tenney wanted to maintain control and "could not let go" of what he had built. Yet, undeniably, having someone in charge who was thoroughly familiar with the myriad unusual features of the situation had its benefits.

Tenney was, in fact, in a difficult position. Until Chapman actually arrived, Dartmouth Medical School was in something of a holding pattern. Nor was it easy to recover from what had been "an impossible situation" and a "long and tangled story," when there were lots of "anguished meetings" with people "talking past each other," to say nothing of the loss of colleagues—the crisis had certainly had its idiosyncratic features. To the extent that the "turmoil" had been about the differences between Ph.D.s and M.D.s, however, Dartmouth was by no means alone. These differences were a widespread problem. Furthermore, it was a time when at "most medical schools, the rapid growth in faculty size, the frenetic chase for grants, and the increasing competitiveness of biomedical research led to a loss of the close association with colleagues that had characterized faculty life before World War II," as historian of medical education Kenneth Ludmerer has noted.[3] But Dartmouth—because of its long history of close community and collegiality—suffered more than others from the ruptures caused by such factors. Without a doubt, when Tenney became Acting Dean in 1966, there were loose ends, residual concerns left from the "upheaval" over molecular biology. But there were also other issues to be taken up, too.

The Two-Year Medical School Saga Continues

Not least among the ongoing concerns was the old issue of whether DMS was finally to become an M.D.-degree-granting institution again. Quite apart from the years of insisting on the merits of remaining (or becoming) the best-possible two-year medical school, a model for the nation, gestures had been made in the four-year direction well before Tenney returned to the dean's office. Most importantly, the desirability of reconsidering "the question of Dartmouth's evolution to a four-year school" (after the new departments of medicine and surgery were satisfactorily in place) had been explicitly posited in the TPC subcommittee's report of May 1965.[4] (This was in sharp contrast to the 1955 TPC statement to the Trustees on the fine future of DMS as a two-year school.)

This was no surprise: In a "Charge" to the Subcommittee two years earlier, Trustee Dudley W. Orr (writing for the TPC) had acknowledged that "there arises, inevitably, the old and difficult question of [turning DMS into] a possible four-year school."[5] Earlier yet, in 1960, President Dickey had included a discussion about the special value of the two-year medical school at a "National Fund for Medical Education" dinner.[6] In a 1961 interview, *Medical World News* quoted Tenney on two-year medical schools thus: "It's my opinion that there will be a renaissance of the two-year school in this country for two reasons; because of the significant role it can play in its own right and because it represents, to a good many people, a four-year medical school of the future."[7] This nicely ambiguous statement left open whether Tenney himself saw DMS's two-year school as a stepping stone toward a four-year DMS. Among the recurrent but obscured themes in all the discussions about possible restoration of the four-year program was whether DMS could or would remain as high-quality a four-year school as it was—all agreed—a two-year school. In 1962, the issue arose in a confidential memo now in the provost's papers: "[T]he question is repeatedly asked when Dartmouth will 'go four years.' The question is realistic historically, since many other two year schools have evolved in that direction within the last two decades. The question is unrealistic to the extent that it presupposes that four years will be a panacea for the School's problems, whether real or imagined."[8]

The base on which that question stood was still the matter of pride in the two-year school. In 1964, Associate Dean Henry L. Heyl concluded an editorial in the newly launched *Dartmouth Medical School Quarterly* by stating his belief that the undertakings he had just described were "part of the opportunity of the two-year school to create and demonstrate a finer program in medical education."[9] On the other hand, by the academic year 1966–1967, only three of the eighty-nine medical schools "in active operation" in the United States were two-year schools: the universities of North Dakota and South Dakota—and DMS. This was not the company Dartmouth was used to keeping.[10]

The subject that had been the basso continuo underlying every discussion about the medical school for half a century became, by early 1966, more nearly the *leitmotiv* of discussions about the medical school's future. In February, the minutes of the executive committee meeting included a record of President Dickey's report "that the question of a four-year program is becoming increasingly relevant with respect to developments involving the Medical School, Hospital, Clinic and White River VA Hospital, including the search for a new Medical School dean."[11] (This was also not a new topic. Thirty years earlier, in a letter to Dean John Bowler, Frederic Lord had posed a question on this very issue: "Is there any chance that in the future, perhaps if and when a four-year school is under weigh [*sic*], of once more effecting a more definite fusion between School and Hospital in the legal aspects of ownership and control?"[12])

A kind of compromise proposal also emerged at the beginning of 1966. Gilbert Mudge wrote to Allan Tisdale (his former Dartmouth colleague, then at the University of Vermont College of Medicine), saying he had "become convinced that the future of Dartmouth-Hitchcock lies in a modification and/or modernization of the two-year school concept"—perhaps in the form of a "small tutorial clerkship for third and fourth year leading to an M.D. degree."[13] That spring, Acting Dean Tenney appointed a committee to review "all aspects" of a planned pilot program leading to the M.D. degree—which, it was beginning to be thought, would not necessarily have to be a four-year program.[14] The media picked up the news in May.[15] Tenney in his memoir recalled that the *New York Times* "reported Trustee approval of the plan to expand the medical curriculum. *Medical World News* took up the story and embellished it with a review of the molecular biology disturbance."[16]

One might be tempted to view the frequent refrain on the importance of the role DMS was playing as a two-year school—or could play by becoming the best-possible two-year school—as a rather desperate maneuver, an attempt to find something worth hanging onto in the flotsam of the past. On the other hand, no less a figure in medical education than Alan Gregg was very much in favor of the idea, as we have seen, because he saw Dartmouth's approach as one of the best ways to reduce the long period of time required to become a physician. For those at Dartmouth, having Gregg's support and focusing on the perceived virtues of the two-year school enabled DMS to see itself as a trendsetter or pioneer, a leader in medical education. No one wanted publicly to acknowledge that DMS was perhaps still a rather weak school, despite its narrow escape from the chopping block, its successful refounding, and its having weathered the molecular biology controversy.

In the end, the decision was made to go ahead. In 1966, the trustees—perhaps anticipating the arrival of Carleton Chapman, with what had been announced as his special interest in matters of medical education—"approved in principle" a proposal "to expand the curriculum, faculty, and plant in order to accommodate an [eventual] enrollment of 168 students." The real significance of this was that a few students were to be included in the third and fourth years, as part of "an experimental tutorial program leading to the M.D. degree"—just as Mudge had written to Tisdale. All this was in keeping with the resolutions the trustees had passed the previous autumn.[17]

The Return of the M.D. Degree

Dean Chapman arrived just in time to take on the responsibility for implementing the new program. Of course what transpired was not the work solely of either the new dean or of the acting dean, Tenney. Before Chapman arrived on campus, for example, Mudge had written to Robert Loeb to report "working on a 4-year curriculum. . . . I have come to think of it as a must."[18] There is every evidence that Chapman agreed with Mudge on this point. A leading feature of the argument Chapman used to push forward on restoration of the four-year curriculum was that changes elsewhere in medical education were going to make it increasingly difficult for students to transfer into another school's third-year class. He may also have had genuine skepticism about the extent to which it was going to be possible for DMS to continue being the outstanding two-year school that those who had been at Dartmouth a long time insisted it was. The tension was between those who thought the days of the two-year school were numbered (for any of several reasons) and those who feared that DMS would be at best a school of middling quality if it jumped to the league where four-year schools played. In any case, though talk about abandoning the two-year concept was in the air, the active "planning and faculty recruitment" for an expanded program "got under way in late 1966"—in other words, under Chapman's deanship.

Perhaps not surprisingly, given the long years in the wilderness of two-year ("incomplete") schools, Dartmouth during this phase of its rebuilding showed that DMS was by no means finished with educational innovations. The trustees were insistent that the restoration of an M.D. degree "brought with it the responsibility for determining the most effective alternatives for implementing such a change." What emerged from a series of faculty retreats early in 1968 was a version of the tutorial idea, a determination to establish an intensive three-year M.D. program that came to be known as "The Dartmouth Plan." The "shortened, more flexible curriculum" called for by the plan was based on an eleven-month school year—yet one more attempt to reduce the amount of time taken to become a physician.[19] It was also agreed that the basic science curriculum would be reorganized and that Ph.D. programs would be "preserved and encouraged," Chapman reported. And then: "Formal faculty action endorsing the program came on 4 March 1968 by a vote of ninety-four to one. The Board of Trustees accepted the faculty action on 13 April [1968], 'subject only to the development of the necessary financing.' "[20]

Chapman's account leaves out any hint of disagreements over the wisdom of going this route as well as any evidence of the tensions that may have existed among leading members of the faculty. More than one person has suggested that Tenney was not wholly in favor of making DMS a four-year school again, but this seems unlikely given some of his remarks to the media (including the interview with *Medical World News* five years earlier). *The Dartmouth*, for instance, reported him saying that the school had been refounded with a belief in the viability of the idea of the two-year school, but that "All during that time, Tenney added, there had been 'continued discussion of when the time was right to once again offer a four year degree.' "[21] Quite apart from whether DMS students were finding transfer to the third-year class at other "top" schools more difficult (by no means everyone agrees on this point), which alone would have been enough to make the future of the two-year school precarious, we are told:

> Fortunately, changes in the surrounding community had been taking place as well. Mary Hitchcock Memorial Hospital had become a major referral center with over 400 beds, serving a population of 300,000 as one of only two academic medical centers in northern New England. . . . The Veterans Administration Hospital . . . affiliated with the Medical School since 1945, provided another 224 beds. The Hitchcock Clinic was recording over 144,000 outpatient visits annually.[22]

Such developments made it clear that this was not the Hanover of yesteryear and that a full-scale medical school was indeed a reasonable prospect. The first phase of serious discussions among Hospital, Clinic, and School that would eventually lead to the official creation of the Dartmouth-Hitchcock Medical Center (DHMC) began during this period. A press release announcing that DMS was establishing a program on such a condensed schedule—"designed to serve as a test model for shortening and modernizing medical education as one means of meeting the nation's need for increased numbers of physicians"—was issued in February 1970, as the first students were being accepted.[23] It was a new world in many ways, as no one could doubt or deny when the first M.D. students (a class of sixteen) entered DMS in September 1970, anticipating the receipt of their degrees from Dartmouth in June 1973. The most recent visit of the CME in 1968 had resulted in no rude surprises—nor would there be any at the time of the next one, in 1972.

By 1970, then, the physical plant of DMS had also been considerably changed—mostly by being enlarged with new buildings (Remsen, Strasenburgh, not long afterward Vail and Dana Library) springing up on the west side of College Street. An important consideration in where to locate the new campus had been proximity to the Mary Hitchcock. As Tenney pointed out in his memoir when discussing plans for the first new building, it was "deemed necessary" that it "should be adjacent to the hospital." This was, he went on, "an important factor in our concept of a medical center (the terminology had already begun to be used) and surely essential if the school decided to re-introduce a four-year program." There also had to be room for expansion.[24]

Along with construction there was also destruction. DMS loyalists and others with a serious interest in history have never gotten over the razing in 1963 of Nathan Smith's "New Medical House" (which had, in the meantime, come to be called the "Old Medical Building"). Despite considerable correspondence with the College treasurer, John F. Meck, former dean John Bowler was not able to influence the decision to demolish the building. The press release that was issued in late April 1962 stressed the structural weaknesses of the building and downplayed the historic significance. The claim that it had been constructed after Smith left Dartmouth is of course not true, and the fact that he had lectured in it was ignored. This lack of sentiment (to say nothing of the lost artifacts) did not sit well with those to whom the building *was* Dartmouth Medical School. Decades later Marsh Tenney, for one, was still sputtering about it. Tears were shed and hearts were broken the day Nathan Smith's "Medical House" came down.[25] The rest of the "old" school finally disappeared (literally) in 1990, when the 1908 Nathan Smith Laboratory was also razed. Even "Medical North"—which although originally President Tucker's home (at 43 College Street) had for some time housed the physiology department and then become a residence for women medical students—ceased having a medical function when it became the home of a Dartmouth sorority.[26]

Other Curricular Changes

For all the good things that seemed to be happening in late 1966 and early 1967—an enthusiastic new dean, the decision to work toward reinstating an M.D. program, the gradual winding down of the molecular biology program (most of the unhappy people left and AAUP involvement fizzled out)—controversy was not altogether a thing of the past. Although the initial correspondence and early memos exchanged between the former dean, Mudge, and the newly arrived dean, Chapman, were friendly and mutually supportive, a dramatic clash occurred in January 1967. Without warning or explanation, Chapman abruptly requested Mudge to resign his chairmanship of the department of medicine.

This was a bafflement and a blow to Mudge. He saw that particular department as one of the main building blocks for revitalizing the Medical School's clinical offerings; however others might have viewed the appointment, Mudge had been pleased at the role that being chair of Medicine would allow him to play at DMS after stepping down from the deanship. It was fully in character, then, for Mudge to refuse to step aside even as he acknowledged Chapman's authority to relieve him of the position. When Chapman did just that, the tension between them reached crisis proportions. Despite the fact that Tenney's letter appointing Mudge Chairman of Medicine is a matter of record, Chapman wrote that period of Mudge's career out of his history of DMS, saying the departments of Medicine and Surgery "existed but lacked chairmen."[27] The relationship between the two deans never recovered.

If Chapman's management style was difficult for some members of the faculty to accept—he has been called "arrogant" and accused of being devious; he also had an occasionally volatile temper—it may nonetheless be that he was exactly the right man for the job. A dean who was self-assured, undeniably brilliant, "handsome and articulate," "effective," "creative," and a "very wise man" (one colleague called him "dangerously" intelligent), he arrived without the putative advantages *or* encumbrances of previous Dartmouth ties. This made another fresh beginning possible. DMS was poised for change, and—for better, for worse—Chapman was both a symbol and an engineer of that change. During his deanship, for instance, student body and faculty alike increased substantially; the building program continued apace; sponsored research nearly doubled. Most of this was tied to the reintroduction of the M.D. program, a plan to which Chapman was deeply committed. He truly believed that two-year schools were a thing of the past; to a considerable extent, he rested his reputation on moving the full four-year program closer to reality. And although there were many developments during the Chapman years, most people would probably agree that the most significant change for DMS was its transformation to being a full-fledged medical school again. Another major reform introduced by Chapman was to award tenure to all Medical School faculty at the associate professor level and up. This change, while less visible from outside the institution, had far-reaching—stabilizing, morale-boosting—consequences inside.

Chapman was fortunate to arrive when the molecular biology crisis was essentially over. Yet turbulence and tension, conflict and controversy had not been eliminated altogether; rebuilding collegiality in the aftermath of that stressful period would have been difficult for anyone. Certainly Chapman made some excellent appointments. Two in particular would prove critical to the future of DMS. In October 1967, James C. Strickler—a 1950 graduate of Dartmouth College and 1951 graduate of DMS (he received his M.D. in 1953 from Cornell)—arrived in Hanover to take up a post as Associate Professor of Medicine and Associate Dean to succeed Philip O. Nice. At the same time, Thomas P. Almy was appointed Professor and Chairman of the Department of Medicine (following Mudge); he was scheduled to take up his appointment at Dartmouth in March 1968. These two physicians would make profoundly important contributions to the Dartmouth Medical School.

Among Strickler's numerous attributes seems to have been an ability to get along with everyone. He understood and worked well with Chapman and those who praised the dean's brilliant leadership; he also understood and worked well with those who found Chapman difficult. ("Both were correct views" of Chapman, Strickler would later say, and the split in opinions about Chapman was not a simple one of clinical vs. basic science faculty.) Probably no one anticipated it when Strickler was hired, but he would in the end be deemed the best candidate to follow Chapman as the next dean (though, as noted already, to fill out the academic year 1972–1973 after Chapman left in 1972, Marsh Tenney was appointed Acting Dean once again). This would give greater continuity to the administration of DMS than it had experienced since the Syvertsen years, something that was badly needed. Strickler soothed bruised egos and wounded spirits alike. (This is a man who, on stepping down from the deanship, took a year to retool and update himself as a practicing physician and who has in subsequent years played a leading and personally active role in international medicine, among other things working in refugee camps in remote and medically underserved areas of the world.[28]) He was also doubtless in the best position to face honestly the fiscal crisis that began to grow under Chapman and that would hit Strickler full force when he became dean.

Almy's appointment marked the real beginning of a clinical-training component for medical students. Up to that point, there had been a good deal of debate and discussion about the shape this part of the curriculum should take, but Almy played a key role in creating what came to be a required fourth-year course—"Health, Society, and the Physician" ("HSP"). An integrated approach to medicine based on a bio-psycho-social model, the popular course used case studies. Almy showed his hand early on another matter, too, presenting an outline of "The Role of Graduate Medical Education in Dartmouth's Expanding Program" in an article published just a few months after he had begun at DMS. "The current developments," he wrote,

> are but the first phase of a long-range plan to enlarge the graduate education program to play its full role in a teaching medical center, and to reshape it to meet changing standards and increasing public demands for medical manpower. The trends in the next few years will be toward closer integration of the internship with the content of the undergraduate curriculum, toward more advanced and research-oriented training in clinical specialties, and toward a new and more effective pattern of training for the family physician.

He closed with a section on "The Family Physician of the Future," a topic that would increasingly become the focus of his efforts at Dartmouth. "While thus populating our ivory tower with skilled specialists and imaginative clinical research workers, we shall bend our efforts to another assignment . . . for which Dartmouth, in its rural setting, is particularly suited. The public clamors loudly (and rightly) for a modern counterpart of the general practitioner."[29]

This all fit well with what Chapman had in mind for the direction he wanted the school to take. Chapman, according to Strickler, "conceptualized the idea for a rural medical school that has carried through." While Strickler was dean, there was a move to abolish the Department of Community Medicine (as it was first known). But Strickler, convinced Chapman had been right, fought to maintain it. Seeing the whole concept of community medicine not only as right but as crucial to the survival of the medical school, Strickler persuaded Tenney—who likened the department's work to fuzzy sociology of medicine—not to fight it. Both Strickler and Almy were unhappy when cutbacks became the cost of its preservation, but future successes of what in 1979 became the Department of Community and Family Medicine at DMS, under Michael Zubkoff, have eliminated any doubts about the wisdom of the Chapman/Strickler support for the idea.[30]

Part of what makes the Strickler years in the deanship interesting is the way this man who later said that "administration is not why I went to medical school" took hold of the administrative reins and—with some creative planning—helped stabilize DMS fiscally. Though Strickler would leave the deanship with a large debt still on the books, he would leave it sufficiently improved for his successor finally to balance the budget. Strickler had signed on to work with Chapman because the challenge of transforming the basic science school into a full M.D. program appealed to him, and nothing during Chapman's tenure changed his mind.

Furthermore, Strickler was convinced that the financial problems facing the school could not be laid wholly at Chapman's feet. Others disagreed, some strongly. Although Strickler has acknowledged that there may have been some unsophisticated financial planning on Chapman's part, he has also insisted that the fiscal crisis was aggravated by changes in federal granting procedures and an energy crisis that helped bring on double-digit inflation. Chapman had tried to warn the trustees of the growing financial problems, but—according to Strickler—he was made the scapegoat "to an extent that . . . was extremely unfair." Thus it may have been a degree of loyalty to Chapman as well as to Dartmouth Medical School that motivated Strickler to accept the additional challenge of being dean himself. Besides, by his own account, he was committed to what had been started. (He shares credit with Chapman for giving a significant boost to efforts at coeducation at DMS, and he worked with notable success to recruit women and minority candidates into administrative positions.) Strickler also thought he knew the problems the School faced as well as anyone, and—only partly in jest—he recollected later that he didn't want to run the risk of working as Associate Dean for someone else.

Nonetheless, 1973 was a very difficult time to take on the top administrative position at Dartmouth Medical School. The Survey Committee appointed to review DMS's situation following Chapman's resignation concluded $20 million was needed to set things right—a daunting amount of money to raise. On the other hand, Strickler knew he had a strong ally in President John Kemeny, with whom he had worked and whom he "admired and revered." Strickler was convinced there was no way Kemeny would let the medical school close on *his* watch. In addition, although several Board of Trustees members believed it was at last time to shut down medical education at Dartmouth after all, Trustee William Morton—a "great champion" of DMS—prevailed. As President Kemeny put it in his remarks to the Alumni Council in June 1973, "the Board of Trustees agreed they were not going to either abolish or weaken the fourth oldest medical school in the country, and that they were prepared to make a long-range commitment to the support of the Medical School if three conditions were met." (We will examine these conditions shortly.)[31]

Four years into his deanship, Strickler had to acknowledge that the School's "current fiscal situation is precarious." He also insisted, however, that the trustees' agreement "to commit College resources to help us while an all-out joint development effort is made on the School's behalf," fortuitously coupled with "encouraging" signs of support from the DMS side of the Dartmouth family, meant "the outlook from the Dean's office" could be a cautious "concerned but confident." A year later things sounded no better, however. Focusing on the high cost of medical education, but trying to put Dartmouth's situation in its national context, Strickler wrote that the "fiscal plight of medical school students as we approach the 1980's is acute."[32]

Among the curricular matters overseen by Strickler during his deanship, one of the most innovative contributions was the program that he and Stanley Aronson, then dean of Brown University's medical school, brought into existence by signing a contract (endorsed by their respective boards of trustees) in 1981 for a joint program, allowing DMS to send some third-year students to Brown. (Implementation would fall to Strickler's successor, Robert McCollum.) Initially, there was concern that having even a few students transfer after the second year would make it look as if DMS were returning to being a two-year school.[33] DMS could not expand its student body beyond the sixty-four clinical students it had at the time using only the facilities of the Medical Center as it existed then. The much larger number of patient beds available for Brown students (some 2,000, about four times what Dartmouth could provide) was part of the appeal. Still in place more than twenty years later, the "Brown–Dartmouth Program" allows what was initially up to one quarter of the DMS second-year class (the number is set at twenty students) to transfer to Brown for their clinical years; those students earn an M.D. degree from Brown University. From the start it was—according to one of its principal architects—"a very congenial relationship."[34]

Meanwhile, the vaunted flexibility of the special three-year program was being explicitly called into question. "The Dartmouth Medical School's three-year M.D. program, once widely hailed as an innovation that set it apart from other schools, might have to undergo significant change. . . . [O]verall the Medical School is doing a good job but . . . the three-year curriculum is trying to achieve too much in too little time," according to a report in the *Dartmouth Alumni Magazine*.[35] And the faculty evaluation of the three-year curriculum concluded that the "unrelenting inflexible 'lock-step' pressure on the students" was the number one limitation of the program.[36] In the autumn of 1980, the transition from the novel three-year M.D. program to the standard four-year curriculum began. The school catalog for that year put a positive spin on the change:

> When DMS returned to the M.D. program in the late 1960s, it adopted the shorter program to help alleviate the national physician shortage and lower the total cost of a medical education. . . . Today the concern is not one of number; it is one of distribution: a need for more physicians providing primary care in rural and inner-city areas.
>
> The curriculum expansion will allow students more time for the study of both the basic sciences and the clinical disciplines.[37]

Student Life

Even as the student body was growing and changing, becoming ever more heterogeneous, two constants could be noted. The first was that the quality of the students stayed at a high level (though precise measurements of "quality of student body" are difficult, and some faculty believed there was initially some falling off). This was important, because a record of outstanding students had been one of "the most influential factors in the decision . . . to refound the Medical School." The second unchanged factor was the close relationship between students and faculty, a long-time characteristic of the school and "one of the most important contributions to high morale."[38] Recalling the beginning of the academic year in 1969, for example, one member of the class of 1971 would later write that "teachers like Elmer Pfefferkorn amazed us by knowing our names and all about us. We had never been in such a personal environment before. The professors set the tone of collegiality for our class and helped us master the basic sciences in such a way that we left DMS with a background that was the envy of our peers in the schools to which we transferred."[39]

For the class of 1981, classes in microbiology and pathology were merged with clinical work in a course called the "Scientific Basis of Medicine." Though this class was still part of the three-year Dartmouth Plan, the days of "lock-step" inflexibility were clearly past, as clerkships "broke the class into five tracks, taking members of the class not only to Mary Hitchcock . . . , but also to the White River Junction VA Hospital, Hartford (Conn.) Hospital, Concord (N.H.) Hospital, and the Brattleboro (Vt.) Retreat. Elective clerkships took class members even further afield [Arizona, Alaska, California]."[40] But a more local note was struck in a press release issued in the spring of that class's last year. Among the then-current candidates for the M.D. degree, thirty-three were New Hampshire men and women. Their presence at DMS and the reasons some of them gave for why they hoped to practice in New Hampshire after completing their training would have made Nathan Smith smile with satisfaction. Yet of course there were also many students from "away." If there ever had been "typical" DMS students, identifying what was typical about those in the latter part of the twentieth century became more difficult as the classes became less and less homogeneous. The wide variety of answers that each of ten students gave (in a 1985 review) to ten questions about why they were studying medicine illustrates this point well. Yet there did seem be one near-constant. A strong social conscience frequently emerged: a concern for the health of rural New Hampshire residents, a desire to improve emergency care in rural areas, an interest in serving ethnic communities.[41]

Perhaps the best additional evidence that a strong social conscience is "typical" of DMS students today comes in the form of reports on their entirely voluntary participation in community service efforts (upward of 80 percent of the students are involved each year). A "brainchild of the DMS student government," the Community Service Committee came into being in the middle of 1990. It "quickly became an integral part of the DMS experience," one that had students working with victims of domestic violence, teaching health in local elementary schools, volunteering in the Good Neighbor Health Clinic in White River Junction, Vermont, or singing in nursing homes and helping elderly patients keep their medications straight. In 1995, after a mere five years of operation, the Community Service Committee accepted for DMS the Paul R. Wright Award from the American Medical Students Association, given to recognize "a medical school whose 'exemplary medical education programs best foster the development of socially responsible physicians.'"[42]

Also beginning in the early 1990s, DMS began offering a course called "Literature and Medicine." An elective course that Senior Advising Dean Joseph O'Donnell (DMS 1971) helped design, it aims at helping "remind students there is more to people than their symptoms and to make them better, more empathetic observers." Students read a range of classics and not-so-well-known books that many will either have missed in their rush to fill pre-med science requirements or read before they decided to study medicine. The course is all part of a movement to teach the humanities as well as science and medicine to future doctors. A course in life drawing is offered, to improve students' hand-eye coordination "and make students more comfortable with the body." A course in improvisation assists students in their ability to "read patients' body language and emotion."[43] And already in the 1970s, DMS had formed a liaison with the College's Ethics Institute, which fosters the study of applied and professional ethics throughout the Dartmouth community in an interdisciplinary way. For DMS faculty, there are thus opportunities to grapple with (and incorporate into their teaching) philosophical issues that present themselves in the decisions physicians must make about patient care.

The availability of such opportunities and the inclusion of such offerings in the DMS curriculum are a dramatic indication of how much Dartmouth Medical School has changed in its second hundred years, roughly since the days when Carleton Pennington Frost was trying out the formula of a separate recitation term (the changes since Nathan Smith's days are of course even more marked). Perhaps a still bigger change is the gradual increase in the presence of women in several different roles at Dartmouth Medical School.

Women Come to Dartmouth

A graph showing women graduates of Dartmouth Medical School between 1960 and 1977 and a bar chart showing the percentage of each first-year class that was female (nationally and at DMS) at five-year intervals between 1972 and 1997 are both up-and-down affairs. Today, men and women take turns making up more than 50 percent of the first-year class, as they have done ever since 1985 when women first went over that mark (54 percent).[44] For the class that entered in the autumn of 1987, the figure was even higher—58 percent female, with 49 women and 35 men.[45] In fact, it appears that DMS was the first medical school in the United States not historically dedicated exclusively to the education of women to reach that milestone. The class that matriculated at DMS in its bicentennial year was 51 percent women and 49 percent men.[46]

This kind of balance was a long time coming. We saw earlier that Dartmouth chose to reject its first woman applicant, Emily Blackwell, in 1852. More than a century passed before Valerie Leval (later Graham) matriculated—in 1960—a solitary woman to join 23 young men in the class of 1962. In 1978 the percentage of women admitted to DMS rose to more than 30 percent (slightly better than the average for all U.S. medical schools), and by 1979 Leval was no longer the only female matriculant, but rather the first of 169. As of that year women finally also constituted 12 percent of the DMS faculty. The early postgraduate doctoral programs—molecular biology while it lasted, physiology-pharmacology, and biochemistry (just started in 1973)—all had women students in them: 36 percent, 28 percent, and 35 percent, respectively, as of 1979.[47] Though the first women started arriving at DMS as students in the 1960s, it is only fair to cite the particularly strong support of Robert McCollum, dean in the 1980s, as a major factor in Dartmouth Medical School having, today, such a strong female presence. In his winter 1988 column for *Dartmouth Medicine*, McCollum wrote:

> This has not been the result of special targeting or of quotas. Rather, it has been the outcome of a fair and competitive admissions process, of increasing numbers of women applicants, and of the recognition that male dominance in medicine over the centuries was largely determined by cultural and societal factors rather than by gender-linked intellect or skills. . . . [A]t DMS there is no doubt that women make a difference and that the difference is good.[48]

Dr. Helen Pittman became the first woman on the Hitchcock Hospital staff in 1928; Dr. Agnes Bartlett was the first woman to complete a residency at the Hitchcock Hospital, in 1950. Elizabeth French, a pathologist who joined the DMS faculty in the 1950s, was the first (and for many years only) woman member of the Hitchcock Clinic.[49] Another forward step for women was taken when Dr. Lisabeth Maloney (DC 1977), an anesthesiologist, was named medical director for the Mary Hitchcock Hospital and the Hitchcock Clinic in 1995.

Other early women on the faculty have been mentioned: Jean Botts, Jane Sands Robb, Frances McCann, Lucile Smith. Both McCann and Smith—who stayed and were each granted *Emerita* status at retirement—have tales to tell of the awkwardness, oddity, and sometimes downright discomfort of working in such an overwhelmingly male enclave. McCann's account of her arrival in Hanover to take up the post she had been offered, and her first encounter with Marsh Tenney, is a lively but sobering tale; a less-intrepid medical scientist might well have given up.[50] Smith tells of attending the lunch (in 1964) where she was to be awarded the honorary Dartmouth degree that went with having been promoted to full professor: "the other candidates (all male) assumed that I had come to serve the lunch and handed me their empty sherry glasses." Perhaps this helps explain her observation more than twenty-five years later that "Since then we've made some progress, but it's been slow."[51]

Having a few women on the faculty and being ahead of the crowd, nationally (and in comparison to Dartmouth College) in opening the student ranks to women did not mean there was sudden equality of opportunity and treatment, as Smith's anecdote makes clear. One among many possible examples is the way women who sought to be surgeons—long considered a profession of singular status for men—were treated at Dartmouth. Helen Pittman, just mentioned as the first woman on the Hitchcock Hospital staff, pioneered in another way as well. Having during her Hitchcock internship performed "a few appendectomies," she was encouraged by Jay Gile to write them up "so that she could use them later . . . in applying to the American College of Surgeons." This kind of support sounds in retrospect quite extraordinary. It "was to be another fifty years before the idea of a woman being a general surgeon was taken seriously enough at Dartmouth to result in the appointment of Dr. Martha McDaniel '77 and Dr. Kathleen Kopach . . . the first women above the intern level on the general surgical house staff." Dr. Joan Lange, halfway through her surgical rotation at that same time, rated her experience a cautious "'So far, so good.'"[52] But at least one female medical student from the time who later became a surgeon felt she had been quite deliberately discouraged from following that path.[53] On a more positive note, while still a student at DMS, Kristina Rosbe (DMS 1993) wrote enthusiastically of her surgery rotation: "When I finished the four weeks of surgery in Hanover, I thought I had found my calling. Never before had I experienced anything like the atmosphere in the OR."[54]

In addition to these former students and house officers, there are women who have joined the DMS faculty without any prior Dartmouth connections and women who have moved from being Dartmouth College students to being Dartmouth Medical School faculty members (and administrators). An example of the former is Constance Brinckerhoff, a

Smith College and SUNY Buffalo graduate in biology and microbiology respectively, who began her research career at DMS in 1972. In the decades since, she has made her presence felt in a variety of ways. Not only has she published widely and taught biochemistry for first-year medical students (an assignment she began in 1984; she became course director in 1990). She has also served on or as chair of numerous committees and in several administrative posts: acting chair of biochemistry, acting provost, associate dean for science education, director of the M.D./Ph.D. program. She also holds the Nathan Smith Professorship in Medicine and Biochemistry. One trusts Smith himself would be pleased at this evidence that his medical school has changed with the times.

Lori Arviso Alvord left Dartmouth College behind for medical school elsewhere and then returned to DMS as a faculty member and administrator. Her career holds additional interest because she is part of the Dartmouth tradition in the education of Native Americans. A member of the College class of 1979, Alvord—the nation's first Navajo woman surgeon—graduated from Stanford Medical School, where she also trained in surgery and served as chief resident. After returning to practice general surgery for six years at the Gallup Medical Center in New Mexico (with mostly Navajo and Zuñi patients), she was persuaded to return to Dartmouth as an assistant professor of surgery and an associate dean of student and minority affairs at DMS. She saw the administrative aspect of the appointment in particular as an opportunity to share something of "the Navajo approach to medicine."[55] As Alvord makes clear in her 1999 autobiography, *The Scalpel and the Silver Bear*, she is a great believer in the possibility of creating "a synthesis of the very best elements of all types of medicine. . . . We may perfect techniques that coax the mind into being a partner with the body in healing."[56]

Dartmouth may seem a surprising choice for a young Navajo woman leaving high school. Yet the College has for historical reasons had a somewhat better record than many institutions of higher learning in paying attention to the educational needs of Native Americans. DMS has a shorter record, to be sure, but one that—as of 1995—had "produced in the last 20 years the highest number of Native American graduates of any public or private medical school in the East." DMS records show twenty-one Native American graduates in the twenty-year period 1975–1994. Dartmouth's relatively good results in this area can be "attributed largely to President John Kemeny, who . . . renewed [the Dartmouth] commitment" to educate America's native people, in 1971. Another who deserves credit for seeing and stressing that the benefits of multiculturalism flow in both directions was George Margolis, a pathology professor in the 1970s who, "when it was a new thing to have minorities in medical lecture halls and labs . . . pushed for minority enrollment and remained a friend and mentor to many" members of minority groups who attended DMS.[57]

Yet Native Americans and women are not the only groups whose acceptance are a measure of an educational institution's success in becoming appropriately heterogeneous for the modern era. Progress is evident, although still perhaps slower than would be ideal, in particular as far as the faculty is concerned. Although the 1970 figure of only two minority students matriculated at DMS had by 1997 increased to the point where 13 percent of the first-year students came from underrepresented minorities—quite a good ratio in light of DMS's northeastern United States, rural setting—the faculty figure was still only 4.6 percent, "below the national availability."[58]

Research Takes Off

In the nineteenth century, DMS (like most other medical schools) had little to show in the way of faculty-generated research. We saw that several Dartmouth Medical School faculty members were authors of or contributors to medical textbooks, and a few founded, edited, and wrote for professional journals. Significant though these contributions were at the time, medicine a century and a half later required much more. Members of the Dartmouth Medical School faculty have increasingly risen to the challenges and joys of engaging in research and encouraging their students to do likewise. The distresses surrounding the research powerhouse in molecular biology notwithstanding, from the time of the refounding of Dartmouth Medical School right up to the present, people at DMS have been vigorously and productively engaged in basic science research. The research program gradually grew to encompass clinical research as well—and a goodly amount of research that cut across the divide between "clinical" and "basic science."

Marking a few points along the continuum by mentioning names and fields of endeavor helps make this clear. During the early 1960s, for example, in biochemistry, Peter von Hippel did important work on protein structure and then on DNA; Lucile Smith studied oxidative phosphorylation and Lafayette Noda studied phosphatases; Mel Simpson worked on protein synthesis and Arnold Wishnia on physical chemistry. Shinya Inoué in anatomy-cytology (who came to Dartmouth with a stellar reputation already established) studied chromosome structure.

Physiology, under Marsh Tenney, was a hotbed of respiratory research, and its reputation in this field continues to this day. The department is known especially for its elucidation of the control of respiration and sudden infant death syndrome (SIDS), with important contributions from Eugene Nattie, Donald Bartlett, James Leiter, Walter St. John, and Andrew Daubenspeck. Heinz Valtin led renal physiology and became well known for developing the Brattleboro rat, an early animal model of diabetes insipidus, and for his textbooks in renal physiology and pathophysiology. When Frances McCann arrived, she settled into work that evolved into elegant electrophysiological studies on the moth heart. Within the endocrine group, Allan Munck developed in vitro studies on the glucocorticoid receptor and later proposed an important theory on the role of glucocorticoids in the response to stress. In the same group. Valerie Galton's interest in the biochemistry of thyroid hormones led to her groundbreaking work on deiodinase enzymes in relation to the actions of thyroid hormones (later significantly expanded by Donald St. Germain, who had originally worked with her as a postdoc and then set up his own lab). In microbiology, Elmer Pfefferkorn arrived with an established reputation in virology and then turned to studying *Toxoplasma*. He also did beautiful work on gamma interferon mechanisms.

Focusing in this manner on a very small selection of the people and projects that helped put and keep DMS on the research map inevitably means omitting others that would serve equally well. Among the examples of the work that sets DMS apart from other institutions where research in the medical sciences is conducted—and one that helped generate an impressive $34 million in research grants and contracts in 1989–1990—is an organization within DHMC that has been an important part of the medical scene in Hanover and in the region since 1972. Under the leadership of Dr. Frank Lane, the Norris Cotton Cancer Center (NCCC) was established that year, largely through the initiative of New Hampshire's senior senator at the time, Norris Cotton (after whom the center was later named). NCCC was one of the first two dozen cancer centers designated by the National Cancer Institute (NCI) as a comprehensive cancer center; it is still the only one in a truly rural area. (To be designated as a "Comprehensive Cancer Center," an organization not only must deliver clinical cancer care but also must conduct research in three areas basic, clinical, and prevention and control—and must support programs that ensure that these three areas are not pursued in isolation from each other. Finally, such a center must provide information, outreach, and education to the lay community as well as to health-care professionals.) NCCC thus serves as a regional resource, with a dozen or more outreach sites scattered across New Hampshire and Vermont. The significance of the "Comprehensive Cancer Center" designation, according to O. Ross McIntyre—the second director of the Cancer Center (he served in that capacity for seventeen years, stepping down in 1992)—is that it meant being recognized as an institution that could " 'deliver the highest quality of cancer treatment' and that had the 'features that constitute a national resource in the effort to reduce cancer incidence and mortality.' "

Around the same time, McIntyre himself was singled out for distinction, having been "elected to a five-year term as chairman of the board of the National Institutes of Health's Cancer and Leukemia Group B (CALGB)—a consortium of twenty-five major cancer centers across the country."[59] In 1991, the Cancer Center began a move to the DHMC campus in Lebanon; the move into a new building was completed in 1995. That same year, Michael Sporn—winner of the American Cancer Society's Medal of Honor in 1994—moved to DMS after a thirty-five-year career at the National Institutes of Health (NIH). Sporn, looking forward to being part of a smaller operation, welcomed the opportunity he saw being offered to him at Dartmouth to plunge into some new work. His collaborative endeavors with Gordon Gribble, a Dartmouth College chemist, for example, fit well with the "multidisciplinary approach" that McIntyre says is the "optimal method of cancer care"—one of the greatest contributions NCCC has made to medicine in the region. The Cancer Center is one of the places where the link between basic bench science and clinical science is most evident.[60]

A firm conviction that the best way to counter cancer is to prevent it led to work that resulted in Sporn being considered the "father of chemoprevention" (he coined the term); for the second half of his NIH career he was chief of the Laboratory of Chemoprevention. In the approach to cancer that he has advocated and practiced, "chemicals are used to combat cancer before it develops—particularly in people who are known to be at high risk." Sporn's NIH lab ran a ten-year study that produced "synthetic derivatives of natural Vitamin A" (dubbed "retinoids" by the lab). Some of the retinoids were already in clinical trials when Sporn joined DMS, where he immediately turned his attention to identifying "new, natural products that could be used to prevent cancer."[61]

NCCC has had national significance; a lowly rat is the centerpiece in a very different kind of research project that has inspired work internationally. In 1961, Dr. Henry Schroeder—an associate professor of clinical physiology at DMS with a laboratory in Brattleboro, Vermont—made a chance discovery of a strain of rats in his colony that had congenital diabetes insipidus. Schroeder turned the rats over to Heinz Valtin, the only nephrologist at DMS at the time; Valtin, collaborating with Dr.

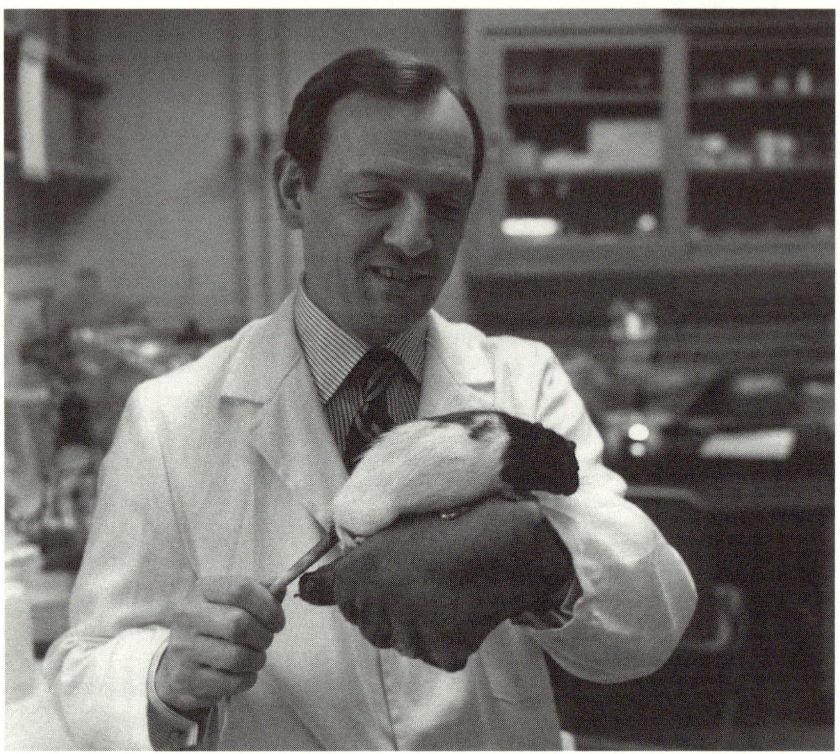

Professor Heinz Valtin and the "Brattleboro Rat," 1974. The rat proved useful when researchers at DSM figured out why it couldn't hold its water. Courtesy of Dartmouth College Archives.

Hilda Sokol (whose background was in comparative endocrinology), used the rats "as a model to elucidate problems concerning the secretion and synthesis of hormones in neurohypophysis . . . and the mechanism of vasopressin."[62] Valtin immortalized Schroeder's role by dubbing the model animal "the Brattleboro Rat" after the lab's location; the name has stuck, even as this particular strain of rat "has become so valuable to medical research that breeding colonies have been established on four continents."[63] In 1981, on the twentieth anniversary of Schroeder's intuition that his rats might be useful in research, Valtin and Sokol hosted an international symposium at Dartmouth dedicated to the Brattleboro Rat. One hundred and fifty scientists from three continents and more than a dozen countries gathered to hear more than one hundred scheduled papers. All because of a sick rat—but one that has done much to help sick human beings.[64]

Working with laboratory rats has a comfortingly old-fashioned ring to it, for all the modern-day importance of the work. Much more "modern" sounding, because it has to do with inventing and patenting scientific processes with commercial value, is the story of Medarex, a biotechnology company bred in Dartmouth labs. The "history of Medarex and its fortunes actually begins with the story of the monoclonal antibody for acute myeloid leukemia (AML) which Edward Ball made at DMS in the early 1980s," according to an article that tells how things got started.[65] Its origins reach back to 1978, when Paul Guyre arrived at DMS as a postdoctoral fellow; then Michael Fanger was brought on board (a few years later) to do research on immunology at Dartmouth. A three-way collaboration developed among Clark Anderson at Rochester and Fanger and Guyre at DMS; they invented a process for purifying molecules, making monoclonal antibodies, and using an assay to figure out which ones were good and which were not. Li Shen, recruited by Fanger, made further progress, developing a bispecific antibody with unique properties.

Fanger, Guyre, and Ball together formed Medarex in 1987; it was "DMS's first effort in the world of corporate-academic partnerships." The prospects were exciting: "In addition to the potential benefits of the liaison, Dartmouth stands to gain from the visibility the venture will give the Medical School in high-tech circles," according to a school publication.[66] The euphoria was quashed by an anonymous letter alleging scientific misconduct and business impropriety sent to the College administration just as a secondary offering of stock was getting under way in the summer of 1992 (the company had gone public with its first sale of stock in 1991). The end of the story is important: Both then and on two subsequent occasions when "similar charges" were made "by the same person or person,"[67] Medarex and all its officers were cleared of all charges. But the excruciatingly slow pace of the investigation and the anonymous nature of the charges left those involved in the basic research that spawned the company in an awkward and unhappy situation. The administration eventually took action—but in a ponderous, insensitive, and legalistic way that seemed designed primarily to spare the institution from damage and left the bewildered targets of the accusations in limbo for some time.

This relative administrative ineffectiveness vis-à-vis the Medical School was baffling to those who had not previously experienced what appeared to be lack of College support for DMS. It was, according to

Guyre looking back years later, very disappointing and dispiriting to those against whom the allegations were made that the College seemed from the outset to be more serious about considering the allegations than it was about pursuing the perpetrators. On the other hand, the principals were gratified by support from many colleagues in conversations, letters, and petitions signed and sent to the College administration. A *Valley News* article in early 1993 ("Medarex Charges Declared Baseless") and a *Dartmouth Medicine* story shortly thereafter ("Investigation finds no merit to charges") provided public vindication; Dean Andrew Wallace was content in 1995 to be quoted simply saying, "'we have no reason to believe that this third, and latest, edition of anonymous allegations warrants any revision of the findings made following the prior reviews.'"[68]

The whole experience had some salutary results. It succeeded in moving the College (and with it the Medical School) to overhaul its policies for reviewing work that has come under fire; it also forced a reassessment of how the College would evaluate efforts by its faculty members to patent their work. More subtly, it served as one more reminder that the faculty and the institution itself would be stronger if the "ethic of community" could be preserved. In addition, each time the College has been called upon to commit itself anew to the Medical School, communication between the College administration and DMS has improved. The Medical School survives precisely because it is an integral part of something larger—of Dartmouth College and of the Dartmouth-Hitchcock Medical Center (about which, more in the next chapter).

Without a doubt, the research projects at DHMC that have received the most publicity—and have had the most direct effect on the way physicians and patients alike think about the practice of medicine—are the numerous studies of variations in health care pioneered by John Wennberg and his colleagues in the Center for the Evaluative Clinical Sciences (CECS). In addition to a steady stream of articles based on the studies undertaken in CECS (Wennberg was another of those whose success in being awarded grants accounted for the huge jump in the amount of funded research received in the 1989–1990 fiscal year), CECS in 1993 began "the nation's first graduate program in the evaluative clinical sciences." Within three years, it was "a model for several other programs," and by 1996 it was offering both M.S. and Ph.D. programs. A whole new field of clinical research—outcomes research—has been influenced and inspired by epidemiologist Wennberg's insistence that it is both possible and important to base medical care on scientific evidence of what actually works best. His pioneering work means that "whenever

Atlas maps out regional variations in health care

By Doug Levy
USA TODAY

DOCTOR DISTRIBUTION, 7D

The kind of medical care you get could have as much to do with where you live as your medical condition, a 10-year study suggests.

The findings, compiled in the *Dartmouth Atlas of Health Care in the United States* (American Hospital Publishing, $350), include data on hospitalization, surgeries and types of doctors from region to region. The main finding: Health care varies enormously from one place to another.

For example, women with breast cancer in the South and Midwest most often undergo breast removal, while women in the Northeast and parts of California get more breast-sparing lumpectomies.

"We find no evidence that people in regions with more (aggressive) care live longer," says Dr. John E. Wennberg, a Dartmouth epidemiologist who led the research.

He wants patients to know that what their doctors advise may not always be the only treatment or that certain procedures may be more common in their area just because it has more specialists of that type.

Among the differences:

▶ Medicare spending per enrollee is more than two times higher in Miami ($6,429) than in Lincoln, Neb. ($2,729). But there's no evidence that people in Miami get better care and the difference is too big to be explained by the cost of living.

▶ Boston and New Haven, Conn., have similar populations, but Boston has more hospital beds. The result: More Bostonians were hospitalized for common conditions.

▶ The number of specialists per 100,000 population ranges from 56 in parts of the Southeast to 209 in urban areas of the Northeast and far West.

"There's an awful lot of random distribution and consumption of resources," says Dr. Jack Lord of the American Hospital Association, which is publishing the atlas.

"It holds up a mirror to the health-care system," Wennberg says.

Those interested can order the report by phoning 800-242-2626 or ask if their library has ordered it. Regional and consumer versions are due within a year.

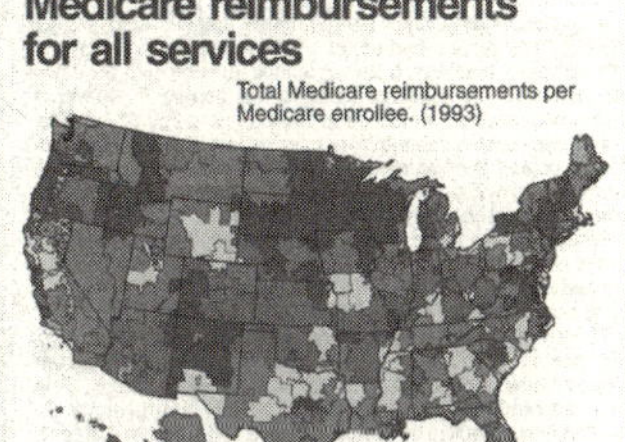

USA Today *was only one of several publications—including the* New York Times *and the* Wall Street Journal*—that picked up the story of the publication of the* Dartmouth Atlas of Health Care, *January 30, 1996.*

expertise in outcomes research is mentioned, Dartmouth's name is at the top of the list."[69]

Wennberg's early work showed that the "amount and cost of hospital treatment in a community have more to do with the number of physicians there, their medical specialties and the procedures they prefer than with the health of the [community's] residents."[70] From there Wennberg moved to helping patients make treatment choices based on information about likely outcomes; an interactive video disk titled "Choosing: Prostatectomy or Watchful Waiting" was the first venture in this direction.[71] Managed care, cost containment, and fear of health care rationing have also come under his scrutiny.[72] Others working in or with CECS have taken on a wide range of topics: John Wasson studied the way physicians staying in touch with elderly patients by phone reduced costs and improved patients' physical health; Joanne Lynn (before leaving DMS to found Americans for Better Care of the Dying, based in Washington, D.C.) published in the *Journal of the American Geriatrics Society* the results of her study on the putatively "wasted" money spent on terminally ill patients; Robert Harbaugh changed his own postoperative practices after analyzing what really determined outcomes for patients recovering from carotid endarterectomies; Elliott Fisher and Gilbert Welch have explored the reality that "as medical care increases, so does the risk of harm."[73] A direct outgrowth of some of the same kind of thinking is the Northern New England Cardiovascular Study Group spearheaded and supported by cardiologist Stephen K. Plume (president of the Hitchcock Clinic at the time the study group was started). A consortium of nine medical centers has made seemingly tiny changes in process, without fancy policy statements, in the way heart surgery is performed. The result of an impressive pattern of collaborative effort, these changes have produced a sustained 25 percent drop in cardiovascular surgical mortality in bypass operations across the region—which now has one of the lowest bypass mortality rates in the country.[74]

But the most sweeping work of CECS, which required processing data that "ran to . . . 24 million discharge records, 70 million enrollment records, and 60 million physician bills," resulted in the publication of *The Dartmouth Atlas of Health Care*. The book contains dozens of maps of the United States—maps that, for instance, "divide the United States into 3,436 hospital service areas, [and] then into 306 hospital referral regions," to show first where people go for acute care and second where they go for specialized services; it is "aimed at a far wider readership than research papers could ever reach." Paul Batalden joined the DMS faculty just in time—as it turned out—to be instrumental in connecting the Wennberg group and the American Hospital Association (AHA) together to jointly publish the *Atlas*. Although the *Atlas* above all "presents a case for global solutions or large-area policy decision that would affect the supply side of health-care services," the hope of Wennberg and others involved in the project is that people on the demand side—patients—will learn from the *Atlas* more about what affects differences in treatment so they can be more informed participants with their physicians in shared decision making.[75]

This sampling of the research being done at DMS pays tribute in a small way to the now thoroughly understood proposition that collaboration and cooperation are critical to the future of the DHMC and each of its components. The whole *is* greater than the sum of its parts, and of course there has to be a "balance" of research and clinical work, both for students and for faculty. Medical education goes hand in hand with medical research and medical practice.

CHAPTER TWELVE

Education for the Future

> Time must be allowed to take our own mental and spiritual pulse, and humanism and medical history give us a point of view so that we are not standing up too close or back too far. —HENRY R. VIETS[1]

Money Matters

IN THE THIRTY-THREE years from 1927 to 1960, Dartmouth Medical School had only two deans; in the six years that followed, there were two deans and two acting deans. Thus, when Carleton Chapman came in 1966 and actually stayed into the 1970s, it was a welcome sign that stabilization was under way (when Chapman left to take up his new responsibilities at the Commonwealth Foundation at the beginning of 1973, Marsh Tenney was acting dean again for a period of a few months). The next three full-time deans each had terms of roughly eight years. The tenures of James Strickler (1973–1981) and Robert McCollum (1982–1990) were separated by Peter Whybrow's six-month stint as acting dean (Whybrow had been executive dean under Strickler from 1980); Andrew Wallace (1990–1998) was dean through the end of DMS's second century. Although each dean could point to particular achievements during his tenure, there was a new kind of seamlessness. Where Tenney's deanship was focused on refounding Dartmouth Medical School, Mudge's became terribly tangled in the molecular biology controversy, and Chapman's was highlighted by the return to an M.D. curriculum. Overlapping endeavors and steady progress marked the years of leadership from Strickler to McCollum to Wallace. Though there were ups and downs during this twenty-five-year period—much of it having to do with financing and with institutional relations—the road ahead was clearer than it had been. There was a new sense of purpose and commitment, a fitting prelude to the beginning of a third century.

Strickler had done much to put DMS on a more stable base, financially speaking. (His successor, McCollum, called what Strickler had achieved the result of "ingenious planning.") Absent Strickler's work, it would not have been even remotely feasible for McCollum to promise to get the Medical School free of debt within three years. That he succeeded—he actually did better than that—is clear from an Overseers Report early in the decade of the 1980s: "The Medical School, in FY'84 as in FY'82 and FY'83, is in fiscal balance." It was an astonishing accomplishment, given what McCollum had inherited: a debt to the College of $2.1 million (he extracted an agreement from the College that the debt would be erased); a deficit that had been running at $800,000 a year and was projected even under improved conditions to be around $400,000 annually; a need to increase the size and the salaries of the faculty; and the need to increase the endowment. The cautionary note that followed the good news in the Overseers Report is hardly surprising: "Although the Medical School now has a degree of financial stability, there remains a scarcity of financial resources or reserves with which to develop new initiatives."[2]

The fiscal problems were thus still considerable. McCollum's understanding was that the College had promised the Medical School a subvention of $20 million—but the new president of the College, David McLaughlin, denied having made such a promise. "That was the end of our $20 million," McCollum recalled years later. Nor was this the only time there was misunderstanding between College and Medical School—though McCollum is also quick to say that President McLaughlin was helpful to DMS on many occasions. Furthermore, the Board of Overseers for the Medical School (appointed by the Board of Trustees to play primarily an advisory role) was helpful in fund raising; Andrew Thompson especially took an unusual degree of interest in the Medical School and gave McCollum a great deal of support. A DMS campaign to raise $55 million helped boost the endowment from $17 million to $60 million.

In anticipation of a trustee retreat in August 1984, Provost Agnar Pytte prepared a background paper on Dartmouth's professional schools and graduate programs. Just how dire the plight of the Medical School had become is clear. Acknowledging that the financial problems facing DMS were "momentous," however, Pytte added that "the opportunities are enormous." There was considerable good news from the Medical School: expansion of faculty, facilities, and clinical training sites; the introduction of one hundred clinical and nonclinical elective courses and two new and "innovative" required courses for fourth-year students ("Health, Society, and the Physician" and "Clinical Therapeutics") that were being reviewed for implementation in other medical schools; a 75 percent increase in the number of student applications as well as an increase in the quantity and quality of minority applicants; a commitment from the Hitchcock Hospital of financial support for graduate medical education; and "an impressive gain (20.8 percent) in the area of sponsored activity [research money]." Yet what lay ahead was still somewhat uncertain. The report continued: "The future of DMS as a four-year medical school is intimately tied to the fortunes of the [hospital and the clinic]. Each unit of the Medical Center is dependent on the others. . . . The President is trying to keep the Medical Center from flying apart altogether, and will give you the latest update at the time of the Trustee Retreat."[3] Clearly, balancing the relationships among the institutions that were increasingly coming to be thought of as part of a "Medical Center" was among the most serious challenges that would face not only McCollum but the next two deans as well.

Institutional Relations

Dartmouth Medical School was never a wholly independent—let alone self-sufficient—institution. From the very beginning, as will be recalled, it was to the "Board of Trust" of Dartmouth College that Nathan Smith wrote, offering in effect to provide the College with a Medical School if they would but allow him to engage in passing on to students what he once referred to as "the Science we have loved and taught."[4] Things had changed dramatically since then, of course, but only partly in jest did James O. Freedman—president of Dartmouth College from 1987 to 1998—once say that "every president curses medical schools." They are always the source of financial problems for their parent institutions.[5] Some outside observers familiar with Dartmouth believe the bridges that Dickey and Tenney had hoped to build between the College and the Dartmouth Medical School have not yet been constructed wholly successfully. Yet without a doubt, DMS today is shaped by the Clinic, the Hitchcock Hospital, and the VA Hospital, as well as by the College.[6]

As for hospitals: The first one in Hanover—Dixi Crosby's nineteenth-century cottage hospital on North College Street—was the creation of a DMS faculty member. The Mary Hitchcock Memorial Hospital itself might well never have come into being without the friendship between its benefactor, Hiram Hitchcock, and two Medical School faculty members—Carlton P. Frost and William T. Smith—who with a third colleague, Gilman D. Frost, comprised its initial staff. And the affiliation with the VA Hospital in 1946 among other things facilitated "the establishment of a residency training program with its various incidental advantages in research opportunities."[7]

Finally, the founding of the Hitchcock Clinic by Dean of the Medical School John P. Bowler and his colleagues is widely believed to have spared the Medical School and the Hitchcock Hospital alike death from a slow wasting disease. Where once—actually more than once—there was a serious question whether the Medical School could survive, where Bowler and his colleagues were seriously concerned about whether the Hospital itself could survive, there is now a true academic medical center. It is unlikely that would have happened had the Clinic not helped stop the medical brain drain that threatened the Medical School in the aftermath of the Flexner report, when DMS was reduced to a two-year school.

The variety and complexity of the issues entailed in building the good working relations responsible for the flowering of DHMC make it impossible to tell anything like the full story here. A few examples, spread over many years, will have to suffice. In Nathan Smith's day, the College was happy to boast that it offered medical courses while letting its professors of medicine depend on student fees alone for compensation. Furthermore, although the School operated under the authority of the Dartmouth College Board of Trustees, the State of New Hampshire owned both the Medical House and the land on which it stood. Throughout the nineteenth century, it is fair to say, the "administrative relationship between the Medical School and the parent institution was undeniably a confused affair. . . . [A]nd relations between the two faculties were often strained."[8] Nor did those remarks apply only in the nineteenth century. In the 1970s, relations were still sufficiently strained that President John Kemeny's insistence that closing the Medical School would be a "disaster" and his firm belief that DMS's problems had to be considered the College's problems were worthy of note. According to Don Penfield, who worked closely with Kemeny as his assistant, Kemeny was able to make others understand that. But it took a well-respected individual like Kemeny—able to get people with tightly crossed arms to relax and start talking to each other—to accomplish that.[9]

A brochure dated "1947–48" and published by the then recently formed Hitchcock Foundation indicates that the idea of a complex combination of institutions had been around for some time. Referring to the "rural medical center which has been evolving over a period of many years," the text goes on to describe (in very brief compass) just how the "three main groups, the Dartmouth Medical School, the Mary Hitchcock Memorial Hospital and the Hitchcock Clinic" are related to and work with each other.[10] A file copy of a March 1957 report titled "Dartmouth Medical School" painted a picture of mutual benefit among these institutions: "The Hitchcock Hospital and Clinic have grown in recent years to become a major center for upper New England. The strong clinical staff has been a major supplement to the [Medical School] faculty, and the wards of the hospital provide ample clinical material for teaching and for clinical research."[11] (This was a far cry from the repeated insistence in earlier years that the "clinical material" was woefully inadequate!)

"Graduate Medical Education," an undated brochure that appears to be from around 1959—basically a sales brochure for a variety of programs (residencies and fellowships, but not Ph.D. programs)—mentions DMS, the Clinic, the Hitchcock Hospital, and the VA Hospital as contributors.[12] On the other hand, reviewing the character of meetings with the Clinic's Staff Board of Governors in 1962 while he was dean, Gilbert Mudge (several years later) wrote that he "would be the first to say that we began with a sequence of misunderstandings on both sides." But, he continued, "despite these difficulties, all of us were in complete agreement that a satisfactory solution had to be found."[13] That some progress was made toward finding a solution can be inferred from a confidential letter written in late December 1963 to then-provost John Masland, by the president of the hospital, Edward Cavaney: "An objective look at the medical complex in Hanover indicates to me that our four organizations have an interdependence upon each other that is becoming more pronounced with the running of time."[14] This view was corroborated nearly a quarter of a century later by Heinz Valtin, retired but serving as chair of the committee planning the school's bicentennial celebration. "[E]ach of the entities of the Dartmouth-Hitchcock Medical Center—the clinic, the hospital and the medical school—is essential to the well-being of the others." He went on to say that the VA Hospital in White River Junction, the Medical Center's fourth component, "contributes equally to patient care and medical education."[15] A "Joint Medical Affairs Committee" held its first meeting on October 12, 1964. (A summary of a meeting called by that committee "to consider joint hospital and Medical School planning" is dated two years later.[16])

In 1964, a "Policy Agreement" spelled out how joint recruitment by the Clinic, the Hitchcock Hospital, and Dartmouth Medical school was to be handled. Mudge, dean at the time, was confident that "the final Policy Agreement was safe, sound, and practical. The key to our future success lay in this basic policy of joint recruitment." He was blunt about it being something of a "novel arrangement," but reported that the kinds of confusions that had arisen earlier were resolved by "the procedures adopted in the Policy Agreement of 1964" as well as "subsequent discussions within the Advisory Board of DMS and the Staff Board of MHMH regarding fund raising." The fundamental issue was the recognition that "four separate [medical] entities were involved," for which "a 'one institution, one purpose' policy" was established.[17] General policy, faculty recruitment, and financial support were the chief recurring areas of concern.[18]

Even though much had been agreed upon, as arguments over whether DMS should return to degree-granting status flared during the early 1970s, Hitchcock Clinic members were divided. "Fortunately," recalled Harry Bird (president of the Clinic from 1984 to 1990), "those of us who favored the academic model prevailed." He was, he said, "quite confident . . . that without the commitment of the . . . full-time clinicians, Dartmouth could never have created an adequate on-site faculty to [do so]."[19]

In preparation for a planned site visit from the Liaison Committee on Medical Education (LCME), in January 1972 Dean Chapman prepared a report. A "Special Note" was appended on "Relations Between Dartmouth Medical School and The Hitchcock Clinic." Chapman admitted that "an orderly system for assignment of function and exchange of funds" had not fully evolved (it was, he said, being worked on and would shortly be in place); his description of the faculty arrangement was remarkably concise:

> Basically all members of the Hitchcock Clinic are part-time members of the Dartmouth Medical School faculty and have the vote in faculty meetings.[20] None is permitted to practice outside the Center and all are on straight salary. There is no incentive system. . . . Administratively, the full-time clinical faculty is paid by the school and is under the jurisdiction of the Dean. The part-time faculty is paid by the Hitchcock Clinic and is under the jurisdiction of its Board of Directors. The two faculty segments are, however, to a significant extent under a unified administration. The Dean and Clinic officials collaborate closely on salary levels and reimbursement principles. In addition, recruitment of new faculty . . . has been by joint mechanism for some time.

Chapman ended this "Special Note" acknowledging that "the existence at Dartmouth of two categories of clinical faculty . . . poses some problems." He insisted none of them was major and that DMS was "unmistakably moving toward the development of a single, unified clinical faculty and [we] anticipate that the most important step in this direction will have been taken by 30 June 1972."[21] The LCME came away apparently convinced that the unusual arrangements they had encountered in Hanover were working. Members of the LCME were particularly struck by the Clinic's policy of equal salaries for members regardless of specialty (based on one of the founding principles of the Clinic, the uniform-salary schedule lasted until 1979). Although they continued to be concerned about whether the Medical School could remain solvent, they were favorably impressed by the results of the affiliation agreement "signed by representatives of the hospital and Dartmouth College on November 23, 1970[, which] established a joint Medical Center Committee." The members of the survey committee also found that "the formal agreement developed by the Hospital and the Medical School provides a framework for facilitating mutual interest while protecting the welfare of each of the parties."[22]

Full agreement on how to proceed was not easily achieved. In June 1972, Chapman sent his colleagues a letter that opened in an anguished tone:

> What follows is a message, a plea if you will, to our clinical faculty, reluctantly and respectfully submitted, in the belief that our common endeavor in the Dartmouth Hitchcock Center is in danger of faltering.
>
> The Faculty of Dartmouth Medical School has, over the last decade, reestablished the M.D. degree, revised its curriculum, and, as part of the Dartmouth-Hitchcock Medical Center has begun to relate constructively and imaginatively to the community of which it is a part. . . . But the organization of the total clinical faculty—full and part-time—has lagged seriously and has now become a very urgent matter.
>
> Our clinical faculty is a house divided, despite hopeful statements to the contrary, and the situation constitutes a serious threat to the Center as a whole: School, Hospital, and Clinic. . . . There is very obviously only one feasible solution to the problem which is to create a truly unified clinical faculty at Hanover.[23]

He was not alone in his assessment that the lack of a "unified clinical faculty" was the central issue. The three-legged stool of research, teaching, and patient care—much talked about, then and now—really needed to be under one administration. And it was not. Trying to get people to understand and accept that any physician hired by the Clinic was going to have to qualify for appointment at DMS and to be granted admitting privileges at the Hospital was no easy task.[24] (The hospital was paymaster to the residents program, which had no ties to the Medical School; the Clinic was paymaster to the clinical staff—most of whom did not want to do research and many of whom seemed to care very little about DMS.)

Mudge responded with a letter of sharp disagreement, both with Chapman's assessment of the situation—he drew attention to what he saw as a contradiction between the LCME's evaluation of the status quo and Chapman's dire predictions of imminent collapse—and with his suggested solution, which Mudge believed was a proposal for "a major administrative reorganization."[25] Full collegiality, even agreeing to disagree, was still some way off (although in 1973 the Dartmouth-Hitchcock Medical Center did officially come into being as an umbrella organization, a point to which we will return).

In May of the following year, 1979, the LCME came calling again.[26] Still very concerned about DMS's "extremely precarious" financial situation, the committee recognized that the School's resources just might be adequate by the mid-1980s (its cautious prediction proved accurate, as we saw, under McCollum). Under the heading "Brief Description of the Dartmouth-Hitchcock Medical Center," the report contained much to say of a very positive nature. "The medical education and medical care situation in Dartmouth is unique in the nation," the committee wrote, in that "it represents the joining together of a developing clinical medical school (DMS), a large community general hospital (MHMH), a large private group (HC), and a federally operated Veterans' Administration hospital (VA)." This claim to uniqueness and the insistence that DMS had a special role to play in medical education for the nation had long been a rallying cry. (Walsh McDermott, in a 1978 consultant's report, had stressed the oft-made point that "if Dartmouth is to survive . . . it must become in some way unique."[27]) But there was more: "It appears that progress has been made in inter-institutional relationships in recent years"; a "situation of mutual need should induce the adoption of bold measure to solve current problems DMS faces in the fiscal arena"; "Relationships between DMS and Dartmouth College are better now than earlier"; "Collaborative efforts with the faculty of Arts and Sciences have recently been intensified with the support of a large institutional (Dartmouth College) grant"; "At the level of Trustees and principal administrators, the interlocking relationship between the separate organizations is centered in the Joint Council of DHMC." Furthermore, the report acknowledged the plans progressing "toward implementation of a four-year curriculum in September 1980." Best of all, in its "Summary and Conclusions," the report ended with the observation that the "improved relationship between the School, Clinic and Hospital, and the recognition of their absolute interdependence, is a most impressive accomplishment since the last LCME visit."[28]

The Dartmouth-Hitchcock Medical Center

The Dartmouth-Hitchcock Medical Center effectively came into being when the constituent organizations moved from an "informal alliance"

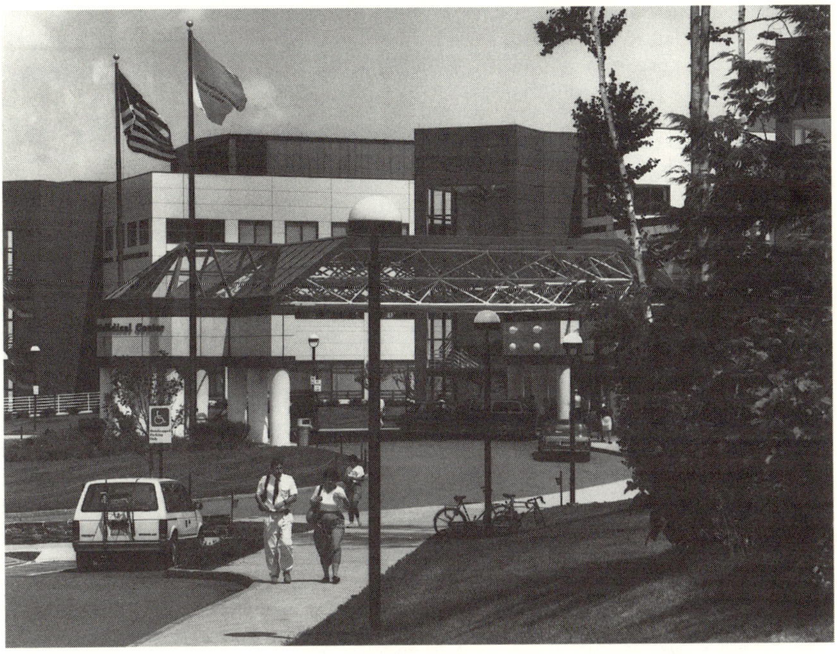

Dartmouth-Hitchcock Medical Center, 1991. Courtesy of Jon Gilbert Fox.

to an "effective confederation" operating under articles of agreement drawn up by the administrative leadership of DMS, the Clinic, and the Mary Hitchcock Memorial Hospital (MHMH). The "first public announcement" was made in a press release of June 19, 1973.[29] A few days prior to that, President Kemeny spoke to the Dartmouth Alumni Council about the creation of "a new body called the Joint Council for the Medical Center" that would initially have "only delegated authority from the three Boards. But it is a Council with the right and the obligation to make plans for the Medical Center as a whole so that we do not have three separate bodies each going its individual way."[30]

By 1980, then, it was de rigueur for the Medical School's main publication to include a diagram illustrating the way the three Hanover-based institutions plus the VA Hospital came together in the Dartmouth-Hitchcock Medical Center governed by a "Joint Council." A prose description of the Medical School accompanied the diagram:

> Dartmouth Medical School is a component of the Dartmouth-Hitchcock Medical Center, an organization established in 1973 to coordinate the work of its

member institutions in patient care, training for medical students and residents, continuing education for health professionals, and biomedical research. Through this body, the members plan and act together for their mutual advantage while each retains its corporate integrity.

The "three other components of the Center"—Mary Hitchcock Memorial Hospital, the Hitchcock Clinic, and the Veterans' Administration Hospital (the latter is often not listed, so that it sometimes appeared there was a total of three "components" rather than four)—were then named and described; in each case the exact relationship with DMS was indicated. The Mary Hitchcock, for example, was identified as "the principal teaching hospital for DMS. It affords clinical instruction in outpatient and inpatient care as well as in operating room and laboratory procedures." (If truth be told, however, when Robert McCollum began serving as dean of the Medical School, the "central organization of Dartmouth-Hitchcock Medical Center was still in its infancy and still just an advisory body, while its individual members were accustomed to acting very much on their own."[31]) On the next page, under "Other Resources," the Norris Cotton Cancer Center, the Dartmouth-Hitchcock Mental Health Center, and the Hitchcock Foundation were also briefly described. Clearly, the Medical School wanted to be seen as an integral part of something much larger and more comprehensive.[32]

It was not always thus. The increased amounts of federal money made available beginning in the 1960s, which greatly enhanced the feasibility of the "refounding" of the medical school, also affected the Clinic. If the Clinic wanted to remain independent of the sometimes-floundering school, it is not altogether surprising. But when talk about reinstating a four-year program at the medical school became earnest, it was clear that there needed to be a renegotiation of the relationship between the Hospital and the Clinic as well as between DMS and the Clinic. Efforts to balance responsibilities and roles of the various players intensified in 1974, but discussions about creating a genuine medical center—an umbrella organization—turned into a further point of tension. The mood at times was "somewhat acrimonious," according to John Collins, CEO of the Clinic for more than three decades. By no means everyone approved the School's expansion, nor was everyone in favor of the concept of a medical center. The benefits of a formal arrangement among the institutions were not intuitively obvious. The Clinic had such a strong ethic of clinical care that the medical school's insistence on the need for research seemed a bit suspect to some; the Medical School argued that good teaching and good clinical practice were both dependent on research. The tensions had to do with what, exactly, an outstanding academic medical center should look like. In well-established centers of the sort Dartmouth emulated, much of the basic research was carried out in clinical departments. But at DMS at the time it was less clear what was expected, what could be achieved. The clinical departments were by and large staffed by clinicians who wanted, hardly surprisingly, to practice clinical medicine. Teaching and doing research on top of that were not always easily accepted (or fully understood) parts of the deal.[33]

By 1983 the Dartmouth-Hitchcock Medical Center, functioning on an ad hoc basis for a decade, was formally incorporated. More than one observer has expressed the view that the prolonged debates worked, in the end, to everyone's advantage. A better balance of power was established than would have resulted if one institution had prevailed in all the bargaining from the outset. The symbiotic relationships among the constituent groups belonging to DHMC—so essential to making the whole enterprise functional—took time to mature. Today, Collins says, the institutions that comprise DHMC are "interdependent" organizations; they take turns "carrying the heavy water," is the way Harry Bird puts it.

Another step beyond incorporation remained, however, before DHMC would be not just theoretically or corporately or administratively an umbrella organization but also physically a unit that all the watching world could see as a significant institution. The move to a new "campus" in Lebanon in 1991 dramatically marked what close observers had known for some time: DMS and the medical center of which it is part had truly come of age. Yet the plan to move did not meet with immediate and total agreement. The VA Hospital remained in White River Junction, Vermont; thus, the new DHMC campus was still not the home for the whole Medical Center. More controversially, the Medical School faculty itself was split.[34] The not-so-old basic science buildings, the source of so much pride and symbol of so much progress when they were constructed in the 1960s and 1970s, found themselves home once again to students only in the first two years of medical school. The clinical years would be spent largely on the Lebanon campus, at the new hospital. (Research would continue to come out of both Hanover and White River Junction; this would be vigorously encouraged and supported in Lebanon. With the occupancy of the Borwell Building, additional excellent research comes also from the DHMC campus in Lebanon.)

The need for the move to Lebanon arose first because Hospital and Clinic alike had simply run out of space. New services in the Hospital "found themselves in odd places; the Intensive Care Nursery was constructed on the roof of the East Wing." And the Clinic was "unable to recruit additional staff members, however much they were needed, because of the shortage of examining rooms." Parking "had become a daily logistical nightmare for patients, staff, and visitors." When the Dewey Field "plan for coping with the problems of the physical space" was developed in 1982 but then turned down by the town of Hanover, something had to give. Once expansion in Hanover was no longer an option, "the unwelcome prospect of splitting operations by developing a second campus was raised."[35] Finally, in the autumn of 1985, the "resolution recommending that Dartmouth College purchase the present Hospital land and buildings; that a unified DHMC move to an off-site location; and that the College work with DHMC on a capital campaign," was passed by the Medical School faculty on a vote of 136 to 3. The Medical School was on board.[36] (The Medical School would nonetheless always be a slightly "different" member of the DHMC, since it is connected to Dartmouth College in a way that the Hospital, the Clinic, and the VA Hospital are not.) A "Memorandum of Understanding" was drawn up between the College and the MHMH on December 19, 1985.[37] The trustees' statement approving the relocation of the Medical School facilities came six months later, on June 8, 1986.[38] A major source of tension was the threat by the Clinic to build its own facility elsewhere (it owned land near where the DHMC was eventually built); not surprisingly, this did not sit well with the Hospital. President McLaughlin's ambitions for College expansion helped tip the balance. Compromises always leave a feeling of frustration or disappointment; however necessary the move may have finally seemed, there is no question that physically separating the basic science faculty was not helpful. Collaborations became more difficult. On the other hand, the new physical complex would not have been possible without the space gained by the move.

The whole enterprise was, of course, enormously complicated; views on the wisdom of the plan ranged from conviction that the move was the right thing to do to the certainty that it was a poor institutional strategy. But in time, as the very real benefits of having more space became evident, even the nay-sayers began to come around. Some of the structure's most novel features—and most satisfying—are the result of the "idea of horizontal adjacency," which "became the organizing theory of the design."[39] Nor was that all. "The trustees, physicians, researchers, nurses, administrators and patients met for months to come up with an overall philosophy for the hospital. Their first thought was to design a hospital with the convenience of those who worked in it every day foremost; but they soon decided to put the patients' needs first," according to hospital spokeswoman Georgia Croft. "'When this began, doctors were told that they would have large offices. They have small offices.'"[40] Within a relatively short time, in part because the bulk of the old hospital on Maynard Street had been razed, no one could imagine returning to the status quo ante. And although the sheer size and gleaming newness of the sprawling complex may be a bit intimidating, the inside is as warm and light and cheerful as a hospital could conceivably be. Certainly it was a change from the dark, twisting, confusing corridors and tunnels of the warren that had evolved from the original and very handsome MHMH. (Not that there weren't moments of nostalgic regret. James Varnum, president of the Mary Hitchcock Memorial Hospital, wrote a letter to all the Hospital and Clinic staff just after the move had been made, acknowledging the mixed feelings shared by many: "There was a joy, an anticipation and an excitement about our move to our new facilities, but at the same time there was a feeling of nostalgia about leaving behind so many memories at Maynard Street."[41])

Moving day—"M-Day" (October 5, 1991)—was a major and dramatic exercise in logistics. Varnum's letter praised employees for their role in making everything go smoothly. The myriad people involved in organizing and carrying out the massive undertaking seem to have thought of everything. "The biggest moving party in northern New England's history—the relocation of Dartmouth-Hitchcock Medical Center and 232 patients from Hanover to new quarters . . . three miles down the road—was held yesterday," wrote one reporter. "Thanks to two years of planning and more than 3,000 movers, the transition proceeded, in the words of a nursing director, 'slick as ice.' "[42]

The dedication celebration—held on a splendid autumn weekend three weeks earlier (September 13 and 14, 1991) and billed "Transferring the Tradition"—was full of symbolic events and gestures. There was substance, too. C. Everett Koop (DC 1937, founder of the C. Everett Koop Institute at Dartmouth, and former U.S. Surgeon General) was the keynote speaker, challenging DHMC to play a leadership role in the problems facing American medicine. A symposium organized by John Wennberg, director of the Center for the Evaluative Clinical Sciences at DMS, had an impressive group of panelists looking critically at health care reform. The symposium's title was both symbolic and descriptive of the serious discussion that emerged: "Moving to New Ground: Reallocating vs. Rationing Medical Care" solved no problems that day, but it brought into focus some of the weaknesses in the delivery of health care in the United States.[43]

The move to DHMC's new home on the Lebanon campus has been both the catalyst and a result of ongoing developments, according to one faculty member. Signage provides visible reminders that the Medical Center is more than a hospital. The full name—Dartmouth-Hitchcock

Medical Center—appears over the main entrance; inside, standing at the information desk in the rotunda, those who raise their eyes can see the individual names of the three constituent parts of DHMC housed on the Lebanon campus emblazoned on the overhead balconies: "Mary Hitchcock Memorial Hospital," "Dartmouth-Hitchcock Clinic," "Dartmouth Medical School." It is a medical center known for its distinctive culture, for having a more collegial environment than most traditional academic medical centers.

Even late in his tenure as dean, Andrew Wallace in 1997 (several years after the formal incorporation of DHMC) still found the relations among the distinct entities that make up the Medical Center among the most challenging matters he had to deal with; the nature of the relationship of each with DMS was, he believed, "never really adequately resolved." (On the other hand, when he was stepping down as dean, one of the individuals he singled out was John Hennessy, chair of the DHMC Board for much of Wallace's term as dean, for "fostering increased harmony among the Center's component institutions.")[44] The bottom line in any case, according to an outside consultant, is that it is impossible to "stress enough how different this place is from most healthcare organizations." DHMC is, she says, "a diamond in the woods."[45] Although there is no actual diamond to be displayed, "in the woods" is quite literally true. The DHMC campus is a largely tree-covered 200 acres.

DMS and Regional Involvement

The Mary Hitchcock Memorial Hospital has long been an important regional resource, a tertiary-care hospital that has saved many a northern New England patient from the need to travel to Boston. The Hitchcock Clinic also served patients beyond Hanover (sometimes well beyond) from its opening day, though as we saw earlier, the founders were concerned that they not seem to be competing with local doctors; they wanted their expertise to be a supplemental benefit to the region. In recent years, for instance, some of the specialists have periodically worked in local hospitals (by invitation), and in the 1970s both the new neonatal unit and the oncology services developed into statewide resources.[46]

But neither the size and importance of the MHMH nor the spread of Hitchcock Clinic sites is the only sign that the DHMC is actively engaged in outreach and has regional importance. As DMS's second century ended in 1997, Dean Andrew Wallace could report that in addition to

DMS's fourteen clinical and basic science departments, the Center for the Evaluative Clinical Sciences, the Norris Cotton Cancer Center, and "other nationally recognized programs," Dartmouth Medical School boasted "some 550 full-time faculty member who secured $49 million in research grants in 1995–96, almost 1,000 part-time and adjunct faculty from throughout northern New England and across the country, and nearly 300 medical and 150 graduate students."[47]

A brief look at some of the curricular changes toward the end of DMS's second century and particularly at the way the Department of Community and Family Medicine (formed in 1971) has evolved will illustrate how far DMS has come since the desperate days when it was put on confidential probation, was staring closure in the face, and needed so desperately to be vigorously and creatively refounded. A reasonable terminus a quo is the recruitment to the faculty of Thomas Almy in 1968. Many have testified to his direct and indirect influence on the shape of the curriculum over the next several decades. From the outset, he was concerned that the Medical School should be more involved in the medical care of the whole region. One of the earliest actions he took was to prepare, with Dean Chapman, a proposal "to establish an integrated relationship between the Medical School and seven (or more) community hospitals in the Upper Connecticut River Valley for the express purposes of upgrading rural medical care and developing a new system for the teaching of medicine at all levels."[48] The Medical School Survey Committee, when it delivered its "Final Report" to the College Trustees in 1973, included some strong language on the subject: "In Northern New England, the Dartmouth Medical School has a mission which extends beyond that of a peer relationship to other excellent medical schools. . . . For a medical school in rural United States, reestablishing an M.D. program in the seventies which attempts to replicate the traditional urban-based medical center would be both anachronistic and unrealistic."

The report went on to say that a rural medical school had no business boasting about the quality of its intramural biomedical activities if it was going to "remain indifferent to the deprivations of medical care experienced by its rural constituency. The rural medical school should accept the challenge of optimizing its resources to develop programs which are of high academic quality and which carry over broad benefits to its rural residents." The point was pounded home: DMS "cannot choose to be an indifferent spectator of the rural health care system. . . . A medical school responsive to the health needs of the surrounding rural communities will lead the way to the reenfranchisement of rural residents in their right to decent medical care."[49]

A brochure about DMS released around that same time, in seeking to clarify the new "Dartmouth Medical Plan" (the "shortened, more flexible curriculum" described earlier), stressed a related commitment: "Through its developing programs in primary care, Dartmouth has taken a strong initiative in responding to the critical need for general practitioners, now an endangered species in the United States. . . . Although this face of education prepares the student for practice in both urban and non-urban environments, an increasing number of students are considering taking up practice in rural communities where they can make the most positive impact."[50]

One of the most explicit demonstrations of this commitment to regional health care came with the announcement in 1977 that the Mellon Foundation had granted Dartmouth Medical school $450,000 "to support an educational program designed to augment students' clinical training in primary care medicine." In particular, the three-year grant was to be "used to refine the Medical School's Rural Outreach Program which extends the education resources of the School and enables students to gain practice experience in teaching sites located in nearby communities in the northern New England region."[51] Much of the credit for "finding office sites where DMS students could be mentored in ambulatory medicine" goes to Almy. His work and that of his colleagues in Community Medicine, like Michael Zubkoff, led to the formation of "a new category of faculty—regional physicians [later adjunct faculty], who took students into their office practices." A year later, with colleague John Wasson, "Almy developed at the VA the first model curriculum to focus on the one-on-one, doctor-patient relationship in primary care."[52]

This was a major step forward from the days in the early 1950s when Jerome Nolan—determined to do a residency in general practice in New England—fell in love with the Mary Hitchcock despite its lack of such a residency (which several other New England hospitals *did* offer). Assured that "something could be arranged"—another example of the vaunted personal touch at Dartmouth—Nolan used the latter part of his rotating internship (1952–1953) at the Hitchcock to set up his own general practice residency for the following year. Although it is to the credit of the Dartmouth doctors that they gave him the go-ahead and were, throughout, very supportive, most of the credit for building that residency program goes to Nolan himself. The "most terrifying part of the entire residency" was when he was pushed into serving as a locum tenens for Dr. Israel Dinerman, in Canaan. "I wondered," he reminisced, "whether I was fit for general practice at all." Yet clearly the program he and the MHMH staff devised was effective; Nolan went on to work as a general practitioner for many years in the Exeter, New Hampshire, Clinic (modeled, apparently, to some extent on the Hitchcock Clinic).[53]

That there was still a real need a quarter of a century later for training aimed more specifically at preparing students for careers in primary care medicine ("primary care" or "generalist" physician and "family practitioner" have replaced "general practitioner" as the preferred nomenclature today) is clear from what one of the new "adjunct faculty" members had to say in an article written in 1979. His autobiographical account of how he "carried the dream of being a rural practitioner through the academic world into reality in a New Hampshire town" illustrates the "inadequacies" of traditional training in internal medicine "for a career in primary care." No wonder he was happy to have his practice in New London, New Hampshire—thirty miles from Dartmouth—become a clerkship practice site for DMS students.[54]

Support for the commitment to rural medicine also came from the Hitchcock Foundation. A 1981 document explaining why the Foundation was seeking an expanded endowment emphasized the opportunity that increased funding would create "to focus on one very special area of clinical research . . . that centering on community health problems which are special to the northern areas of New England." (Examples of projects already under way at the time were a comprehensive evaluation of hundreds of members of an extended family with a high incidence of thyroid cancer and one involving the rehabilitation of stroke patients.)[55]

That DMS wanted its connection to the region to be seen as part of its program is also clear from several different kinds of evidence. In 1976, a press release reported a bequest to DMS in memory of New Hampshire native Edward Carlton Atwood (DC 1871) that made explicit reference to how DMS's "location, in the North Country of New England" made "family practice in rural surroundings . . . a natural part of the clinical experience for students."[56] On another occasion, a press release was issued to make a point of how many New Hampshire residents were studying at DMS, and then-dean James Strickler was quoted as saying that " 'The school makes a special effort, as New Hampshire's only school of medicine, to help this state.' "[57] One example of very practical help for Vermont as well as New Hampshire is the Dartmouth-Hitchcock Air Response Team (DHART), a helicopter ambulance service introduced in 1994. In a little more than three years of operation, more than 1,000 flights (many different sorts of life-saving transports) convinced even early skeptics of the service's value.[58]

Some of these activities and programs have to do more directly with the Hitchock Hospital than with DMS, but drawing a rigid line between the two is virtually impossible and would be pointless in any case, given that both are part of DHMC. In the late 1980s, with the primary care clerkship already a decade old, DMS was in prime position to make adjustments to its clinical curriculum to take into account the growing realization that more and more medicine is likely to be practiced in outpatient settings. In the autumn of 1989, the new clinical curriculum significantly increased "the intensity and the quality of outpatient clinical training for medical students."[59] Within two years, there were five more weeks of clerkships available to students than there had been, and Dean Andrew Wallace was stressing the "need to free up some time for students to go out and ask questions and find the answers"—as opposed to sitting in lecture halls. While acknowledging that DMS, like other medical schools, needed constantly to reevaluate the curriculum of the first two years, he also was convinced that Dartmouth was "ahead of its time." He explained:

> For many years, our second-year Scientific Basis of Medicine (SBM) course has epitomized what everyone is saying the system needs. . . . SBM still has a fair amount of lecture time, but it does an excellent job of weaving together basic science knowledge, clinical problems, and physical diagnosis skills in ways that are targeted towards understanding *real* problems that *real* physicians have to solve, rather than cutting medicine up neatly into the basic sciences here and the clinical sciences there.[60]

The stage was set for the curriculum revision that would come to be called "New Directions." By September of 1994, the Office of Admissions for the Medical School was able to talk about the available clinical facilities (DHMC), the range of patient populations and health-care settings that DMS students could be exposed to (the clerkships set up by the Department of Community and Family Medicine), the College's C. Everett Koop Institute (CEKI) founded the previous year ("dedicated to influencing, on a national level, the practice of medicine, health-care delivery, and medical education"), as well as the "New Directions" curriculum, the first stages of which were being introduced that autumn. The program was described thus for prospective students:

> DMS has entered an exciting period of curricular examination and revision. The broad framework of our newly revised curriculum, called "New Directions," is designed to integrate the study of basic and clinical sciences throughout medical school while supporting close working relationships between students and the faculty. A hallmark of the curriculum is the Longitudinal Clinical Experience, a required course that pairs students with faculty practitioners in local communities. Clinical training in the LCE, which begins shortly after matriculation, alternates with biweekly tutorials. . . .
>
> Curricular revision at DMS also supports small-group and independent learning opportunities. Study in the second year, for example, has evolved in recent years from 80 percent lectures to 60 percent seminars.[61]

The document's few brief paragraphs on the "New Directions" curriculum and the passing reference to the CEKI belied the enormous amount of time and energy that went into their creation. A planning grant from the Robert Wood Johnson (RWJ) Foundation was used to explore these ventures. The goals of the RWJ grant were ambitious; the curricular revision was aimed specifically at increasing the number of primary care physicians. The interface between the intellectual content of the courses and the social-change agenda of the CEKI was the institutional context of what was to be taught. The curricular reform was already in progress when Koop returned to Dartmouth. Driven "in part by the desire of students at DMS to have clinical training be more integrated with basic science" and in part by "the students' own growing commitment to community service," the changes implicit in the "New Directions" curriculum looked like exactly the kinds of changes that "could put form around Koop's ideas." (The Koop Institute's "stock-in-trade," it has been said, "is ideas.") DMS was interested in trying to hold a middle ground where all its students would develop the attitudes of the generalist even if they chose to become specialists; this fit well with Koop's championing the "call for a return to the family doctor concept of care."

CEKI may not have worked out quite the way some people envisioned it; among the disillusioned was John Duffy, director of the Institute for its first year and a half. (Koop himself from the outset held the title of "Senior Scholar.") When Duffy stepped down, it was out of frustration over inability to get programs off paper and into place. CEKI remains "little more than an intriguing idea," we are told Duffy thought.[62] Yet it is an experiment that has withstood the test of time, evolving as so much else does when ideas about educational reform are what is at issue. CEKI has ties to the College, the Tuck School of Business Administration, and the Thayer School of Engineering as well. And as Koop's central place in the program at the DHMC dedication testifies, he and his institute are still very much part of the DMS picture. The institute has, we are told, "concentrated on programs in social service and education and on technology projects and initiatives." Particularly well received by students are two programs: "Partners in Health Education" (students in their first two years of medical school are "paired with K–12 classroom teachers throughout the . . . region to teach health education in the public schools") and "Healing and the Arts" (which includes the course in life drawing mentioned earlier and "hands-on cooperation between medical students and pediatric and adolescent patients" at DHMC "in such activities as painting, puppetry, ceramics and model making"). Another initiative of CEKI is "World Wide Web-based teaching, yet another step in the pioneering use of telemedicine at DMS."[63]

Koop's own reflections include the belief that some of the attitude changes initiated at DMS—especially the attitude of faculty and administration toward students—were unique among medical schools at the time; if such improvements are now visible elsewhere as well, that should be a source of considerable satisfaction. The work of CEKI continues, "not only locally," but within the framework of a consortium of more than a dozen medical schools. A longitudinal study aimed at finding out "what happens to medical student thinking during their years of study" set out to devise more accurate means of choosing the students among medical school candidates "those who will serve their patients well."[64]

At the end of two hundred years of uninterrupted teaching, DMS was once again being innovative, as it "rolled out a new plan for the third year of the curriculum." The main thrust was to make a few "specific improvements" in the traditional third-year clerkships and then to "bundle" them to make explicit the way some topics are shared across clerkships, and to teach those shared topics more efficiently. "In the spirit of overall quality improvement that we've applied to the whole curriculum, the stimulus was to take something that we were doing pretty well and do it even better," according to David Nierenberg, the associate dean for medical education who also oversees the New Directions curriculum. Koop himself likes to quote the saying that it is easier to move a graveyard than to change a curriculum. That DMS has been willing so often to engage in a reevaluation of its curriculum (this was very much a team effort) is a sign of its strength and stability.

CEKI and CECS (with which CEKI has been closely allied) between them rank high in the "media mentions" that come DMS's way. Both have worked with the Department of Community and Family Medicine, which is—appropriately—the home base of many of the efforts to increase the number and percentage of students going into primary care medicine. The Dartmouth Primary Care Cooperative Project (Dartmouth COOP) makes it possible for the community doctors, the adjunct faculty, to come together for mutual support; this program, unique to DMS, has proved to be an effective and productive alliance that coordinates primary care research and teaching across northern New England. The family medicine clerkship, where those adjunct faculty really come into their own, has been rated by students as the best required clerkship experience year after year. Before the late Thomas Almy's retirement, it could perhaps have been said that the Department of Community and Family Medicine covered the medical school curriculum (there are required courses in the department for students in each of the four years) from A (Almy) to Z (Zubkoff).

Only at Dartmouth

Just before arriving in Hanover to take up the post of dean, Andrew Wallace wrote to the DMS faculty to "set out . . . two goals." In his final "From the Dean" column in *Dartmouth Medicine*, eight years later (in 1998), he reminded his readers of what those two goals were: "One was to make [DMS] an even more *distinguished* institution—to increase its recognition nationally; the other was to make it more *distinguishable*—to identify and capitalize on the things that make DMS discernibly different." He went on to say he thought significant progress had been made in both of those areas, and to express his gratitude to "everybody who has helped to move DMS ever closer to achieving its potential to be one of America's best medical schools, in a unique, Dartmouth sort of way."[65]

Some of what might be meant by a "unique, Dartmouth sort of way" can be deduced from the story told in the preceding pages. The very history of the school, from its unusual beginning as the brainchild of a single entrepreneurial physician, through the trials and tribulations of the post-Flexner period, to the refounding under the guidance of Stephen Marsh Tenney, to the reinstatement of the full M.D. program (the work of many, but carried out under the leadership of Carleton B. Chapman), sets it apart. Its small size (at some times *very* small) and rural location (DMS is the only medical school in the country that is part of a major medical center with a teaching hospital in a municipality as small as Lebanon, New Hampshire) have always been part of what makes Dartmouth Medical School different. And then there is that elusive factor of the "culture." Pressed on the use of the word, staff and faculty members connected with DHMC persist: Yes, they say, the culture difference at Dartmouth-Hitchcock is very real. The most recent past president of the Clinic—cardiothoracic surgeon Stephen K. Plume—calls it "the Dartmouth flavor."

Part of that flavor comes from the fact that research has for a long time been a vital component of life at Dartmouth Medical School. A relaxed spirit and a welcoming culture at Dartmouth Medical School (different from the high-pressure, hypercompetitive atmosphere of many institutions) has encouraged research of all kinds—in basic and clinical sciences. To cite just one of several benchmarks along the way that could be singled out: In the 1988–1989 funding year, DMS income from sponsored research reached a record high of $25 million; a year later, a staggering 36 percent jump in grants and contracts brought the total to $34 million (mentioned in the previous chapter).[66] Teaching has always been considered an important activity, but one that complements, and is complemented by, research. That research at DMS is of both the clinical- and the bench-science sort makes sense. Many of the basic-science researchers were (and are) practicing physicians with clinical commitments. Though each has a research base in a basic-science department, some of them have a primary appointment in a clinical department.

Of course another way to mark out what makes a place "distinguishable" is to talk about its innovations, special achievements, or programs it was the first to produce. The matter of priority is not always one of great importance; there is too much evidence that new knowledge often surfaces in several places more or less simultaneously. Yet DMS does have a number of "firsts" or near-firsts of a wide variety to its credit. With no claim to completeness or comprehensiveness, the examples given next illustrate the point.

A nineteenth-century story (for which we do not have the exact dates) tells of a little-known "first." Dartmouth faculty member Dixi Crosby was sued by a patient whose broken leg he had set. When subsequent abscess and gangrene resulted in a shortening of the patient's leg, the patient decided to sue—eight years later! The verdict initially went against Crosby (for $800), but he won on appeal. According to James Spalding, who relates the story, the case "attracted attention throughout the entire nation, because . . . it was the first case in which a consulting surgeon had ever been sued for malpractice." Furthermore, "it was the first suit in which so long a period elapsed after the date of the original visit before proceedings were completed." When it was all over, "Dr. Dixi received congratulations from the entire medical profession in this country, and many kind letters from Europe."[67] But this belongs to the category of amusing tidbits from the past. A much more important piece of history took place at Dartmouth, on February 4, 1896. Just eight days after the New York *Sun* published a story about Wilhelm Conrad Roentgen's breakthrough discovery of x-rays, a Hanover photographer named H. H. Langill brought the matter to the attention of Frank Austin, an assistant in Dartmouth College's physics department. They in turn enlisted physics department professor Edwin Frost—who like Langill and Austin belonged to the Dartmouth Scientific Association. Though Austin is almost certainly the one who found the tube that would work, Edwin Frost was the one who "took charge of the crucial clinical experiment" (and later wrote it up for publication), which entailed x-raying the broken arm of a patient brought to the physics lab by Frost's brother, Gilman Dubois Frost of the Medical School. Thus it was a "town-and-gown thing," according to Peter Spiegel, chair of DMS's

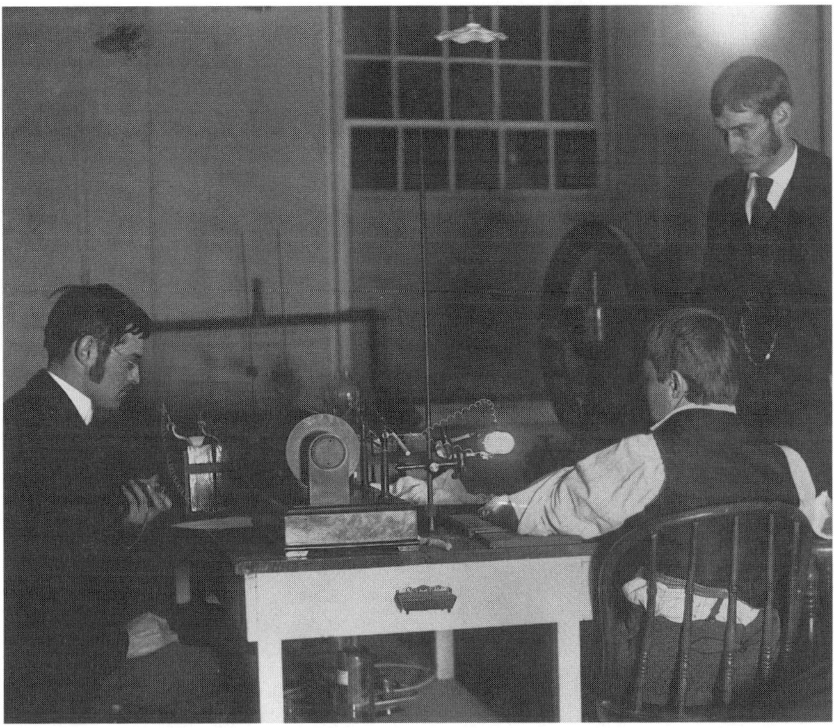

First x-ray taken for medical diagnosis, 1896. Courtesy of Dartmouth College Archives.

radiology department.[68] The x-ray taken that wintry day is significant in that it was the first clinical x-ray, taken for diagnostic purposes, in the United States.[69]

Probably less well known but extremely important for subsequent developments in the practice of hospital medicine was the development in 1955 by William T. Mosenthal at MHMH of the nation's first intensive care unit, facilitating more efficient care for acutely ill patients (and less disruption for other patients). Two years later, in 1957, Radford Tanzer—founder of the plastic surgery program at DHMC—developed what became the standard technique for total ear reconstruction. He is recognized internationally as the "Father of Ear Surgery." In an earlier piece of ingenious reconstructive surgery, done while he was in Utah during World War II, Tanzer constructed a thumb out of one finger for a patient who had cut his thumb off. Although his superior advised against the novel and time-consuming surgery, Tanzer insisted—on the grounds that some degree of opposed digits, even if inelegant and not completely "normal," would be more useful for a man than a hand with four fingers and no thumb at all. (He was right, as it turned out; his reconstruction worked well.)[70] This echoes nicely the attitude of Nathan Smith, exemplified by his advice to students that if "you can save one finger it will be best to save it. . . . A part of a hand would be of great use" to a man.[71]

Nathan Smith's first faculty assistant—also his friend, apprentice, and protégé—Lyman Spalding was, in 1820 (shortly before his early death), the author of the first U.S. pharmacopoeia. This alone is enough to secure Spalding's place in American medical history. (The significance of that publication is easy to underestimate today, when national and international pharmaceutical agreements and standards are largely taken for granted. In the first decades of the nineteenth century, it had not yet been fully grasped why it might be important to consolidate and standardize epidemiological or therapeutic information.) A latter-day Lyman Spalding at DMS is Robert Gosselin, founder of DHMC's poison control project and coauthor of what has widely been called the "bible" of poison information hotlines. The *Clinical Toxicology of Commercial Products*, first published in 1957, has gone through numerous editions.[72]

Important though scientific discoveries are—and they are being made at DMS—it may be that what truly sets Dartmouth apart, the more striking characteristics of the place, are of a rather different sort. Two examples of activities having to do with DMS's regional involvement, mentioned earlier, deserve special mention. The Primary Care Cooperative Project that allowed "physicians throughout a large and essentially rural area to take a close common look at the quality of health care they provide" was a first of its kind in the nation.[73] A decade or so later, the state of New Hampshire and DMS forged an agreement for the provision of mental health services in the state—a first in the nation.[74]

If Dartmouth is different, if Dartmouth has unique qualities, some of the difference and some of the uniqueness can probably best be found in cooperative enterprises like this. Whether they really add up to making Dartmouth a different place in an important way, however, remains to some extent a matter of interpretation. Former dean Marsh Tenney once said that although medical schools like to advertise their differences and stress how their curricular objectives are somehow distinctive, it is not clear how significant that is; the real differences tend not to emerge until the years of postgraduate education. This did not deter Tenney from helping to initiate some of the different things that have been done at DMS. Furthermore, at the time of the School's bicentennial celebration, a veritable catalogue of "The Dartmouth Difference" was compiled in an article with that title; three sidebars gave the views of Nathan

Smith's 1806 student William Tully, DMS faculty member (since 1959) Frances McCann, and ten graduates scattered through every decade from the 1940s. For all the variety in reasons these individuals gave for being at Dartmouth, there is still reason to think that for those students who have chosen to be part of the DMS community over a period of two centuries, "Something about Dartmouth made a difference."[75]

What makes a place seem different is bound to be subjective; what counts as especially noteworthy is also dependent on point of view. A few more examples make clear that DMS today is far more concerned with making delivery of health care, teaching, and basic research mesh than with what may have been done first at DHMC or how Dartmouth is—or isn't—"different."

Constance Brinckerhoff started as a postdoc with Edward (Ted) Harris, an outstanding physician-scientist and rheumatologist, in medicine; she went on to clone the collegenase enzyme and has done outstanding work on inflammatory processes. The Department of Medicine gradually introduced more basic researchers: Lester Salans, working in endocrinology and metabolism, was active clinically and had a significant basic research program going. He worked on insulin mechanisms with Samuel Cushman (another postdoc), who in turn collaborated with Gustav Lienhard in biochemistry on work that eventually led Cushman to the discovery of the glucose transporter after he moved to the NIH. Lienhard later discovered one of the insulin receptor subtrates' (IRS), important components of the metabolic response to insulin.

In biochemistry, outstanding work has been done by Bernard Trumpower on oxidative phosphorylation, by Oscar Scornik on protein degradation, by T. Y. Chang on cholesterol metabolism, by Jay Dunlap and Jennifer Loros on clock genes, and by William Wickner on transport across cell membranes. Kendall Smith, after spending some time at the NIH, conducted research at Dartmouth in immunology; he made significant contributions to understanding the role of interleukin-2 (originally called T-cell growth factor, or TCGF) in the immune response. He and Allan Munck collaborated in research on the glucocorticoid receptors Munck had discovered in the 1960s (mentioned earlier) in patients with leukemia and lymphoma who were undergoing treatment with glucocorticoids. Charles Wira, one of the first Ph.D.'s from the graduate program in physiology, joined the DMS faculty in the early 1970s. He has studied the immunology of the female reproductive tract in both rats and humans, collaborating with researchers from physiology, obbstetrics and bynecology, pathology, and microbiology.

Anikó and Géza Fejes-Tóth discovered an enzyme called 11-beta hydroxysteroid dehydrogenase type 2, which plays a crucial role in allowing aldosterone to get to receptors in its target cells. Leslie Henderson has carried out penetrating electrophysiological studies on how anabolic androgenic steroids act to regulate neurotransmitter receptors. Paul Guyre was the first to observe an effect of gamma interferon on Fc receptors (a discovery for which he is rarely credited, because at the time he did not identify it as gamma interferon and instead called it Fc Receptor Activating Factor, or FRAF).

All of which brings us back to the important and close relationship between research—bench or clinical—and practice. Along with teaching, all of these continue to be critical to DMS today.

"Forward to the Past"

Is it too far-fetched to see DMS today as an extension of Nathan Smith's dream? The students are, happily, no longer just northern New England "boys"—and much else has changed. Indeed, more has changed than has remained the same. Yet the renewed emphasis on serving the region, the efforts to teach medical students to think like doctors rather than merely to cram them full of information, the projects aimed at putting students in the best-possible position to develop the best-possible doctor–patient relationships—these are all implicit in the way Nathan Smith practiced medicine and taught his students. He was a pioneer in patient-centered medical and surgical practice, even if he did not use today's phrases like "shared decision-making" and "watchful waiting." We have no reason to think he would disapprove at all of the way teaching, patient care, and biomedical research—all clearly here to stay in the "new DMS"—work together.

Indirect tributes to Nathan Smith and the lessons to be learned from the past were to be expected in the school's bicentennial year, 1997, especially. Jordan Cohen, president of the Association of American Medical Colleges, the Class Day speaker who addressed the students graduating in Dartmouth Medical School's 200th year, put a novel spin on the historic occasion by titling his talk "Forward to the Past." As President Freedman would say in his opening address at the school's main bicentennial celebration event—the symposium on "Great Issues for Medicine in the Twenty-first Century"—"progress is not inevitable," "progress is not without challenge." And therein lies the tension that any medical student and any medical school must learn to use productively. "As we contemplate the role of medical education in the American future," Freedman said in closing his remarks, "I am confident that Dartmouth Medical School will not succumb in the critical years that lie ahead; that it will remain identifiable to us as an integral part of Dartmouth's liberal arts environment; and that as it ventures forth into its third century, . . . it will prove still again the indisputable truth of progress."[76]

Indisputably, there has been progress at DMS. Some of the changes that were mentioned at the time of another bicentennial event—the "Birthday Party" itself—seem almost quaint. It is difficult to imagine DMS without its M.D. program, without the development of programs in family medicine and community health care, without its Board of Overseers, without ties to the Ethics Institute, minus the DHMC "umbrella," without the vast improvement in endowment that resulted from DMS's outstanding contribution to the College's five-year "Will to Excel Campaign," without women students, without vigorous involvement in volunteer community service on the part of 80 percent of the DMS student body. Yet each of these was at one point an innovation; none of this progress was inevitable. Shortly before Andrew Wallace arrived as dean in 1990, he wrote the faculty, saying, "I begin this new adventure with you convinced that no school in America provides a better atmosphere, a higher sense of values, and as appropriate a balance as Dartmouth."[77] In the course of giving the Alan Gregg Lecture at the American Association of Medical Colleges' 1996 national meeting, Wallace touched on that theme again in an oblique way: "When I came to Hanover as dean, an important part of my rationale was that I felt Dartmouth was a place that could turn out the kind of doctors our country needs most." In quoting from President Freedman's book *Idealism and Liberal Education*, Wallace aligned himself both with Freedman and—aptly, under the circumstances—with Alan Gregg. Gregg, like Freedman, would have endorsed Wallace's expressed conviction that "a liberal education is the soundest platform for our profession."[78] Wedded to the idea that Dartmouth College and Dartmouth Medical School were in a mutually beneficial relationship, Wallace—as he approached the end of his decanal service in DMS's bicentennial year—seems to have sensed that the venerable medical school was poised for the future. In the letter to "Friends of DMS" in which he publicly announced that he would be stepping down at the end of his second four-year term, he confirmed that: "We approach both DMS's third century and the new millennium full of hope and promise, confident that Dartmouth Medical School will continue to make a difference."[79]

APPENDIXES

APPENDIX A

*Dartmouth Medical School Deans**

William Thayer Smith	1896–1909
John Martin Gile	1910–1925
Colin Campbell Stewart II (Acting)	1925–1927
John Pollard Bowler	1927–1945
Rolf Christian Syvertsen	1945–1960
Stephen Marsh Tenney	1960–1962
Gilbert H. Mudge	1962–1965
Ralph W. Hunter (Acting)	Sept.–Dec. 1965
Stephen Marsh Tenney (Acting)	Jan.–Sept. 1966
Carleton B. Chapman	1966–1973
Stephen Marsh Tenney (Acting)	Jan.–June 1973
James C. Strickler	1973–1981
Peter C. Whybrow (Acting)	July 1981–Dec. 1981
Robert W. McCollum	1982–1990
Andrew G. Wallace	1990–1998

*Nathan Smith was not only the sole faculty member, initially, of the medical school he had founded, but as such he did all the work for which a dean or other officer of the school might have been considered responsible. Not until Reuben Dimond Mussey became secretary and treasurer of Dartmouth Medical School did the institution have an appointed officer. Mussey (1814–1820) was followed in sequence by James Freeman Dana (1820–1826), Daniel Oliver (1826–1839), Oliver Payson Hubbard (1839–1845), Edmund Randolph Peaslee (1845–1859), Albert Smith (1859–1869), Lyman Bartlett How (1869–1872), and Carlton Pennington Frost (1872–1896).

Frost is often incorrectly referred to as the first dean—a testimony to the length of time he held the dual office of secretary and treasurer as well as to the importance to DMS of his leadership. A dean—William Thayer Smith—finally was formally appointed when the senior Frost died. His son Gilman Dubois Frost became secretary and treasurer (1896–1904) until the treasurer of the College took over the responsibility of being medical school treasurer as well. Gilman Frost continued as secretary until 1909. From William Smith's time forward, the secretary was no longer the chief officer of the school.

APPENDIX B

*Examination Questions. Session of 1888.**

ANATOMY. NO. 1.

1. Describe a serous and a mucous membrane, with the various kinds of epithelium on each.
2. All you know about the neck of the Femur.
3. Name all the muscles and ligaments attached to the Clavicle.
4. Name all the muscles attached to the Humerus. (25).
5. Origin and Insertion of the Supinator Longus, Subscapularis, Trans versalis.
6. Describe the Large Intestine, its subdivisions and anatomical relations, and the relation of the Peritoneum to each part.
7. Course of the arch of the Aorta, and name its branches in order.
8. Give the anatomical directions for tying the Right Common Carotid.
9. Describe the Inguinal Canal.

ANATOMY. NO. 2.

1. In diseases of the mammary gland what lymphatic glands may become affected? Ditto of uterus, of lungs, of the ileum?
2. Trace a white blood-corpuscle from the left ventricle to the skin on the inner side of the knee and back to its starting point, naming every vessel it goes through. Also tell how it may return by the lymphatics, naming every vessel and set of glands.
3. Origin and insertion and nerve supply of these muscles; Adductor Longus, Rectus Femoris, Soleus.
4. Describe the Phrenic nerve—its course, relations and function.
5. Ditto the Great Sciatic.
6. Describe the Trachea.
7. Describe an air cell.
8. Name all the structures of a Root of a Lung.
9. Describe the True Vocal Bands and name the muscles that separate and that make them tense.

PHYSIOLOGY.

1. Which are the most abundant chemical elements in the body, and under what forms are they taken in?

*DMS, *Records*, DA-3, Box 7:6, DCA.

2. Origin of animal heat and modes of its regulation in the body.
3. What articles of food would you give to a diabetic? State the reasons.
4. Describe arterial pressure and state the factors that enter into it.
5. What is lymph, and what are its uses?
6. Describe the contents of the duodenum after a meal and the changes that take place in them.
7. How does the spinal cord act as a nerve center, and what are its functions as such?
8. Distribution and functions of the fifth cranial nerve.

CHEMISTRY.

1. What is meant by monobasic, isometric, homologous, deliquescent, univalent?
2. How do red and yellow phosphorus differ?
3. Given As_2O_3, HNO_3, H_2O and heat what As compounds can be made?
4. Why is the molecular weight of a gas twice the vapor density?
5. What are some of the properties *common* to all forms of carbon?
6. Preparation and properties of CO.
7. Give formulae and methods of preparation of four compounds of Mg.
8. What are some of the characteristics of $CHCl_3$, CHI_3, $KMnO_4$, CaO?
9. Give some of the properties of Cu, K, Ag, Pb.
10. What is caustic soda, lunar caustic, blue vitriol, lime water, saltpetre?
11. What is vaseline, woodspirit, soap, chloral hydrate, cream tartar?
12. Preparation and properties of ordinary ether.
13. What are the fatty acids, source and properties of acetic acid?
14. Explain the principle of the hypobromite of soda test for the quantity of urea.

THERAPEUTICS.

1. Sources of danger in use of *Opium* in pneumonia, and method of safe use in this disease.
2. How use *Belladonna* in general and local hyperhydrosis?

3(*a*). Compare impressions of *Opium*, *Conicum* and *Aconite* on the nervous system.

3(*b*). Give chief uses of *Cannabis Indica*.

4. Give mean adult dose of (1) Pulv. Opii., (2) Laudanum, (3) Tr. Bel ladon., (4) Atropiæ Sulph., (5) Ext. Physostig., (6) Choral [*sic*] Hydr., (7) Tr. Aconite Rad., (8) Fl. Ext. Cannab. Ind., (9) Aloes as cathartic. (10) Pulv. Ipecac, as emetic.

5(*a*). Give special advantages of *Sodium Brom.* over *Potassic* and the other inorganic Bromides.

5(*b*). What difference, in general terms, is there between the therapeutic action and application of the *Inorganic Bromides* and the *Inorganic Iodides*?

6. What special dangers attend the use of *Opium* in Infancy?
7. What cathartic can we give in chronic constipation where *Aloes* is contraindicated?

8. What *Cathartics* are energized by the addition of an alkali? And why? What by the addition of nux vomica? And why?

9(*a*). Give composition of *Rhubarb*. What evidence have we of the action of four of its constituents on the system?

9(*b*). Compare the emetic action of *Apomorphia* with that of *Ipecac.*

10. Give the principal indications for the use of *Oleum Terebinth.*

10(*b*). Neurosal cardiac states—and their causes—indicating *Digitalis.*

GYNECOLOGY.

1. Varieties of Dysmenorrhea.
2. Symptoms and dangers of the Menopause.
3. Causes of Sexual Disease in the Female.
4. Varieties of Uterine Fibroids.
5. Ligaments of the Uterus.
6. Treatment of Congestion and Inflammation of the Ovaries.
7. Causes and Treatment of Menorrhagia and Metrorrhagia.
8. Varieties of Uterine Cancer.
9. Varieties and Treatment of Uuterine Catarrh.
10. Varieties of Utierine Displacements.

SURGERY.

1. *Gangrene.* Causes, Varieties, Treatment.
2. *Amputations*—Varieties, Causes of Death after.
3. *Hæmorrhoids*—Varieties, Diagnosis, Treatment.
4. *Foreign Bodies in Air Passage*—Diagnosis, Prognosis, Treatment.
5. *Cancer of Breast*—Diagnosis, Treatment.
6. *Penetrating Wound of Abdomen*—Diagnosis, Prognosis, Treatment.
7. *Pott's Fracture*—Diagnosis, Prognosis, Treatment.

OBSTETRICS.

1. Describe the placenta.
2. Give the treatment of inevitable abortion.
3. Give the management of a breech delivery.
4. Describe fully the use of the forceps in a R.O.P. position of the Vertex.
5. Give the causes and the treatment of post-partum hemorrhage.
6. Give the premonitory symptoms and the treatment of Eclampsia.
7. Give the pathology and the treatment of Phlegmasia Alba Dolens.

PRACTICE. NO. I.

1. Describe your ideal room for person sick with Acute Infectious Disease, as Scarlatina, Typhoid Fever, etc.

2. Give Differential Diagnosis between Scarlet Fever and Measles. Describe a case of each disease with such complications as are especially related to it.
3. Anatomical Characters of Typhoid Fever and Symptoms attendant upon them.
4. Define Empyema. Diagnosis and treatment.
5. Cerebral Embolism. How caused, and what are its symptoms?
6. Describe the processes of Inflammation in the order of their occurrence. Give the products of Inflammation in the different tissues.

PRACTICE. NO. 2.

1. Symptoms, Physical Signs and Treatment of Capillary Bronchitis.
2. Define Bronchial, Puerile and Senile Respiration. Subcrepitant and crepitant rales, when produced.
3. Cerebral Hemorrhage. Causes and consequences.
4. Endocarditis. Cause and Sequelae.
5. Give stages of Pneumonia and Diagnosis from Pleurisy, with and without effusion.
6. Symptoms of Cerebral Meningitis.

APPENDIX C

*President's Letter to the Alumni of Dartmouth Medical School, April 30, 1913**

To the Alumni of the Dartmouth Medical School,—

The Trustees of Dartmouth College, after most careful consideration, have come to feel that it is wise, temporarily at least, for the institution to discontinue granting the degree of Doctor of Medicine. In order to make clear the reasons for such action, this communication is sent to the alumni of the Medical School.

The problem of preparing young men for the profession of medicine has, in recent years, become one of the most difficult of those that confront the educator. The discovery of the scientific basis for all infectious processes, and the now rapidly growing knowledge of physiological chemistry, have, of necessity, greatly lengthened the period required for gaining an education in medicine. More important still, they have completely changed the methods of instruction; for, whereas formerly a room where lectures could be given was virtually a sufficient plant, there is now the demand for great laboratories expensively manned and elaborately equipped. The increase has, further, involved the necessity for better elementary preparation in science and in scientific habits of thought; in other words, for raising the standards of admission to the medical school. This has been accomplished by making from one to four years of college work the essential preliminary to medical training.

But this has not been all. In addition to the demand for more thorough scientific training, there has been a steadily growing consciousness of the fact that the public health is too important an asset to be entrusted to any but those completely equipped: in short, that, unlike the representative of any other profession or occupation, the medical man must leave the school a finished product, not only in scientific theory, but also in the highest practical application of that theory. To meet this unique situation, the hospital as well as the laboratory must become an integral part of medical school equipment, if the school would meet what appears to be the demand of the time.

Dartmouth College has been a leader in accepting the call for improved preparation, a longer course, and the providing and equipping of laboratories for medical training. It has found more difficult the supplying of full clinical facilities in the hospital. Situated as Dartmouth is, far from centers of population, a large out-patient department is clearly impossible; children's diseases, contagious cases, and important examples under general medicine cannot be secured in numbers sufficient for extensive study. The tendency of surgical cases toward the hospital makes that type of clinic amply large; the size of the medical clinic is limited by a geographical location which takes the matter out of the control of the Hitchcock Hospital or the Dartmouth Medical School.

*DC Office of the President, *Records*, DP-10 (Nichols), Box 15:39.

Outside influences must also be taken into account in any present consideration of medical education at Dartmouth. Such influences are exerted chiefly by state boards of medical registration, and by the educational council of the American Medical Association. The latter organization, in its investigation and rating of the medical schools of the country, has always commended the Dartmouth Medical School for its academic ideals and its readiness to advance its standards; yet it has insisted that the clinical facilities of the School did not entitle it to first rank. Leaving aside the question of the justice or the injustice of this attitude, to be ranked in second or third class by such a body as the American Medical Association would seriously reduce the ability of the school to attract desirable students. Still more prejudicial would be the refusal of state boards of registration to accept Dartmouth graduates for examination. The danger of such refusal, based on the assumed lack of clinical facilities, has of late been imminent.

It is in view of these considerations that the Trustees have decided upon the action announced in this statement. The Medical School will continue as a department of Dartmouth College. It will, however, give only the first two years of medical work, which may be elected by undergraduates in the College. Courses will be so arranged that upon completion of them the student may, without loss of time, make transfer to the school of his choice, where he may find satisfactory clinical opportunities.

It is the sincere hope of the Trustees that the alumni of the Dartmouth Medical School will agree with them as to the wisdom of the action taken. Graduates of the School will, as in the past, be cordially granted the use of the school laboratories, hospital facilities, and clinics, in the conduct of which their advice and coöperation is earnestly invited.

DARTMOUTH COLLEGE,
PRESIDENT'S OFFICE,
APRIL 30, 1913

APPENDIX D

*Medical School Revives M.D. Degree**

In June 1965, a subcommittee on the Medical School appointed by the Board of Trustees submitted its final report. The most significant recommendation was as follows:

> Dartmouth Medical School has been fulfilling satisfactorily its educational mission in medicine as a two-year school. Problems remain with the clinical subjects, but there is every expectation that they will be resolved with the establishment of the new departments of medicine and surgery. When these new departments are developed, and after the present hospital expansion is accomplished the question of Dartmouth's evolution to a four-year school should be reconsidered. In view of potential developments on the national scene which will greatly increase the demand for trained physicians, this committee considers that it is feasible within the scope of these plans, to expand the number of medical students in the two-year program to 128 (64 per class).

On October 9, 1965, the Board of Trustees approved the Subcommittee's report and included the following statement:

> The Medical School should proceed for the foreseeable future on the assumption that it will continue at the undergraduate level of medical education to offer the first two years of the M.D. program. The Board is prepared to consider at an appropriate time the establishment of a pilot program in clinical instruction beyond the first two years in which selected students would be given a tutorial clinical education leading to the M.D. degree. Prior to the consideration of a Medical Scientist (M.D.–Ph.D) offering, a program leading to the M.D. degree must be more fully developed.

In mid-February 1966, Acting Dean Marsh Tenney appointed an ad hoc Planning Committee for the Four-Year Program, and on June 24, 1966, it submitted a preliminary report recommending that:

> The Dartmouth Medical School inaugurate a program leading to the M.D. degree, that the program be of a highly tutorial nature,

*The excerpts that follow (with introductory statements in which the wording has in places been slightly revised), come from Carleton B. Chapman, *Report of the Dean: Dartmouth Medical School 1966–67 to 1971–72* (Hanover, N.H.: Reporter Press, Oct. 1972), 10–14; DC Trustees, *Records*, DA-1, Box 23:56, DCA.

> that present planning be based on the admission of 16 students per class, and that the program be initiated as soon as the necessary facilities and faculty become available. . . .

On March 4, 1968, the following motion was introduced at a regular meeting of the medical school faculty:

> *Resolved*: that the faculty of Dartmouth Medical School endorse the development of an experimental curriculum leading to the M.D. degree for a limited number of students. The provisional date for the acceptance of the first third-year class is 1971.

On April 13, 1968, the Board of Trustees:

> *Voted* to accept, subject only to development of the necessary financing, the objective set forth in the resolution adopted by the Medical School faculty, March 4, 1968. . . .

On January 22, 1970, the Medical School faculty issued the following statement:

> *Resolved*: that the faculty go on record as enthusiastically endorsing the following statement from [Chairman of the Dartmouth College Board of Trustees] Lloyd Brace's letter to Mr. Robert L. Belsley of N.I.H., thus committing the faculty fully to conversion from a basic science medical school to a full M.D. degree program.
>
> "The Board of Trustees of Dartmouth has repeatedly confirmed its support for the return to a full M.D. program at Dartmouth Medical School. The School is authorized to accept 16 candidates for the M.D. degree in September, 1970 and to expand the number of candidates to a total of 64 as rapidly as resources will permit.
>
> "The Trustees expect the full program of expansion to be completed by 1975–76 and are anxious to facilitate the completion of the expansion of the program in every way open to them.
>
> "The commitment is to the program as stated, within the time limits set by law pertaining to such grants, barring catastrophic shortage of funds."

Notes

Abbreviations

BOOKS, JOURNALS, AND NEWSPAPERS

For the most part, the names of journals will be self-evident or can be quickly deciphered. Other abbreviations are listed below.

BG	*Boston Globe*
DAB	*Dictionary of American Biography*
DAM	*Darthmouth Alumni Magazine*
DM	*Dartmouth Medicine*
DMSAM	*Dartmouth Medical School Alumni Magazine*
DMSAN&N	*Dartmouth Medical School Alumni News & Notes*
DMSQ	*Dartmouth Medical School Quarterly*
JAMA	*Journal of the American Medical Association*
NEJM	*New England Journal of Medicine*
NYT	*New York Times*
VN	*Valley News[Lebanon, N.H.]*

PUBLISHERS

CUP	Cambridge University Press
OUP	Oxford University Press
UPNE	University Press of New England

LIBRARIES AND OTHER INSTITUTIONS

BRBML	Beinecke Rare Book and Manuscript Library, Yale University
CLM	Francis A. Countway Library of Medicine, Harvard University
M&A, YUL	Manuscripts and Archives, Yale University Library
MHS	Massachusetts Historical Society
NHHS	New Hampshire Historical Society
NYAM	New York Academy of Medicine

PERSONS

For Dartmouth graduates, "(DC 1930, DMS 1932)" indicates the year of graduation from the College and graduation from the Medical School, respectively.

I have frequently used initials only for individuals whose names come up repeatedly in the notes. They are as follows:

JPB	John Pollard Bowler
CBC	Carleton B. Chapman
PD	Philip Denenfeld
JSD	John Sloan Dickey
RCF	R. Clinton Fuller
SI	Shinya lonué
RWMcC	Robert W. McCollum
GHM	Gilbert H. Mudge
DHM	Donald H. Morrison
LN	Lafayette Noda
GCS	George Cheyne Shattuck
JCS	James C. Strickler
LS	Lyman Spaulding
NS	Nathan Smith
SMT	Stephen Marsh Tenney

Chapter 1. In the Beginning

1. Oliver P. Hubbard, *Dartmouth Medical College and Nathan Smith: An Historical Discourse* (Washington, D.C.: Globe Printing and Publ., 1880), 12.

2. William Allen, *An Address Occasioned by the Death of Nathan Smith, M.D.* (Brunswick [Maine]: G. Griffen, 1829): 13.

3. Henry N. Andrews, Jr., "The King's Pines," *Historical New Hampshire* (Jan. Suppl., [194?]), [1].

4. The 1786 figure comes from a 1977 "Regional Land Use Plan" put out by the Upper Valley–Lake Sunapee Council. See also Evarts B. Greene and Virginia D. Harrington, *American Population before the Federal Census of 1790* (Baltimore, Md.: Genealogical Publ. Co., 1993), 81; and Ronald Vern Jackson, *First Census of the United States* (Bountiful, Utah: Accelerating Indexing Systems, 1978), 9.

5. The new building was called simply "The College" for nearly forty years; only after Thornton and Wilder halls were built did the central edifice in the triptych come to be known as "Dartmouth Hall." Francis Lane Childs, "Dartmouth Hall—Old and New," *DAM* 28, no. 4 (Jan. 1936): 7–17, at 9.

6. Frederick Chase, *A History of Dartmouth College and the Town of Hanover, New Hampshire* (John K. Lord, ed.), 2 vols. (Cambridge, Mass.: John Wilson, 1891), I: 616.

7. A lively account of the history of Dartmouth Medical School given in the "Inaugural Talk of the Dartmouth Medical Student Lecture Series," on which one is tempted to rely for many miscellaneous details, is Frederic P. Lord's "The Very Old and the Old," *DAM* 54, no. 5 (Feb. 1962): 23–28. Lord's account does contain errors. Nathan Smith did not, for example, "early" come "to live in New Hampshire, not far from Hanover." Nor was it in New Hampshire, as Lord seems to imply, that the seminal event persuading Smith he wanted to be a physician transpired.

8. For evidence of this and other civic activities of John Smith, see Town Records: Chester, Windsor County, Vt., 1772–1775, Vol. A., pp. 19, 20, 22, 24, 26, 28, 31, 33, 35, 39, 40.

9. Rehoboth, Massachusetts, has also been called the birthplace of public education.

10. The accounts of this event are numerous, many of them full of fanciful details that cannot be known for certain. Directly or indirectly, the original source for all of them was Goodhue's letter (see *infra*, n11)—itself perhaps not wholly reliable, since it was written years after the event.

11. Goodhue, Josiah. Letter to George Cheyne Shattuck, 4 Mar. 1829. George Cheyne Shattuck Papers, MHS.

12. On Warren's lectures, see Henry K. Beecher and Mark D. Altschule, *Medicine at Harvard: The First Three Hundred Years* (Hanover, N.H.: UPNE, 1977), 34, 35, 39, and Edward Warren, *The Life of John Warren, M.D.* (Boston: Noyes, Holmes, 1874), 225–26. On Smith at Harvard, see *Harvard University: Quinquennial Catalogue of the Officers and Graduates, 1636–1930* (Cambridge, Mass.: Published by the University, 1930), 851, and Thomas Francis Harrington, *The Harvard Medical School: A History, Narrative and Documentary, 1782–1905*, 3 vols. (New York: Lewis Publ., 1905), 1: 335–54; Harrington's ch. 13 is devoted wholly to Nathan Smith.

13. Nathan Smith's dissertation appeared in *Mass. Mag.* 3, no. 1 (Jan. 1791): 33–35, and 3, no. 2 (Feb. 1791): 81–83. "Dr. Smith's Reply" was published the next year in *Mass. Mag.* 4, no. 5 (May 1792): 314–15, and "Dr. Smith's Replication to Philozetemia" in *Mass. Mag.* 5, no. 4 (Apr. 1793): 218–21.

14. NS, *A Practical Essay on Typhous Fever* (New York: E. Bliss and E. White, 1824).

15. Oliver P. Hubbard to M. D. Bisbee, 24 June 1897; Mss. 897374, DCA.

16. For a brief account of Gallup's life and insights into his career, see Oliver S. Hayward, "Jo Gallup, New England Epidemiologist," *NEJM* 269 (7 Nov. 1963): 1015–18; reprinted in *DMSAM* (Fall 1981): 30–32, 44.

17. A. B. Crosby, in his *Contribution to the Medical History of New Hampshire* (Nashua, N.H.: Moore and Langley, 1870), 11, implies that the idea of starting a medical school in New Hampshire came from a consensus among members of the Medical Society that "the young men of the state should have systematic didactic instruction, and that this could be accomplished only by the foundation of a regularly chartered medical college." Crosby gives full credit to Smith for actually executing the plan ("This plan was eventually reduced to a demonstration through the energy and talents of one man . . . Nathan Smith"). As far as I have been able to ascertain, he is the only person who has intimated that the idea was not wholly original with Smith.

18. NS to Board of Trustees, 25 Aug. 1796; Mss. 796475, DCA.

19. NS, "Proposal for [a] Medical Institution," [n.d.] Aug. 1796; Mss. 796490.2, DCA.

20. NS to Board of Trustees, 25 Aug. 1796; Mss. 796475, DCA.

21. See Oliver S. Hayward and Constance E. Putnam, *Improve, Perfect, & Perpetuate: Dr. Nathan Smith and Early American Medical Education* (Hanover, N. H.: UPNE, 1998), 40–41, and 286–87n31, for a discussion of how Smith paid for the trip.

22. *The Med. Repository* 2 (1799): 337.

23. NS to GCS, 20 [*sic*: postmarked 15] Apr. 1811; Mss. 811265, DCA.

24. Meeting Minutes, Vol. I, p. 211 (21, 25, and 26 Aug. 1796); DC Trustees, *Records*, DA-1, DCA. See also Extract from Minutes, Annual Mtg. of Board of Trustees (Dartmouth College), B. Woodward, secretary, [n.d.] Aug. 1796; Mss. 796490, DCA.

25. John Wheelock to the Rev. Samuel Peters, 7 Nov. 1796; Mss. 796607, DCA.

26. For some details of the relationship and the insights it gives into Smith's life, see Hayward and Putnam, *Improve*, especially 124–26.

27. Phineas Sanborn Conner, *Address: Dartmouth Medical College Centennial Exercises, . . . 1897* [Hanover, N. H.: Dartmouth Press, 1907], 27. Given on 29 June 1897, Conner's address was not published until a decade later (a bill from "The Dartmouth Press" makes this clear; see DMS, DA-3, Box 14:4, DCA) and then in a much-expanded version.

28. See DMS, DA-3, Box 7:11, DCA.

29. See DMS, DA-3, Box 7:24, DCA.

30. Eugene Orsenigo, "The Medical School at Dartmouth College, Hanover, N.H." [unpubl., bound ms., 11 June 1934], p. 23; DCA.

31. The two articles on this period by Robert E. Nye, Jr., both titled with questions: "Nathan Smith's Trip to Edinburgh: A Waste of Time?" *DMSAM* [8, no. 1] (Fall 1983): 24–27, and—two years later—"Nathan Smith's Time in London: A Better Investment?" in *DMSAM* [10, no. 1] (Fall 1985): 12–15, remained the most valuable source of information on Smith's trip abroad for Hayward and Putnam, *Improve*, more than twenty years later.

32. Oliver S. Hayward and Elizabeth H. Thomson, eds., *The Journal of William Tully, Medical Student at Dartmouth 1808–1809* (New York: Science History Publications, 1977), 75–76.

33. NS to Sally Smith, [n.d.] Feb. 1797; quoted in Emily A. Smith, *The Life and Letters of Nathan Smith, M.B. M.D.* (New Haven: Yale Univ. Press, 1914): 19–20. Various writers have claimed Smith learned a lot from his trip abroad. See, for example, Orsenigo, "The Medical School," p. 2: Smith, in "his travels of less than a year . . . acquired a great deal of valuable information on medical subjects." But Orsenigo, like others who have made similar observations, gave no evidence to support this claim.

34. Smith, Nathan. Letter to John Warren, 4 May 1797. John Collins Warren Papers, MHS.

35. Arnold A. Bank, review of George Washington Corner, *Two Centuries of Medicine: A History of the School of Medicine University of Pennsylvania* (Philadelphia: Lippincott, 1965), in *Arch. Intern. Med.* 116 (Nov. 1965): 800.

36. NS, "Observations on the Position of Patients in the Operation for Lithotomy, with a Case," in *Memoirs of the Medical Society of London* 6 (1805): 227–31; and "On the medicinal properties of sanguinaria Canadensis, or Blood Root," *Transactions of the Medical Society of London* 1, part 1 (1810): 179–85. The latter piece was reprinted twice: *Annales cliniques ou Journal des sciences médicales* (Montpelier) 26 (1811): 394–95 (in French); *Edinburgh Medical and Surgical Journal* 8, no. 30 (Apr. 1812): 216–17.

37. Meeting Minutes, Vol. I, pp. 222–23 (23 Aug. 1798) and p. 229 (28 Aug. 1798); DC Trustees, *Records*, DA-1, DCA. See also Mss. 798490, DCA.

38. Meeting Minutes, Vol. I, p. 222 (22 Aug. 1798); DC Trustees, *Records*, DA-1, DCA. See also Mss. 798490, DCA. Awarding the M.B. to Lyman Spalding

was like awarding the A.M. to Nathan Smith; the trustees presumably thought that Spalding ought to have a Dartmouth degree if he was going to teach at Dartmouth.

39. Meeting Minutes, Vol. I, pp. 227–29 (28 Aug. 1798); DC Trustees, *Records*, DA-1, DCA. Emphasis in the original.

40. Jonathan Knight, in his *Eulogium on Nathan Smith* (New Haven: Hezekiah Howe, 1829), 7, attributed the sentiment to Josiah Goodhue. Quoted in Nathan R. Smith, ed., *Medical and Surgical Memoirs* (Baltimore: Wm. A. Francis, 1831), 16, and in Hayward and Putnam, *Improve*, 9.

41. The content of this chapter relies heavily on the opening four chapters ("Part I: The Road to Dartmouth") of Hayward and Putnam, *Improve*, where more information on virtually every aspect of this chapter can be found.

Chapter 2. Pressing Forward

1. Harvey Cushing, *The Medical Career: An Address in The Ideals, Opportunities, and Difficulties of the Medical Profession* (Hanover, N.H.: Dartmouth College, 1929), 37–38.

2. Samuel Elder, fragment of undated letter (addressee unknown); Mss. 000676, DCA. We know when Elder was at Dartmouth (though not when he wrote the letter) because he dated the notes he took of the lectures that term. See his "Medical Notebook, containing notes of lectures by Nathan Smith and Cyrus Perkins at Dartmouth Medical College" [NS lectures from 27 November 1811 through 9 December 1811] (ca. 100 pp.); Vault Mss., DCA.

3. A. T. Lowe to Oliver P. Hubbard, 7 Apr. 1879; Mss. 879257, DCA.

4. A. B. Crosby, *A Contribution to the Medical History of New Hampshire* (Nashua, N.H.: Moore and Langley, 1870): 26. The "system" to which Crosby referred was very like what is sometimes referred to as the "Bigelow Maneuver." But Smith never wrote it up, and it was left to Henry Jacob Bigelow to get credit for demonstrating the importance of the iliofemoral (Y-)ligament and the use of flexion for reducing dislocated hips, when he published *The Mechanism of Dislocation and Fracture of the Hip with the Reduction of the Dislocation by the Flexion Method* (Philadelphia: Henry C. Lea, 1869), forty years after Smith's death.

5. Robert McCollum to Gov. Lane Dwinell, 29 Apr. 1996, personal communication. McCollum's permission to quote from the letter is gratefully acknowledged.

6. Thomas Almy, 21 June 1996, personal communication.

7. NS, "Dissertation on scirrhous & Cancerous affections," unpublished ms., ca. 1808 (48 pp.); BRBML (typescript copy in CLM). The next three quoted passages come from this paper.

8. William Frederick Norwood, *Medical Education in the United States Before the Civil War* (Philadelphia: Univ. of Penn. Press, 1944), 186, 202.

9. Leonard K. Eaton, *New England Hospitals: 1790–1833* (Ann Arbor: Univ. of Mich. Press, 1957), 173.

10. George W. Corner, *Two Centuries of Medicine: A History of the School of Medicine, University of Pennsylvania* (New York: Lippincott, 1965), 57.

11. NS to LS, 5 May 1819; Mss. 819254, DCA.

12. Rather than writing out the words, Smith used the common apothecary signs and abbreviations for these measures.

13. NS to John Powers, [no date]; Mss. 000650, DCA.

14. NS to LS, 19 Nov. 1796; Mss. 796619.1, DCA. In James A. Spalding, *The Life of Dr. Lyman Spalding* (Boston: W. M. Leonard, 1916), 6. In general, see Oliver S. Hayward and Constance E. Putnam, *Improve, Perfect, & Perpetuate: Dr. Nathan Smith and Early American Medical Education* (Hanover, N.H.: UPNE, 1998), 40–41 and 286n30). See "Nathan Smith in account with Lyman Spalding"; DMS, DA-3, Box 15 (Accounts Relating to DMS Folder), DCA.

15. On Lyman Spalding's education, see Spalding, *The Life*, 3, 11 (plus note); see also LS, *A new nomenclature of chemistry, proposed by Messers. De Morveau, Lavoisier, Berthollet, and Fourcroy; with additions and improvements* (Hanover, N.H.: Moses Davis, 1799). For additional discussion of Spalding's brief career at Dartmouth, based in part on these sources, see Hayward and Putnam, *Improve*, 75–76 *et passim.*

16. See Denis I. Duveen and Herbert S. Klickstein, "The Introduction of Lavoisier's Chemical Nomenclature into America," *Isis* 45 (1954): 278–92.

17. For more on what was available in Edinburgh to students of chemistry, see R. G. W. Anderson, *The Playfair Collection and the Teaching of Chemistry at the University of Edinburgh, 1713–1858* (Edinburgh: Royal Scottish Museums, 1978).

18. Oliver S. Hayward and Elizabeth H. Thomson, eds., *The Journal of William Tully, Medical Student at Dartmouth 1808–1809* (New York: Science History Pubs., 1977), 53.

19. Andrew Mack, "Journal Kept during a course of chemical Lectures D[artmouth] College Oct. 4, 1810, by Dr Smith"; Vault Mss., DCA.

20. A. B. Crosby, *Contribution*, 21.

21. Isaac Patterson to Oliver P. Hubbard, 13 Oct. 1879; Mss. 879563, DCA.

22. Ezekiel Dodge Cushing to Nathaniel Cushing, 30 Oct. 1809. Ezekiel Dodge Cushing Papers (Folder 1). M&A, YUL. For more on Smith's attempts to put and keep chemistry in the curriculum, see Hayward and Putnam, *Improve*, 74–77.

23. Meeting Minutes, Vol. I, p. 229 (25 Aug. 1798); DC Trustees, *Records*, DA-1, DCA.

24. LS to Samuel Brown, 1 Apr. 1799; Mss. 799251.1, DCA.

25. L. B. Richardson, writing a piece on the "Shattuck Observatory," in *DAM* 36, no. 3 (Dec. 1943), claimed chemistry was not taught to undergraduates until 1816, when James Freeman Dana joined the faculty; this appears to be false.

26. Hayward and Thomson, eds., *Tully*, 48.

27. See especially letters from Ezekiel Dodge Cushing to his mother, his father, and his sister; he frequently reported in detail and with great excitement on the trips he and other students made with Smith. Ezekiel Dodge Cushing Papers, M&A, YUL. Several of these are quoted in Hayward and Putnam, *Improve*.

28. [Robert E. Nye], "Notes from Dartmouth Archives," *DMSQ* (Spring 1969): 96.

29. Calvin Gorham, "Extracts from Nathan Smith's Lectures Delivered at Dartmouth University, AD 1811–12, [etc.]"; Vault Mss., DCA.

30. Isaac Patterson to Oliver P. Hubbard, 13 Oct. 1879; Mss. 879563, DCA. For several examples of the way real cases were inserted in the lectures, see Hayward and Putnam, *Improve, 66 et seq.*

31. For further information about the use of student notebooks at the time, see Hayward and Putnam, *Improve*, which also includes as complete a bibliography of student notebooks containing notes from Smith's lectures as was established at the time of that book's publication (pp. 339–42; two more have been located since). Much work on both Smith's style and the actual content of his lectures remains to be done.

32. Untitled student notebook, pp. [91–92, or first two pages of the second of several notebooks bound together]; DMS *Records*, DA-3, Box 8:5, DCA. This is one of the two student notebooks not listed in Hayward and Putnam, *Improve*, 339–42.

33. The best source on Ramsay's unusual career is G. P. Bradley, "Biographical Sketch of Alexander Ramsay, M.D., of Parsonsfield," in *Maine Med. Assoc. Trans.* 8, no. 1 (1883): 161–82. See also Hayward and Putnam, *Improve*, 88–95 *et passim.*

34. NS to LS, 9 Oct. 1808; Mss. 808559, DCA. In Spalding, *The Life*, 150. Also, NS to LS, 22 Sept. 1808; LS Papers, NHHS. In Spalding, *The Life*, 149–50. The ad appeared in the *Portsmouth [N.H.] Oracle* 19, no. 52 (1 Oct. 1808): [3].

35. A very helpful piece of work on Perkins can be found in Robert E. Nye, Jr., "Cyrus Perkins, M.D. (1778–1849)," in *DMSQ* 3, no. 2 (Autumn 1966): 28–34. See also Hayward and Putnam, *Improve*, 137–39.

36. Meeting Minutes, Vol. I, p. 348 (24 Aug. 1810); DC Trustees, *Records*, DA-1, DCA.

37. Nathan Smith gave a note to Perkins for $951.00 on 28 Oct. 1813, in what was apparently a final settlement of the assets of the partnership; DMS, DA-3, Box 15 (N-Perkins Folder).

38. *Dartmouth College General Catalog, 1769–1940* (Hanover, N.H.: DC Pubs., 1940), 830.

39. Hayward and Thomson, eds., *Tully*, 58.

40. Malthus A. Ward to Ezra Bartlett, 19 Nov. 1814, quoted in William Barlow and David O. Powell, "Student Views of the Medical Institution at Dartmouth in 1813 and 1814," *Historical New Hampshire* 31, no. 3 (Fall 1976): 105.

41. *Dartmouth College v. Woodward*, 17 U.S. (4 Wheat.) 518 (1819).

42. President William Jewett Tucker, eighty years after the case was settled, dismissed the idea that Dartmouth was a university (or even could be) on the grounds that a modern university necessarily implied "advanced scholarship and investigation . . . regardless of its practical outcome," and "large funds to support it." Robert French Leavens and Arthur Hardy Lord, *Dr. Tucker's Dartmouth* (Hanover, N.H.: Dartmouth Pubs., 1965), 166. The issue would rear its head again at DMS.

43. For more details, see, e.g., Baxter Perry Smith, *The History of Dartmouth College* (Boston: Houghton, Osgood, 1878), Ch. XII, and Wilder Dwight Quint, *The Story of Dartmouth* (Boston: Little, Brown, 1914), Ch. VI.

44. Nathan Crosby, *The First Half Century of Dartmouth College, Being Historical Collections and Personal Reminiscences* (Hanover, N.H.: J. B. Parker, 1876): 44. A brief account of how that worked can be found in [Robert E. Nye,

Jr.,] "Notes from the Dartmouth Archives," *DMSQ* 4, no. 1 (Summer 1967): 14–15. See also (among the sources cited there) the [Hanover, New Hampshire] *Dartmouth Gazette* for 3, 10, 17, and 24 Sept. as well as 8 Oct. 1817.

45. [John Wheelock], *Sketches of the History of Dartmouth College and Moor's Charity School, with a Particular Account of Some Late Remarkable Proceedings of the Board of Trustees* [n.p., 1815], 73. D.C. History, LCCN: 07000349.

46. Part of the explanation for Wheelock's difficulties—the source of the trouble between him and the "Board of Trust," according to one writer—was his religious "liberality" (Smith, *History*, 89), a point alluded to earlier. Precisely that aspect of his thinking no doubt was part of what made Wheelock congenial to Smith, who ran into difficulties of his own over *his* religious views when he was moving to Yale. See Hayward and Putnam, *Improve*, 197, 211.

47. Francis Brown to NS, 12 Aug. 1817; Mss. 817462, DCA.

48. NS to Francis Brown, 21 Aug. 1817; Mss. 817471, DCA.

49. NS to Mills Olcott, 14 Aug. 1817; Mss. 817464, DCA.

50. NS to Mills Olcott [mailed on 22] Mar. 1817; Mss. 817240.1, DCA.

51. Bryant Tolles, "Early Medical School Architecture in Northern New England," *Vermont Hist.* 42, no. 4 (Fall 1974): 258.

52. For more on the story of the "New Medical House," see Hayward and Putnam, *Improve*, 126–34.

53. That honor today goes to the University of Maryland Medical School. Founded later than DMS, it nonetheless has a building that dates from 1812—Davidge Hall—still used as a medical teaching facility. See "Raising the Roof: New Clues to Uncover in Davidge Hall," in *Univ. of Maryland Bull.* (Fall 1999): 14–15.

54. See, e.g., Frederick C. Waite, "Three Episodes in Medical Education at Middlebury College [1810–1837]," *NEJM* 206, no. 14 (7 Apr. 1932): 733–35.

55. See Hayward and Putnam, *Improve*, 106.

56. Frederick Clayton Waite, *The Story of a Country Medical School: A History of the Clinical School of Medicine and The Vermont Medical College Woodstock Vermont 1927–1856* (Montpelier, Vt.: Vermont Hist. Soc., 1945), 87, 90.

57. Waite, *Story*, 90.

58. Waite, Frederick Clayton, *The First Medical College in Vermont: Castleton, 1818–1862* (Montpelier, Vt.: Vermont Hist. Soc., 1949): 41, 42, 55.

59. Among them were Josiah Noyes (DC 1801, DMS 1806), Reuben Dimond Mussey and George Cheyne Shattuck (both DC 1803, DMS 1806), and James Hadley, Sr. (DC 1809); see *Dartmouth . . . General Catalog*, 91, 92, 93, 99. See also Jane W. Dieffenbacher, *This Green and Pleasant Land: Fairfield, New York* (Fairfield, N.Y.: Town of Fairfield, 1996), 235–36.

60. James A. Spalding, *Maine Physicians of 1820* (Lewiston, Maine: [privately publ.], 1928), 159–61.

Chapter 3. Creating Shadows of Their Own

1. Joyce Horner, *Flag and Feather* (Elizabeth Alden Green and B. L. Reid, eds.), ([So. Hadley, Mass.]: Mount Holyoke College, 1986), 42.

2. "No account of the College can omit so dramatic a story," wrote L. B. Richardson in his *The History of Dartmouth College*, 2 vols. (Hanover, N.H.: Dartmouth Pubs., 1932), I: 334. He then quoted the version given by Professor Goodrich of Yale and used by Rufus Choate at Webster's funeral. Goodrich's letter to Choate is also quoted in Wilder Dwight Quint, *The Story of Dartmouth* (Boston: Little, Brown, 1914), 110.

3. Today, those not in the know may call the institution "Dartmouth University." Despite the fact that its official name is still "Dartmouth College," only the most sentimental continue to insist that Dartmouth is not a university. James Wright, who became president of the College in 1998, used his inaugural address as an occasion to stress publicly that "Dartmouth College is a university in all but name." James Wright, "Dartmouth: Forever New," *VOX of Dartmouth* 17, no. 7s (23 Sept. 1998): 2.

4. Meeting Minutes, Vol. II, p. 144 (22 Aug. 1820); DC Trustees, *Records*, DA-1, DCA.

5. "Records of the faculty of Medicine in Dartmouth College, 1819–1838," p. 4 (26 Sept. 1820); DMS, *Records*, DA-3, Box 12:1, DCA.

6. Seebert J. Goldowsky, *Yankee Surgeon: The Life and Times of Usher Parsons (1788–1866)* (Boston: Countway Library, 1988), *passim* (especially ch. 2 "Surgeon's Mate, U.S.N." and ch. 3 "The Grand Battle," 19–61). See also *Dartmouth College and Associated Schools General Catalog, 1769–1940* (Hanover, N.H.: Dartmouth Pubs., 1940), 830.

7. Meeting Minutes, Vol. II, p. 153 ([4th Wed. of] Oct. 1820); DC Trustees, *Records*, DA-1, DCA.

8. LS to Samuel Brown, 1 Apr. 1799; Mss. 799251.1, DCA. See also Oliver S. Hayward and Constance E. Putnam, *Improve, Perfect, & Perpetuate: Dr. Nathan Smith and Early American Medical Education* (Hanover, N.H.: UPNE, 1998), 52.

9. William Frederick Norwood, *Medical Education in the United States Before the Civil War* (Philadelphia: Univ. of Penn. Press, 1944), 190, quoting Richardson, *History*, I: 380. Richardson, however, stressed James Freeman Dana's scientific research talents.

10. Meeting Minutes, Vol. II, p. 208 (20 Aug. 1822); DC Trustees, *Records*, DA-1, DCA. Also, *Dartmouth . . . General Catalog* (Hanover, N.H.: Dartmouth Pubs., 1940), 830.

11. Carleton B. Chapman, *Dartmouth Medical School: The First 175 Years* (Hanover, N.H.: UPNE, 1973), 27. See also Meeting Minutes, Vol. II, p. 209 (19 Aug. 1823); DC Trustees, *Records*, DA-1, DCA. Oliver's inaugural address as a professor (on 19 May 1825) was later published by Jacob B. Moore, in Concord, N.H., in 1825.

12. Kenneth C. Cramer, "Dusting the DMS Archives," *DMSAM* (Fall 1982): 29, provides that information. We know Oliver worked with John Pickering to translate the Greek lexicon of Cornelis Schrevel (1608–1664) into English ("with many additions"); the resulting *Greek Lexicon of Schrevelius*—published in Boston by Cummings, Hilliard in 1826—is strong evidence of serious scholarship. A second edition, titled simply *A Greek and English Lexicon*, was published by Hilliard, Gray, Little, and Wilkins in Boston, three years later.

13. Chapman, *175 Years*, 28.

14. Daniel Oliver, *First Lines of Physiology: Designed for the use of students of medicine* (Philadelphia: Hooker, 1840; 1841; Boston: Ticknor, 1844).

15. Daniel Oliver, *An address, delivered before the New-Hampshire medical society* (Concord, N.H.: Marsh, Capen & Lyon, 1833).

16. Emily A. Smith, *The Life and Letters of Nathan Smith, M.B. M.D.* (New Haven: Yale Univ. Press, 1914), 140; see also Hayward and Putnam, *Improve*, 260.

17. Robert Graham, "A Firm Foundation," *DMSAM* 16, no. 1 (Fall 1991): 17.

18. Reuben D. Mussey, "Experiments and Observations on Cutaneous Absorption," *Philadelphia Med. and Physical Jrnl.*, Third Suppl. (May 1809): 288–302, at 302.

19. R. D. Mussey, "Fracture of the Neck of the Thigh-Bone," *Amer. Jrnl. of the Med. Sciences* no. 66 (Apr. 1857): 299–313, and [Letter to the Editor] "The Bi-Lateral Operation for Lithotomy.—Osteo-sarcoma," *Boston Med. and Surg. Jrnl.* 33, no. 16 (19 Nov. 1845): 322–23.

20. See "N. Hampshire Medical Institution," *Boston Telegraph* 1, no. 36 (2 Sept. 1824 [dateline 30 July 1824]): [2].

21. Frederic P. Lord, "The Very Old and the Old," *DAM* 54, no. 5 (Feb. 1962): 23–28, at 24.

22. Lord, "The Very Old," 24.

23. See, for example, R. D. Mussey, "Essay on Ardent Spirits, . . . ," *Temperance Prize Essays* (Washington [D.C.]: D. Green, 1835); *An Essay on the Influence of Tobacco Upon Life and Health* (Boston: Perkins & Marvin, 1836)—which appeared in at least two subsequent editions; and *Health: Its Friends and Its Foes* (Boston: Gould and Lincoln; New York: Sheldon and Co., etc., 1862).

24. Phineas S. Conner, *Historical Address: Dartmouth Medical College Centennial Exercises, . . . 1897* [Hanover, N.H.: Dartmouth Press, 1907], 20. The brief resolution in the trustees' minutes on this point gives no indication that the idea was Mussey's, however. Meeting Minutes, Vol. II, p. 141 (22 Aug. 1820); DC Trustees, *Records*, DA-1, DCA.

25. "Records of the faculty of Medicine in Dartmouth College, 1845–1862," p. 14 (16 Sept. 1845); DMS, *Records*, DA-3, Box 12:3, DCA. For discussion of the importance of the secretary's position, see Appendix A, p. 293, and Rosemary Lunardini, "A Century of Minutes," *DM* 17, no. 2 (Winter 1992): 38.

26. Meeting Minutes, Vol. II, p. 346 (25 July 1838); DC Trustees, *Records*, DA-1, DCA.

27. Meeting Minutes, Vol. II, p. 14 (9 Nov. 1814); DC Trustees, *Records*, DA-1, DCA.

28. Meeting Minutes, Vol. II, p. 106 (26 Aug. 1817); DC Trustees, *Records*, DA-1, DCA.

29. *Dartmouth College . . . General Catalog*, 92.

30. A. B. Crosby, *A Contribution to the Medical History of New Hampshire* (Nashua, N.H.: Moore and Langley, 1870), 28.

31. See *Dartmouth College Medical School Catalog 1825–97;* DC Hist. R 747.D37, DCA. See also *Dartmouth College . . . Catalog*, 830–32.

32. Marilyn Tobias, *Old Dartmouth on Trial: The Transformation of the Academic Community in Nineteenth-Century America* (New York: New York Univ. Press, 1982, 2002): 29.

33. O. W. Holmes to R. D. Mussey, 12 July 1838; Mss. 838412.1, DCA. Cited and quoted in Chapman, *175 Years*, 30.

34. Meeting Minutes, Vol. II, p. 347 (25 July 1838); DC Trustees, *Records*, DA-1, DCA.

35. O. W. Holmes to Usher Parsons, 7 Aug. 1838; Mss. 838457, DCA. Mentioned in Chapman, *175 Years*, 30.

36. Oliver Wendell Holmes, *First and Second Introductory Lectures, 1839 and 1840, Dartmouth Medical School* (photostats); Vault 4, DCA. The originals are at the Houghton Library, Harvard University: bMS Am 1241 *47M-368 (400) and (428), Misc. Mss and Notebooks (391–637).

37. Mss. 839458.2, DCA.

38. Meeting Minutes, Vol. III, p. 2 ([2nd Tues. of] Jan. 1841); DC Trustees, *Records*, DA-1, DCA.

39. O. W. Holmes to Dixi Crosby, 3 May 1839; Dixi Crosby, "Letters to him concerning medical school & family matters," DCA. Quoted in Chapman, *175 Years*, 32.

40. Conner, *Historical Address*, 17.

41. Gilman D. Frost, "Introductory Lecture to the 99th Annual Course delivered at the Dart. Med. School July 16, 1895" (hand-written and apparently unpublished ms.), p. 7; Mss. 895416.1, DCA. (See also Wilbert F. Chambers, "Oliver Wendell Holmes: Poet—Physician—Anatomist," *DMSAM* (Fall 1980), 20–23, at 20, 22. As for evidence that the public sometimes attended lectures other than the introductory ones, see the ticket signed by James Dana admitting "Mr Olcott & Ladies of his Family" to the "Chymical Lectures" for the term beginning 3 Oct. 1819. Papers of the Olcott Family; Box 3:48a, DCA.

42. See, e.g., Lyman Allen, "A Sketch of Vermont's Early Medical History," *NEJM* 209, no. 16 (19 Oct. 1933): 795; Gertrude L. Annan, "Advice of Nathan Smith, 1762–1829, on the Conduct of the Accoucheur," *Bull. NYAM*, 2d series, 12, no. 9 (Sept. 1936): 528; William A. R. Chapin and Lyman Allen, eds., *History: University of Vermont College of Medicine* (Hanover, N.H.: Dartmouth Printing, 1951), 31; Gordon A. Donaldson, "The First All-New England Surgeon," *Am. Jrnl. Surg.* 135, no. 4 (Apr. 1978): 474; [Charles F. Painter], "Dr. Nathan Smith, 1762–1829," *NEJM* 199, no. 2 (12 July 1928): 104; and Lee D. Van Antwerp, "Nathan Smith and Early American Medical Education," *Annals of Med. Hist.* n.s. 9, no. 5 (Sept. 1937): 457. Also: Leonard K. Eaton, *New England Hospitals: 1790–1833* (Ann Arbor: Univ. of Mich. Pr., 1957), works in the remark—with a most unsatisfactory footnote ("*passim*" rather than a page number) to Emily A. Smith, *Life and Letters* (New Haven: Yale Univ. Press, 1914). She quotes the phrase on p. 77, quite typically giving no source. Since she has so often been the primary (if not exclusive) source for writers on Smith, she may well be the reason so many have passed on the remark in the same undocumented manner.

43. Oliver Wendell Holmes, *Addresses and Exercises at the One Hundredth Anniversary of the Foundation of the Medical School of Harvard University, October 17, 1883* (Cambridge, Mass.: John Wilson and Son, Univ. Press, 1884), 6. This is the only record I uncovered, after diligent search, of Holmes actually making the remark. I found it thanks to the citation given by Thomas Edward Moore, Jr., "The Early Years of the Harvard Medical School," *Bull. Hist. Med.* 7, no. 6 (Nov.–Dec. 1953): 542. Yet Moore, despite having located the evidence that Holmes's remark was about von Haller, erroneously claimed that it was made about John Warren at Harvard. In any case—not about Nathan Smith!

44. The first record of my attempt to track down this Holmesian bon mot appeared in my "To promote useful science," *DM* 22, no. 1 (Summer–Fall 1997): 22–29, at 22. A portion of the story also appears in Hayward and Putnam, *Improve*, 136 and 309n63.

45. At least one writer has claimed Holmes applied the remark to himself; see Robert S. Blum, "Oliver Wendell Holmes Slept—and Taught—Here," *DAM* 48, no. 8 (May 1956): 13. Smith, Holmes, and their medical colleagues were not the only ones who taught a wide range of courses in those days; the traditional emphasis on the tour-de-force nature of Nathan Smith's performance is a bit misleading in this regard. In his own time, at Dartmouth, other examples can be found. Peyton R. Freeman, *A Refutation of Sundry Aspersions in the "Vindication" of the Present Trustees of Dartmouth College* . . . (Portsmouth, N.H.: Beck & Foster, 1816), 6.

46. Richardson, "The Gifted Crosbys," *DAM* 36, no. 1 (Oct. 1943): 12–13, 15, is the source of much of the information given here on the Crosby family; this remark is on p. 13. But see Sheila M. Rothman, *Living in the Shadow of Death: Tuberculosis and the Social Experience of Illness in American History* (New York: BasicBooks, 1994), *passim* (esp. ch. 2 "Manhood and Invalidism," ch. 3 "The Pursuit of Health," and ch. 4 "Body and Soul," pp. 26–74).

47. For the story of John Derby Smith (as well as Smith's other sons), see E. A. Smith, *Life and Letters*, 160; also Hayward and Putnam, *Improve*, 257.

48. Mss. 838360.2, DCA.

49. F. P. Lord to O. S. Hayward, 15 Aug. 1962, personal communication.

50. Richardson, "Crosbys," 13.

51. Conner, *Historical Address*, 7, somewhat disparagingly referred to it as a "so-called hospital," saying it had been "carried on as a private enterprise by the elder Crosby."

52. "N. Hampshire Medical Institution," *Boston Telegraph* 1, no. 36 (2 Sept. 1824): [2].

53. Lord, "The Very Old," 24–25.

54. Chapman, *175 Years*, 34.

55. Meeting Minutes, Vol. III. p. 325 (23 July 1863); DC Trustees, *Records*, DA-1, DCA.

56. Meeting Minutes, Vol. IV, p. 20 (22 July 1868); DC Trustees, *Records*, DA-1, DCA.

57. J.W.B. [probably a former student], "Obituary of Dr. Dixi Crosby," *NY Med. Jrnl.* 18, no. 5 (Nov. 1873): 556–60, at 558.

58. A. B. Crosby, *Contribution*, front cover.

59. Cramer, "Dusting," 30; Richardson, "Crosbys," 13. See also *Dartmouth College . . . Catalog*, 830, 831.

60. Meeting Minutes, Vol. II, p. 229 (24 Jan. 1827); DC Trustees, *Records*, DA-1, DCA.

61. Meeting Minutes, Vol. II, pp. 325, 326 (29 July 1835); DC Trustees, *Records*, DA-1, DCA.

62. These three essays, bound together in one volume, can be found in the Gilman collection in the DCA, under the title *Remarks on a pamphlet* . . . and the (putative) authorship of Daniel Oliver. Who decided, and on what basis, that Oliver was behind the pseudonym "Investigator" is unclear.

63. A. B. Crosby, *Contribution*, 29. The story is reminiscent of what happened to Nathan Smith when he was contemplating his move from Hanover to

New Haven. Dartmouth had left him and his religious views alone—though John Wheelock did not escape harassment, as we saw earlier—but Yale was as stringent then as Dartmouth became at the time of the Hale case; Smith is said to have had to announce publicly that he had achieved a new "state of grace" as a good Congregationalist (despite his long-time membership in the Episcopal Church in Cornish, New Hampshire) before he was acceptable to the president and trustees at Yale. See Hayward and Putnam, *Improve*, 197, 251.

64. Carlton P. Frost is often considered to have been the first dean, on the strength of his having held the two offices of secretary and treasurer for twenty-two years. Faculty records show, however, that he still identified himself simply as "Secretary" when he signed faculty minutes as late as the end of 1895. (On the other hand, examples of 1882 letterhead reading "C. P. Frost, M.D., Dean" have also been found.) Not until Frost died in 1896 was anyone officially appointed dean. "Records of the faculty of medicine in Dartmouth College, 1863–1925," [n.p.] (14 Oct. 1895) and (9 Sept. 1896), respectively; DMS, *Records*, DA-3, Box 12:5, DCA. Further indication that Frost was never officially appointed dean can be found in *Dartmouth College . . . Catalog*, 832; the first name to appear in the list of "Deans" (under "Officers of Government and Instruction, Dartmouth Medical School" is that of William Thayer Smith ("Dean 1896–1909")—various claims to the contrary notwithstanding. See, e.g., Chapman, *175 Years*, 34 and 35 (where two different dates for Frost's having been "appointed" as Dean are given). Conner, *Historical Address*, 75, also refers to Frost as the first dean.

65. "Records of the faculty of medicine in Dartmouth College, 1863–1925," p. 9 (30 Oct. 1863); DMS, *Records*, DA-3, Box 12:5, DCA.

66. See Oliver P. Hubbard, *Dartmouth Medical College and Nathan Smith: An Historical Discourse . . .* (Concord, N.H.: Evans, Sleeper & Evans, 1879).

67. For the discrepancies in his reported title and differences between his rank in the Medical School and in the College, see *Dartmouth College . . . Catalog*, 830 and 994. Also, Meeting Minutes, Vol. II, p. 331 (6 July 1836); DC Trustees, *Records*, DA-1, DCA.

68. The donation was significant, comprising some $5,000 worth of mineral specimens (in 1844, Hall gave the remainder of his collection) and $5,000 in cash to be left "to accumulate until it was large enough for the endowment of a professorship of geology and mineralogy." Tobias, *Old Dartmouth*, 107. The importance of the gift can be seen from the decision to abolish the former professorship of mineralogy and geology and to "denominate" the new one as "The Hall Professorship of Mineralogy and Geology" immediately. The sources disagree about the exact wording of Hubbard's title. Much of the confusion seems to arise from the fact that Hubbard had separate but overlapping appointments in the College and the Medical School; he was not officially given full status as "Professor of Chemistry & Pharmacy in the Medical College" until 1871. See Meeting Minutes, Vol. IV, p. 77 ([19 July 1871]); DC Trustees, *Records*, DA-1, DCA. The *Dartmouth College . . . Catalog*, p. 830, is quite explicit about Hubbard having been promoted in 1838. A three-page hand-written letter signed by the Crosbys, *père et fils*, "to the Revd President and Honorable Board of Trustees of Dartmouth College," concerning "the matter of the Chair of Chemistry in the Medical Department of Dartmouth College," betrays some feeling that administrative decisions had been made without the full consultation of the medical faculty. The letter ends with a plea that, "In view of the above facts and others

that might be adduced the undersigned respectfully pray that the President will postpone the appointment of a Professor of Chemistry until some future time." Dixi Crosby and A. B. Crosby to President [Asa Dodge Smith], 16 Aug. 1869; DC Trustees, *Records*, DA-1, Box 32:24, DCA. The Crosbys apparently got their way; this letter precedes Hubbard's appointment—as recorded in the trustees' records—by two years.

69. Meeting Minutes, Vol. III, p. 1 ([2nd Tuesday of] Jan. 1841); DC Trustees, *Records*, DA-1, DCA.

70. Meeting Minutes, Vol. III, p. 57 (13 Jan. 1846); DC Trustees, *Records*, DA-1, DCA.

71. Meeting Minutes, Vol. III, p. 60 (28 July 1846); DC Trustees, *Records*, DA-1, DCA.

72. Meeting Minutes, Vol. III, p. 70 (29 July 1846); DC Trustees, *Records*, DA-1, DCA.

73. The report begins on page 72 and concludes with a resolution on page 77. All the material (including the quotations) in the discussion of Hubbard's complaint comes from those pages. See Meeting Minutes, Vol. III, pp. 72–77 (29 July 1846); DC Trustees, *Records*, DA-1, DCA.

74. Meeting Minutes, Vol. III, p. 103 (15 Aug. 1849); DC Trustees, *Records*, DA-1, DCA.

75. Meeting Minutes, Vol. III, p. 116 (30 July 1851); DC Trustees, *Records*, DA-1, DCA.

76. Meeting Minutes, Vol. III, p. 365 (17 July 1865); DC Trustees, *Records*, DA-1, DCA.

77. A special meeting of the faculty was called to take action on the gift. "Records of the faculty of medicine in Dartmouth College, 1863–1925," [n.p.] (3 May 1871); DMS, *Records*, DA-3, Box 12:5, DCA. Stoughton's letter to Phelps of 30 May 1871 is quoted on the following pages (and a typed copy of it is in DC Office of the President, *Records*, DP-10 (Nichols), Box 2:12). See also Chapman, *175 Years*, 36–37, and Conner, *Historical Address*, 7.

78. See Spalding, *Maine*, 51.

79. DMS, *Records*, DA-3, Box 14:6, DCA.

80. NS to GCS, 22 June 1806/1807 (both dates appear in the letter—one inside and one outside); M&A, YUL. Also in Emily A. Smith, *Life and Letters*, 36 (she dates it, erroneously, 22 Jan. 1806). For a longer excerpt from this letter of NS to GCS and a brief discussion of Nathan Smith's attitude toward the medical school's (or his?) library, see Hayward and Putnam, *Improve*, 203.

81. These quotations (as well as most of the rest of the information given here on Knowlton) come from Parker G. Marden, "A Man Ahead of His Time," *DAM* 59, no. 4 (Jan. 1967): 21–23.

82. For more on Knowlton and his career, in capsule form, see "The Life and Work of Knowlton and His *Fruits of Philosophy*," in S. Chandrasekhar, "*A Dirty, Filthy Book*" (Berkeley, Calif.: Univ. of California Press, 1981), 21–25.

83. See Oliver S. Hayward and Elizabeth H. Thomson, eds., *The Journal of William Tully, Medical Student at Dartmouth 1808–1809* (New York: Science History Pubs., 1977), 21, 22, 23 (diary entries for 24 and 25 Sept. 1808).

84. Leonard Spaulding to James Farrar, Jr., 15 Aug. 1842; Mss. 842465, DCA.

85. See Hayward and Thomson, eds., *Tully*, e.g., 52, 53, 67, 68, 69.

86. Leonard Spaulding to James Farrar, Jr., 15 Aug. 1842; Mss. 842465,

DCA. Another interesting point of contrast is the change in schedule of lectures between Tully's time as a student and Spaulding's, though that may have been chance rather than part of a clear-cut shift in policy. See Hayward and Thomson, eds., *Tully*, 54.

87. See *Dartmouth College . . . Catalog*, 907, where Spaulding is listed as a nongraduate of the 1842 class; his name there is spelled "Spalding."

88. Albert Boyden—grandson of Wyatt Boyden—in a letter to the "Secretary of the College" dated 22 Aug. 1848, confirms the pencilled (and difficult to read) date on the Charles Boyden letter (of which he was making a gift to the College) as "no doubt" 1848, since it was about that time that "Uncle Charles left for the gold fields with the other Forty-niners." Diligent searching has not turned up the present location in the DCA of this letter.

89. Charles Boyden to his parents (Mr. and Mrs. Wyatt C. Boyden), 9 Nov. [1848]. From an original letter at DCA. Current location not known. A transcribed copy of the letter is in C. Putnam's files.

90. This segment of Child's 22 Sept. 1862 letter was among the excerpts (and other letters) quoted in Mark Travis, "Wild Dreamer of Bath," *DM* 24, no. 4 (Summer 1999): 33–39, at 35. William Child himself wrote a massive *History of the Fifth Regiment of New Hampshire Volunteers in the American Civil War* (Bristol, N.H.: R. W. Musgrove, 1893).

91. Flanders's letter to Frost (7 June 1881) and Frost's to Henry (13 June 1881) are filed with Henry's numerous letters; see MS 586, DCA.

92. Simpson was an 1857 DMS graduate. *Dartmouth College . . . Catalog*, 857.

93. Allen had begun his medical studies at DMS, in 1878; he earned his M.D. from the University of Vermont in 1881. *Dartmouth College . . . Catalog*, 918.

94. Millers River Hospital, Winchendon, Massachusetts, accepted its first patients in 1907 and was incorporated in 1915. For more on John G. Henry and his hospital, see Lois Stevenson Greenwood, *Winchendon Years: 1764–1964* (Winchendon, Mass.: Town of Winchendon, 1970).

95. Eugene Orsenigo, "The Medical School at Dartmouth College, Hanover, N.H." [unpubl. ms., dated 11 June 1934], p. 7; DCA.

Chapter 4. Curricular Change

1. Sir Frederick W. Andrewes, *The Birth and Growth of Science in Medicine—The Harveiean Oration: 1920* (London: Allard and Son and West Newman, 1920), 14.

2. *Dartmouth College and Associated Schools General Catalog, 1769–1940* (Hanover, N.H.: Dartmouth Pubs., 1940), 839.

3. "Part of Delegates Report on the Examinations of 1845"; DMS, *Records*, DA-3, Box 9:1, DCA. Emphases in the original.

4. Besides Dartmouth there were six or eight, depending on what counts as a "medical school" (as opposed to a "department") and on who is doing the counting. See, e.g., N. S. Davis, *Contributions to the History of Medical Education and Medical Institutions in the United States of America, 1776–1876* (Washington, D.C.: GPO, 1877); Martin Kaufman, *American Medical Education: The Formative Years, 1765–1920* (Westport, Conn.: Greenwood Press,

1976); and Henry Burnell Shafer, *The American Medical Profession, 1783–1850* (New York: Columbia Univ. Press, 1936). An "Appendix" to William Allen, *An Address Occasioned by the Death of Nathan Smith, M.D.* (Brunswick [Maine]: G. Griffin, 1829), 31, lists seven (including Dartmouth) through 1812.

5. These quotations from Jackson's committee report of 16 June 1812 can be found in A. B. Crosby, *A Contribution to the Medical History of New Hampshire* (Nashua, N.H.: Moore and Langley, 1870), 18, 19, 20.

6. L. B. Richardson, "Shattuck Observatory," in *DAM* 36, no. 3 (Dec. 1943): 72.

7. Oliver Hubbard to Benjamin Silliman, 27 Feb. 1836; Mss. 836177.1, DCA. Emphasis in the original.

8. Henry K. Beecher and Mark D. Altschule, *Medicine at Harvard: The First Three Hundred Years* (Hanover, N.H.: UPNE, 1977), 68, 101–2, 103.

9. Kenneth M. Ludmerer, *Learning to Heal: The Development of American Medical Education* (Baltimore: Johns Hopkins Univ. Press, 1996 [BasicBooks, 1985], 12, 48, quoting from the *Annual Report of the President and Treasurer of Harvard College (1869–70)*, 18.

10. Charles W. Eliot, "The Inaugural Address" (19 Oct. 1869), in William Allan Neilson, ed., *Charles W. Eliot: The Man and His Beliefs*, 2 vols. (New York: Harper & Brothers, 1926), I: 6.

11. Robert T. Edes, *Text-Book of Therapeutics and Materia Medica intended for the Use of Students and Practitioners* (Philadelphia: Lea Bros., 1887), [viii].

12. Meeting Minutes, Vol. III, p. 414 (17 July 1867); DC Trustees, *Records*, DA-1, DCA.

13. Meeting Minutes, Vol. IV, p. 41 (17 Aug. 1869); DC Trustees, *Records*, DA-1, DCA.

14. E. W. Dimond to Asa D. Smith, 25 Jan. 1869; Mss. 869125.1, DCA.

15. Carleton B. Chapman, *Dartmouth Medical School: The First 175 Years* (Hanover, N.H.: UPNE, 1973), 70.

16. Meeting Minutes, Vol. IV, p. 208 (19 Feb. 1878); DC Trustees, *Records* DA-1, DCA.

17. Edwin J. Bartlett, "Materies Medici," *DAM* 16, no. 8 (June 1924): 674.

18. Meeting Minutes, Vol. IV, p. 330 (19 Apr. 1883); DC Trustees, *Records*, DA-1, DCA.

19. Meeting Minutes, Vol. IV, p. 570 (4 Apr. 1892); DC Trustees, *Records*, DA-1, DCA.

20. Meeting Minutes, Vol. IV, p. 516 (26 Dec. 1890); DC Trustees, *Records*, DA-1, DCA.

21. Meeting Minutes, Vol. V, p. 53 (3 May 1893); DC Trustees, *Records*, DA-1, DCA.

22. Meeting Minutes, Vol. II, p. 144 (22 Aug. 1820); DC Trustees, *Records*, DA-1, DCA. See also *Dartmouth . . . General Catalog*, 830.

23. John Duffy, *From Humors to Medical Science*, 2nd ed. (Urbana/Chicago: Univ. of Illinois Press), 81.

24. See Charles E. Rosenberg, "The Therapeutic Revolution: Medicine, Meaning, and Social Change in Nineteenth-Century America," in Morris J. Vogel and Charles E. Rosenberg, eds., *The Therapeutic Revolution: Essays in the Social History of American Medicine* (Philadelphia: Univ. of Penn. Press, 1979),

for a useful discussion of these shifts in attitude and practice. See also William G. Rothstein, *American Physicians in the 19th Century: From Sects to Science* (Baltimore: Johns Hopkins Univ. Press, 1992 [1972], especially ch. 7, "The Thomsonian Movement."

25. Eli Ives at Yale was way ahead; he was a pioneer in teaching the diseases of children as a separate course in 1813, antedating other pediatric-specific courses by more than half a century. See Howard A. Pearson, "Preface," in Pearson, ed., *Eli Ives, M.D., Lectures on the Diseases of Children* (New Haven, Conn.: [privately publ.], 1986), 6.

26. E. R. Peaslee, *Human Histology* (Philadelphia: Blanchard and Lea, 1857). Phineas S. Conner, in his *Historical Address: Dartmouth Medical College Centennial Exercises* [Hanover, N.H.: Dartmouth Press, 1907], 17, is one of those who says Peaslee's text was the first of its kind in English.

27. Edmund R. Peaslee, *Ovarian Tumors: Their pathology, diagnosis and treatment, especially by ovariotomy* (New York: D. Appleton, 1872; London: H. K. Lewis, 1873).

28. Meeting Minutes, Vol. IV, p. 291 (3 Oct. 1881); DC Trustees, *Records*, DA-1, DCA.

29. Chapman, *175 Years*, 71, said "hygiene and public health were introduced" in 1880. Evidence for the claim is in "Medical College," 1880–81, p. 50, in *Dartmouth College Catalogue 1866–81*; DC Hist. LD1427. D3, DCA. Whether it happened is less clear.

30. L. B. How to C. P. Frost, 4 May 1881; DMS, *Records* DA-3, Box 9:7, DCA. They did not get (John Shaw?) Billings.

31. A memo attesting to this vote on 26 June 1895 is in DMS, *Records*, DA-3, Box 9:16. Conn had begun as a lecturer in 1886.

32. Thayer Adams Smith, Jr., and Dorothy Priscilla Schuman, *The Smith–Parkhurst Story* (Los Angeles: Transamerica Press, 1967), 22. It would be W. T. Smith who would perform the first surgical operation after the Mary Hitchcock Memorial Hospital opened in 1893.

33. A fuller review of who was hired when, what each taught, and when in turn those persons resigned—for the period from Nathan Smith to 1870—can be found in A. B. Crosby, *A Contribution to the Medical History of New Hampshire* (Nashua, N.H.: Moore and Langley, 1870), 21–24. For the period up to the Civil War, see also the concise but helpful chapter on "The Medical Department of Dartmouth College" in William Frederick Norwood, *Medical Education in the United States Before the Civil War* (Philadelphia: Univ. of Penn. Press, 1944), 186–91.

34. A. B. Crosby, *Contribution*, 8. Crosby was no doubt moved to this rhetoric by the passage in 1869 of "An Act for the Advancement of Anatomical and Surgical Science," which specified the conditions under which the bodies of wards of the state, etc., could be used by instructors in medical schools for instructional purposes. See New Hampshire Laws of 1869, ch. 40; this was reaffirmed in the 1891 Public Statutes, ch. 136. The only change was to make the *privilege* of granting permission to take a body into a *duty* on the county commissioner.

35. Frederick C. Waite, "Grave Robbing in New England," *Bull. of the Med. Lib. Assoc.* 33, no. 3 (July 1945): 272–94, at 275.

36. See Oliver S. Hayward and Constance E. Putnam, *Improve, Perfect, &*

Perpetuate: Dr. Nathan Smith and Early American Medical Education (Hanover, N.H.: UPNE, 1998), ch. 6 "Trouble in the Anatomy Department" (especially student Ezekiel Dodge Cushing's account of how he fended off the sheriff's men on one occasion, pp. 96–97). Also, in 1826, a Dartmouth student wrote to his brother that the "town has been in a terrible state of excitement the winter past. Subjects have been dug up." John Willard to Augustus Willard, 25 Mar. 1826; Mss. 826255, DCA. See also "Dartmouth Undying," *DAM* 81, no. 2 (Oct. 1988): 96. The DCA contain numerous accounts of episodes involving DMS students.

37. Gilman D. Frost, "Introductory Lecture to the 99th Annual Course delivered at the Dart. Med. School July 16, 1895" (hand-written, apparently an unpublished manuscript), 5–6; Mss. 895416.1, DCA. Emphasis in original.

38. "Records of the faculty of medicine in Dartmouth College, 1845–1862," p. 50 (5 Sept. 1846); DMS, *Records*, DA-3, Box 12:3, DCA.

39. Conner, *Historical Address*, 23.

40. L. B. How to C. P. Frost, 6 Feb. 1880; DMS, *Records*, DA-3, Box 9:6, DCA.

41. L. B. How to C. P. Frost, 4 May 1881; DMS, *Records*, DA-3, Box 9:7, DCA.

42. John Ordronaux, an 1850 graduate of the College, taught medical jurisprudence. His name rather than the subject may have been inserted on the chart because the allotted space did not permit two words.

43. L. B. How to C. P. Frost, 14 Mar. 1878; DMS, *Records*, DA-3, Box 9: 4, DCA. How's proposal did not prevail. The vote taken at the faculty's annual meeting in September approved a different order of courses, one that permitted repeating several sets of special lectures that had been "highly valuable & much appreciated by the class." "Records of the faculty of medicine in Dartmouth College, 1863–1925," [n.p.] (16 Sept. 1879); DMS, *Records*, DA-3, Box 12:5, DCA. Emphases in original.

44. "Records of the faculty of medicine in Dartmouth College, 1845–1862," pp. 44–45 (14 Aug. 1846); DMS, *Records*, DA-3, Box 12:3, DCA.

45. *Boston Med. & Surg. Jrnl.* (22 June 1842): 321.

46. Louis Elsberg to C. P. Frost, 19 Apr. 1881; DMS, *Records*, DA-3, Box 9:7, DCA. Emphasis in original.

47. David Webster to C. P. Frost, 21 Feb. 1890, and C. L. Dana to C. P. Frost, 16 Aug. 1891; DMS, *Records*, DA-3, Box 9:14, DCA.

48. Edwin J. Bartlett, "Materies," 675.

49. C. P. Frost to Faculty (memo and letter), 21 Nov. 1884; DMS, *Records*, DA-3, Box 9:10, DCA. Emphasis in original. All propositions except the one on increasing the course length received majority votes and presumably were implemented. A subsequent vote to extend the course to twenty weeks did pass. "Records of the faculty of medicine in Dartmouth College, 1863–1925," [n.p.] (2 Sept. 1885); DMS, *Records*, DA-3, Box 12:5, DCA, which is reflected in the explicit statement in the 1886 catalog that the lecture course would last twenty weeks. The dates given for the spring course indicate that the twenty-week course may already have begun then. See *Dartmouth College Medical School Catalog 1825–97* (1885, p. 5; 1886, p. 3); DC Hist. R 747.D37, DCA.

50. The documents cited and quoted in the next two paragraphs have been bound together in a volume titled *Dartmouth College Medical School Catalogue 1825–97*; DC Hist. R747 .D37, DCA.

51. Among the textbooks listed were two by Dartmouth faculty: Mundé's *Minor Gynecology* [actual title: *Minor Gynecological Surgery*] (New York: William Wood, 1880) and Ordronaux's *Medical Jurisprudence* [actual title *The Jurisprudence of Medicine*] (Philadelphia: T. & J. W. Johnson, 1869).

52. Jesse Little, [Lecture Notebook]; Vault Mss., DCA. Lewis Emmons, "Medical Notebook 1827–1830"; Vault Mss., DCA.

53. Paul Fortunatus Mundé, "Lecture Notes on Gynecology," [n.d., but see the inserted date "1885"]; Vault Mss., DCA.

54. A sheet indicating what topics were covered in the seventeen hours of instruction in obstetrics given by John Osborn Polak in 1904 is in DMS, *Records*, DA-3, Box 7:24. Polak's *Pelvic Inflammation in Women*, for example, was published in both New York and London by D. Appleton, in 1921, 1922, and again in 1931.

55. "Dr. Hill" may have been Thomas Prentiss Hill, who was practicing in Hanover at the time young Boyden was writing. There was no "Hill" in Wyatt Boyden's class, either in the College or in the Medical School.

56. Low though the fees for medical education seem from today's perspective, the need to earn money between terms was a real one for many of the students—and had been for many years. In 1809, one College faculty member wrote to George Cheyne Shattuck that the students were "as usual at this season of the year, considerably scattered over the country, discharging the humble but useful office of Pedagogues." Adams, Ebenezer. Letter to George Cheyne Shattuck, 6 Dec. 1809. George Cheyne Shattuck Papers, MHS. Twenty years later, in 1828, one of the medical students wrote to a doctor—quite probably his preceptor—that he had been teaching school at "Salisbury Villedge" and at Northfield. Parsons Whidden to Edward B. Moore, M.D.; Mss. 828525, DCA. (Whidden is listed as a member of the class of 1836. *Dartmouth . . . General Catalog*, 848.)

57. Charles Boyden to his parents (Mr. and Mrs. Wyatt C. Boyden), 9 Nov. [1848]. A transcribed copy of the letter is in C. Putnam's files.

58. I am indebted to Robert E. Nye, Jr., for compiling these figures and sharing them with me.

59. Parsons Whidden to Edward B. Moore, M.D.; Mss. 828525, DCA.

60. "Natural theology" is the attempt to establish the existence and nature of God solely by reliance on reason and experience.

61. Oliver S. Hayward and Elizabeth H. Thomson, eds., *The Journal of William Tully, Medical Student at Dartmouth 1808–1809* (New York: Science History Pubs., 1977), 66–67.

62. Mundé, when he gave the Introductory Lecture in 1882, spoke of the "custom of the Medical Faculty," according to which it was the "duty . . . [of] the youngest and last-appointed professor to deliver the introductory address." Evidence exists, however, that this "custom" was honored as much in the breach as in its execution.

63. "Records of the faculty of medicine in Dartmouth College, 1863–1925," [n.p.] (3 Aug. 1880); DMS, *Records*, DA-3, Box 12:5, DCA.

64. "Records of the faculty of Medicine in Dartmouth College, 1845–1862," p. 136 (10 Aug. 1852); DMS, *Records*, DA-3, Box 12:1, DCA.

65. Virginia G. Drachman, *Hospital with a Heart* (Ithaca, N.Y.: Cornell Univ. Press, 1984), 30. Rosemary Lunardini, "A Century of Minutes," *DM* 17, no. 2 (Winter 1992): 35–36.

66. Meeting Minutes, Vol. IV, p. 93 (28 June 1872); DC Trustees, *Records*, DA-1, DCA.

67. Bliss Forbush, "Moses Sheppard & Mental Illness," in *Crosscurrents in Psychiatry and Psychoanalysis* (Philadelphia: Lippincott, 1967), 15.

68. "Records of the faculty of medicine in Dartmouth College, 1845–1862," p. 58 (29 Oct. 1846), p. 129 (4 Sept. 1851), and p. 152 (26 Jan. 1854); DMS, *Records*, DA-3, Box 12:3, DCA.

69. James A. Spalding, *Maine Physicians of 1820* (Lewiston, Maine: [privately published], 1928), *passim* and 82. Also quoted in Samuel R. Webber, "Early Days in Maine Surgery," *NEJM* 260 (22 Jan. 1959): 168.

70. These and many other examples—as well as numerous grade sheets—can be found in DMS, *Records*, DA-3, Box 7:9 (also, e.g., 7:10 and 7:22), DCA. A few miscellaneous test papers (including early "blue books"), grade sheets, and hand-written sheets with examination questions, mostly in medicine and obstetrics, can be found in DMS, *Records*, DA-3, Box 7:12 through Box 7:25, DCA.

71. "Results of Examinations of Candidates for the Degree of MD. At the end of each term. Commencing with the Year 1841." The 1856 examination results (11 Nov. 1856) begin on page [151]. For Hunt, see p. [162]; Merrill, p. [163]; and Gove (9 Nov. 1858), p. [181]; DMS, *Records*, DA-3, Box 7:5, DCA. Emphases in original.

72. "Results of Examinations of Candidates for the degree of M.D. at the end of each term, Commencing with the year 1861," 30 and 31 Oct. 1871, pp. [174 and 175] respectively; DMS, *Records*, DA-3, Box 7:6, DCA. Hamlin, accordingly, is listed as a nongraduate in 1876; Leete returned, successfully passed, and graduated in 1877.

73. L. B. How to C. P. Frost, 21 July 1881; DMS, *Records*, DA-3, Box 7:9, DCA.

74. *Dartmouth . . . General Catalog*, 869.

75. L. B. How memo, [n.d.] Sept. 1881; DMS, *Records*, DA-3, Box 7:10, DCA.

76. Bartlett, "Materies," 677.

77. *Dartmouth College Medical School Catalogs (1825–97)*, 7; DC Hist. R 747.D37, DCA.

78. Meeting Minutes, Vol. I, p. 349 (24 Aug. 1810); DC Trustees, *Records*, DA-1, DCA.

79. Meeting Minutes, Vol. 1, p. 370 (25 Aug. 1812); DC Trustees, *Records*, DA-1, DCA.

80. Meeting Minutes, Vol. II, pp. 155–57, ([4th Wed. of] Oct. 1820); DC Trustees, *Records*, DA-1, DCA.

81. "Statutes of the Medical Institution of Dartmouth College," pp. 1–2 (Aug. 1842); DMS, *Records*, DA-3, Box 8:13, DCA.

82. "Records of the faculty of medicine in Dartmouth College, 1845–1862," p. 36 (7 Nov. 1845); DMS, *Records*, DA-3, Box 12:3, DCA. Emphasis in original.

83. Bartlett, "Materies," 676.

Chapter 5. Shaping the Institution

1. Thomas Coar, trans. [into Latin and English], *The Aphorisms of Hippocrates* (New York: Classics of Medicine Library, Gryphon Editions, 1982 [London: A. J. Valpy, 1822]), 1.

2. William T. Smith, Edwin J. Bartlett, and Gilman D. Frost to the "Faculty of Dartmouth Medical College," 30 May 1896; DMS, *Records*, DA-3, Box 9: 16, DCA.

3. L. B. How to "Dear Doctor [Frost]," 14 Aug. 1877; DMS, *Records*, DA-3, Box 9:3, DCA. Emphasis in the original.

4. Henry Field to "Dear Doctor [Frost]," 14 Nov. 1872; DMS, *Records*, DA-3, Box 9:2, DCA. Emphases in the original.

5. A. B. Crosby to "My dear Dr. [Frost]," 2 Mar. 1875; DMS, *Records*, DA-3, Box 9:2, DCA.

6. L. B. How to C. P. Frost, 14 Mar. 1878; DMS, *Records*, DA-3, Box 9:4, DCA.

7. E. S. Dunster to C. P. Frost, 23 Nov. 1886; DMS, *Records*, DA-3, Box 9: 11, DCA.

8. Diligent detective work has not made it possible to identify "Dr. Chamberlin." Conceivably it was DMS graduate (1880) George Washington Chamberlin, born in Bradford, Vermont. But neither the Bradford nor the nearby Newbury (Vermont) historical society was able to produce information about him. If he was the person How had in mind, he would not have turned out to be a good choice—despite his sensitivity, education, and experience. He died a mere year later—in 1888—in Yellow Springs, Nebraska.

9. L. B. How to C. P. Frost, 30 Jan. 1887; DMS, *Records*, DA-3, Box 9:12, DCA.

10. "Records of the faculty of Medicine in Dartmouth College, 1845–1862," p. 90 (5 Oct. 1848); DMS, *Records*, DA-3, Box 12:3, DCA.

11. "Records of the faculty of medicine in Dartmouth College, 1863–1925," [n.p.] (23 Oct. 1877); DMS, *Records*, DA-3, Box 12:5, DCA.

12. "Records of the faculty of medicine in Dartmouth College, 1863–1925," [n.p.] ([n.d.] Sept. 1888); DMS, *Records*, DA-3, Box 12:5, DCA.

13. Edward Preble on Elsberg, *DAB* VI: 119.

14. "Records of the faculty of medicine in Dartmouth College, 1863–1925," [n.p.] (3 Sept. 1885); DMS, *Records*, DA-3, Box 12:5, DCA. In general, on Elsberg, see letters to Frost in DMS, *Records*, DA-3, Box 9:7, DCA.

15. Paul Fortunatus Mundé, *Minor Gynecological Surgery* (New York: William Wood, 1880) [v].

16. He once held faculty appointments concurrently at Medical School of Maine (Bowdoin) and Albany Medical College as well as at Dartmouth and both New York Medical College and Bellevue Hospital Medical College. Herbert S. Reichle on Peaslee, *DAB* XIV: 371.

17. Phineas S. Conner, Historical Address: Dartmouth Medical College Centennial Exercises, . . . 1897 [Hanover, N. H.: Dartmouth Press, 1907], 17. Conner's praise for Peaslee might seem excessive, but it simply echoes the eight-page memorial testimony to this "Vir bonus et sapiens." "Records of the faculty of medicine in Dartmouth College, 1863–1925," [n.p.] (22 Feb. 1878); DMS, *Records*, DA-3, Box 12:5, DCA. For Peaslee's contributions to professional literature, see Marilyn Tobias, *Old Dartmouth on Trial: The Transformation of the*

Academic Community in Nineteenth-Century America (New York: New York Univ. Press, 1982, 2002), 29.

18. William B. Atkinson, *The Physicians and Surgeons of the United States* (Philadelphia: Charles Robson, 1878), 356. Conner (*Historical Address*, 17) said this book represented a "marvel of research."

19. Carleton B. Chapman, "Development 1797–1968: The Next Logical Step," *DMSQ* 5, no. 1 (Summer 1968): 19; also in Carleton B. Chapman, *Dartmouth Medical School: The First 175 Years* (Hanover, N.H.: UPNE, 1973), 36.

20. Edwin J. Bartlett, "Materies Medici," *DAM* 16, no. 8 (June 1924): 675.

21. Chapman, *175 Years*, 38–39.

22. This concise account of how the system worked and how it changed is based largely on Chapman, *175 Years*, 34–36.

23. Frederic P. Lord, "The Very Old and the Old," *DAM* 54, no. 5 (Feb. 1962): 23–28, at 25. Lord, a student in the College when Frost died, described him as looking "like Michelangelo's painting of God in the Sistine Chapel, with his flowing white beard and great dignity," but reported that "this somewhat fearsome atmosphere" disappeared when Frost visited the sickbed.

24. I am indebted to Robert E. Nye, Jr., for sharing with me his extracts from the course catalogues, some of which I have used in what follows. In general, also, see sections devoted to the Medical School in *Dartmouth College Catalogue 1866–81*; DC Hist. LD1427 .D3, DCA.

25. "Medical College," 1876–77, p. 70, in *Dartmonth College Catalogue* 1866–81; DC Hist. LD1427.D3, DCA. Emphasis in the original.

26. Recall Lyman How's concern over whether there would be room for a course on hygiene if all these special topics were added. Hygiene and public health do seem to have been added to the offerings that year. On the other hand, a rather different picture emerges when one peruses the *Dartmouth College and Associated Schools General Catalog, 1769–1940* (Hanover, N.H.: Dartmouth College Publications, 1940). There we see cconfirmed that Conn—in 1886—was the first lecturer in hygiene (p. 832).

27. "Medical College," 1889–90, p. 61, in *Dartmouth College Catalogue 1881–94*; DC Hist. LD1427 .D3, DCA.

28. Albert Smith to Asa Smith, 30 Oct. 1867; the entire letter is quoted in [Robert E. Nye, Jr.], "Notes from Dartmouth Archives," *DMSQ* (Autumn 1967): 30. See also "Records of the faculty of medicine in Dartmouth College, 1863–1925," p. 44 (14 Sept. 1868); DMS, *Records*, DA-3, Box 12:5, DCA.

29. Not that there hadn't been major efforts in this direction earlier. A case in point is the long report submitted to the medical faculty (by whose members it was unanimously adopted) by a committee comprising Albert Smith and E. E. Phelps, who had been charged with the task of "establishing an exact order for the course of Medical Lectures," already three decades before. See "Records of the faculty of Medicine in Dartmouth College, 1845–1862," p. 166 (7 Nov. 1855); DMS, *Records*, DA-3, Box 12:3, DCA.

30. "Medical College," 1893–94, pp. 109, 110, in *Dartmouth College Catalogue 1881–94*; DC Hist. LD1427 .D3, DCA. Yet already in 1857, the faculty had approved the purchase of an oxyhydrogen microscope for E. E. Phelps. "Records of the faculty of Medicine in Dartmouth College, 1845–1862," p. 179 (6 Nov. 1857); DMS, *Records*, DA-3, Box 12:3, DCA. That same year, E. R. Peaslee published a histology textbook. Thus it seems unlikely that microscopy

and histology were not being taught until the 1890s, even though they were first listed then.

31. The information on the classes of 1855 and 1875 comes from "The Medical Classes in the N. Hampshire Medical Institution, Commencing with the Class of 1855"; DMS, *Records*, DA-3, Box 7:2, DCA; the separate untitled notebook (with class lists from 1878 to 1904), pp. 162–69; DMS, *Records*, DA-3, Box 7:4, DCA; and the "Register of Medical students 1876–1895," pp. 54–57 and 110–119; DMS, *Records*, DA-3, Box 8:15. Similar registers for other years are in separate folders in the same box.

32. Chapman, *175 Years*, 37–38.

33. DC Trustees, *Records*, Vol. II, p. 155 ([mtg. beginning 4th Wed. of] Oct. 1820), DA-1, DCA.

34. In fact, although a few changes were voted by the Trustees at their August 1831 meeting—DC Trustees, *Records*, Vol. II, p. 292 ([last Wed. of] Aug. 1831); DA-1, DCA—remarkably little in the way of alterations had been made slightly more than two decades later. See "Statutes of the Medical Institution of Dartmouth College" (Aug. 1842); DMS, *Records*, DA-3, Box 8:13, DCA.

35. DC Trustees, *Records*, Vol. III, p. 8 ([Tues. before last Thurs. of] July 1841); DA-1, DCA.

36. "Records of the faculty of medicine in Dartmouth College, 1845–1862," p. 13 (16 Sept. 1845); DMS, *Records*, DA-3, Box 12:3, DCA.

37. "Records of the faculty of medicine in Dartmouth College, 1845–1862," p. 47 (21 Aug. 1845); DMS, *Records*, DA-3, Box 12:3, DCA. Emphases in the original.

38. "Records of the faculty of medicine in Dartmouth College, 1845–1862," p. 37 (7 Nov. 1845); DMS, *Records*, DA-3, Box 12:3, DCA.

39. "Records of the faculty of medicine in Dartmouth College, 1845–1862," p. 200 (2 Sept. 1862); DMS, *Records*, DA-3, Box 12:3, DCA.

40. DC Trustees, *Records*, Vol. III, p. 346 (20 Nov. 1863); DA-1, DCA.

41. DC Trustees, *Records*, Vol. IV, pp. 13 and 23 (22 and 24 July 1868); DA-1, DCA.

42. "Records of the faculty of medicine in Dartmouth College, 1863–1925," [n.p.] (16 Sept. 1870); DMS, *Records*, DA-3, Box 12:5, DCA.

43. DC Trustees, *Records*, Vol. IV, p. 66 (22 July 1870); DA-1, DCA.

44. DC Trustees, *Records*, Vol. IV, p. 208 (19 Feb. 1878) and pp. 211, 213 (25 June 1878), DA-1, DCA.

45. DC Trustees, *Records*, Vol. IV, p. 241 (26 June 1879), DA-1, DCA.

46. DC Trustees, *Records*, Vol. IV, p. 270 (7 Apr. 1881), DA-1, DCA.

47. DC Trustees, *Records*, Vol. V, p. 101 (23 Mar. 1893), DA-1, DCA.

48. DC Trustees, *Records*, Vol. V, pp. 137–38 (30 Nov. 1894), DA-1, DCA.

49. DC Trustees, *Records*, Vol. IV, p. 516 (26 Dec. 1890), DA-1, DCA.

50. DC Trustees, *Records*, Vol. V, p. 2 (28 June 1892), DA-1, DCA.

51. DC Trustees, *Records*, Vol. V, p. 81 (30 June 1893), DA-1, DCA.

52. DC Trustees, *Records*, Vol. V, pp. 96–97 (1 Dec. 1893), DA-1, DCA.

53. DC Trustees, *Records*, Vol. V, pp. 151–52 (25 June 1895), DA-1, DCA. A "true copy" of the regulations as voted on, dated 15 July 1895, is in DMS, *Records*, DA-3, Box 9:16, DCA.

54. Robert Graham, "A Firm Foundation," *DMSAM* (Fall 1991): 18.

55. DC Trustees, *Records*, Vol. I, p. 233 (29 Aug. 1799), DA-1, DCA.

56. It is not clear how many structures were included in this plural, but probably Culver Hall—which contained the chemistry laboratory—was being counted, along with the Medical House itself.

57. DC Trustees, *Records*, Vol. III, p. 44 (24 July 1844), DA-1, DCA.

58. "Part of Delegates Report on the Examinations of 1845"; DMS, *Records*, DA-3, Box 9:1, DCA.

59. E. R. Peaslee to C. P. Frost, 10 Feb. 1872; DMS, *Records*, DA-3, Box 9:2, DCA.

60. Chapman, *175 Years*, 36. See also Conner, *Historical Address*, 6.

61. "The Library of the Medical School," *DAM* 7, no. 6 (Apr. 1915): 222. (Tears were shed when the building was razed in 1963.

62. Chapman, *175 Years*, 37, says the Stoughton gift was $12,000 and "did not entirely cover the costs of the pathological museum and the alterations."

63. By "Faculty of the College" Frost clearly means the medical faculty only, for they alone were still paid in part by lecture receipts. *College* faculty were on salary.

64. One writer has observed that having the state own the building, which might superficially have seemed disadvantageous, "was of undoubted value to the college, as it was an added reason for the unwillingness to establish a literary institution in some other place than Hanover." Eugene Orsenigo, "The Medical School at Dartmouth College, Hanover, N.H." [unpubl. ms., dated 11 June 1934], p. 6; DCA.

65. "Records of the faculty of medicine in Dartmouth College, 1863–1925," [n.p.] (28 Aug. 1874); DMS, *Records*, DA-3, Box 12:5, DCA. The temptation to direct that the balance of the $5,000 grant should be used to reimburse the faculty for the roughly $1,400 they had collectively donated for repairs was apparently resisted. In December of 1894, a unanimous vote was recorded authorizing Frost to use the balance of the "N. H. State Fund" instead to help pay for work required at that time "to properly finish and equip for service the new dissecting room built on the south end of the medical college"—a half-basement room added in 1895. "Records of the faculty of medicine in Dartmouth College, 1863–1925," [n.p.] (11 Dec. 1894 [inserted before the 19 Nov. minutes]); DMS, *Records*, DA-3, Box 12:5, DCA. The work was completed at a cost of about $2,200, according to a marginal note. Conner, *Historical Address*, 6, gives the cost as $1,700.

66. "Records of the faculty of medicine in Dartmouth College, 1863–1925," p. 20 (11 Sept. 1865); DMS, *Records*, DA-3, Box 12:5, DCA.

67. "Records of the faculty of Medicine in Dartmouth College, 1845–1862," pp. 95–96 (8 Nov. 1848); DMS, *Records*, DA-3, Box 12:3, DCA. See also Rosemary Lunardini, "A Century of Minutes," *DM* 16, no. 2 (Winter 1992): 35, and *Dartmouth . . . General Catalog*, 854.

68. "Records of the faculty of Medicine in Dartmouth College, 1845–1862," p. 139 (1 Nov. 1852); DMS, *Records*, DA-3, Box 12:3, DCA.

69. "Records of the faculty of Medicine in Dartmouth College, 1845–1862," p. 73 (25 Aug. 1847); DMS, *Records*, DA-3, Box 12:3, DCA.

70. "Records of the faculty of Medicine in Dartmouth College, 1845–1862," p. 32 (28 Oct. 1845); DMS, *Records*, DA-3, Box 12:3, DCA. "Records of the faculty of Medicine in Dartmouth College, 1845–1862," p. 63 (12 May 1847); DMS, *Records*, DA-3, Box 12:3, DCA. Also Records of N. H. Med. Society, May 1846.

71. "Records of the faculty of Medicine in Dartmouth College, 1845–1862," p. 75 (24 Sept. 1847); DMS, *Records*, DA-3, Box 12:3, DCA.

72. "Records of the faculty of medicine in Dartmouth College, 1863–1925," p. 24 (29 Sept. 1845) as well as pp. 27, 28–29, 29–30, and 31–32 (21, 23, 24, and 28 Oct. 1845.); DMS, *Records*, DA-3, Box 12:5, DCA. See also *Dartmouth . . . General Catalog*, 853.

73. G. P. Conn to C. P. Frost, 12 Sept. 1887; DMS, *Records*, DA-3, Box 9: 12, DCA.

74. The allusion is to Rolf Syvertsen's famous "rescues." See ch. 7 for a few of the myriad "Sy stories" still being told forty years after his death.

Chapter 6. The (Carnegie) Inspector Calls

1. Francis Bacon, *The Essays or Counsels, Civil and Moral* (Mount Vernon, N.Y.: Peter Pauper Press, [n.d.]), 83.

2. *The Daily Dartmouth*, 30 June 1897, p. [2]. An enthusiastic review—presumably more original—of the concert that was part of the centenary celebration appeared on the same page.

3. Phineas S. Conner, *Historical Address: Dartmouth Medical College Centennial Exercises, . . . 1897* [Hanover, N. H.: Dartmouth Press, 1907], 23. Quoted also in ch. 3.

4. Meeting Minutes, Vol. V, p. 201 (8 May 1897); DC Trustees, *Records*, Vault Mss., DCA.

5. Two of William Thayer Smith's sons became doctors and had Dartmouth degrees: Morris K. Smith (DC 1907, DMS 1911) and Thayer A. Smith (DC 1910). Of Thayer's nine children, three with Dartmouth College degrees became doctors (Thayer, Jr., 1944; Donald W., 1951, and Samuel G., 1958). See *DMSAN&N* 3, no. 1 (Fall 1999): 6; also Thayer Adams Smith, Jr., and Dorothy Priscilla Schuman, *The Smith–Parkhurst Story* (Los Angeles:Transamerica Press, 1967).

6. Meeting Minutes, Vol. V, p. 201 (8 May 1897); DC Trustees, *Records*, Vault Mss., DCA.

7. Louis B. Matthews, "Who Was Mary Hitchcock?" *DM* 14, no. 3 (Spring 1990): 33.

8. Carleton B. Chapman, *Dartmouth Medical School: The First 175 Years* (Hanover, N.H.: UPNE, 1973), 39.

9. Robert Graham, "A Firm Foundation," *DM* 16, no. 1 (Fall 1991): 18. Some of the information about the hospital's founding is also from this article.

10. "Records of the faculty of medicine in Dartmouth College, 1863–1925," [n.p.] (1 June 1897); DMS, *Records*, DA-3, Box 12:5, DCA.

11. See 1897 N.H. Laws Chap. 63, pp. 53–54.

12. This policy lasted essentially until the four-year curriculum was reinstated in the 1970s. Many students took advantage of it, to save both time and money.

13. "Records of the faculty of medicine in Dartmouth College, 1863–1925," [n.p.] (13 and 20 July 1898); DMS, *Records*, DA-3, Box 12:5, DCA.

14. "Medical School," 1899–1900, pp. 162 and 163, *Dartmouth College Catalogue 1898–99*; DC Hist. LD1427 .D3, DCA.

15. "Medical School," 1899–1900, pp. 157–71, *Dartmouth College Catalogue 1898–99*; DC Hist. LD1427 .D3, DCA.

16. Abraham Flexner, *Medical Education in the United States and Canada: A Report to the Carnegie Foundation for the Advancement of Teaching* (New York: Carnegie Foundation for the Advancement of Teaching, 1910), 12.

17. "Medical School," 1897–98, p. 128, *Dartmouth College Catalogue 1894–98*; DC Hist. LD1427 .D3, DCA.

18. William W. Keen and J. William White, eds., *An American Text-book of Surgery: for Practitioners and Students* 3rd ed., 2 vols. (Philadelphia: W. B. Saunders, 1899).

19. First published by T. & J. W. Johnson in Philadelphia in 1869, the book was reissued by Arno Press in New York, in 1973, in the *Mental Illness and Social Policy: The American Experience* series. See also Charles Sumner Lobingier on Redfield, *DAB*: XV, 439–40, and G. Adler Blumer (who clearly knew Ordronaux personally) on Ordronaux, *DAB*: XIV, 50–51.

20. Charles B. Nancrède, *Essentials of Anatomy . . . prepared especially for students of medicine*, [1st ed.] (Philadelphia and London: Saunders, 1888); *Lectures upon the Principles of Surgery, delivered at the University of Michigan* (Philadelphia and London: Saunders, 1899); 2nd ed. (Philadelphia and London: Saunders, 1905, p. [9]. See also James M. Phalen on Nancrède, *DAB*: XIII, 379–80.

21. "Records of the faculty of medicine in Dartmouth College, 1863–1925," [n.p.] (10 Feb. 1908); DMS, *Records*, DA-3, Box 12:5, DCA (a copy of the recommendations in the faculty minutes is in Box 9:19.) See also Meeting Minutes, Vol. V, p. 484 (30 Aug. 1908); DC Trustees, *Records*, Vault Mss., DCA.

22. W. J. Tucker to W. T. Smith, 24 Dec. 1900; DMS, *Records*, DA-3, Box 9:17, DCA. Emphasis in the original.

23. Meeting Minutes, Vol. V, p. 295 (24 May 1901); DC Trustees, *Records*, Vault Mss., DCA.

24. Meeting Minutes, Vol. V, pp. 312–12 (30 May 1902); DC Trustees, *Records*, Vault Mss., DCA.

25. See Richard Harrison Shryock, "Medical Licensure in America: Past and Present," *The National Board Examiner* 13, no. 8 (May 1966): [1].

26. Robert E. Kohler, *From Medical Chemistry to Biochemistry: The Making of a Biomedical Discipline* (Cambridge: CUP, 1982), 123–24, 128.

27. [Willard C. Rappleye, Dir. of Study], *Final Report, of the Commission on Medical Education* (New York: Office of the Director of Study, 1932), 10. This later (AAMC) "Commission" is not to be confused with the "Council" on Medical Education (CME).

28. Shryock, "Medical Licensure," [3]. On the European influence on medical education in the United States, see, for example, Thomas Neville Bonner, *Becoming a Physician* (New York: OUP, 1995) and John Harley Warner, *Against the Spirit of System: The French Impulse in Nineteenth-Century American Medicine* (Princeton: Princeton Univ. Press, 1998).

29. Richard Harrison Shryock, *The Unique Influence of the Johns Hopkins University on American Medical Education* (Copenhagen: Ejnar Munksgaard, 1953), 31–32.

30. See Eliot Freidson, *Profession of Medicine: A Study of the Sociology of*

Applied Knowledge (Chicago: Univ. of Chicago Press, 1988 [1970]), 23–24, 71–72, *et passim.*

31. N. P. Colwell, "The Need, Methods and Value of Medical College Inspection," and [Editorial], "The Influence of the Carnegie Foundation on Medical Education," *JAMA* 53, no. 7 (14 Aug. 1909): 512–14 and 559–60, at 559.

32. Formerly president of M.I.T., Pritchett was the one who made the suggestion to Andrew Carnegie that resulted in his endowing the Carnegie Foundation for the Advancement of Teaching. Pritchett was its first president; he held the position from 1906 to 1930. Abraham Flexner, *I Remember* (New York: Simon & Schuster, 1940), 114.

33. Henry S. Pritchett, "Introduction," in Flexner, *Report*, vii, x, xi, xvi.

34. Abraham Flexner, *Abraham Flexner: An Autobiography* (New York: Simon & Schuster, 1960), 71. In the 1940 version of the book (*I Remember*), the wording is exactly the same.

35. Flexner, *I Remember*, 115.

36. Flexner, *I Remember*, 115.

37. Abraham Flexner to Ernest Fox Nichols, 4 May 1910; DC Office of the President, *Records*, DP-10 (Nichols), Box 2:12, DCA.

38. Flexner, *I Remember*, 115.

39. Flexner, *Report*, 262–63.

40. Flexner, *Report*, 15.

41. Flexner, *Report*, 264.

42. Colin C. Stewart to Ernest Fox Nichols, [n.d.]; DC Office of the President, *Records*, DP-10 (Nichols), Box 2:12, DCA.

43. Flexner, *Report*, 264.

44. Flexner, *Report*, 264.

45. Flexner, *Report*, 123, 124.

46. Flexner, *Report*, 147. Once again, three of Nathan Smith's four medical schools came in for direct criticism; only Yale passed muster.

47. Flexner, *Report*, 16, 17, 46.

48. Flexner, *Report*, 93.

49. For a discussion of changes going on elsewhere at the time, see Kenneth M. Ludmerer, *Time to Heal* (New York: OUP, 1999), 17–21.

50. "Medical School," 1905–06, pp. 281–89, in *Dartmouth College Catalogue 1903–06*; DC Hist. LD1427 .D3, DCA.

51. [William Thayer Smith], "Report to the Faculty of the Medical School at the Annual Meeting," pp. 2–3 (12 Sept. 1905); DMS, *Records*, DA-3, Box 9:18, DCA.

52. "Records of the faculty of medicine in Dartmouth College, 1863–1925," [n.p.] (17 Sept. 1906); DMS, *Records*, DA-3, Box 12:5, DCA.

53. The original of these recommendations from the "Faculty of the Dartmouth Medical School" (voted on and reported to the trustees 10 Feb. 1908), is in DMS, *Records*, DA-3, Box 9:19, DCA.

54. DC Office of the President, *Records*, DP-9 (Tucker), Box 5:28, DCA.

55. "Records of the faculty of medicine in Dartmouth College, 1863–1925," [n.p.] (11 Sept. 1908 and 16 Oct. 1908); DMS, *Records*, DA-3, Box 12:5, DCA.

56. In 1909, the population of Hanover was 1,797. "Medical Colleges of the United States" (Statistics 1908–1909), *JAMA* 53, no. 7 (14 Aug. 1909): 536. A year later it had increased to 1,951. Flexner, *Report*, 263.

57. N. P. Colwell to Ernest Fox Nichols, 7 Feb. 1910; DC Office of the President, *Records*, DP-10 (Nichols), Box 2:12, DCA. See also "Records of the faculty of medicine in Dartmouth College, 1863–1925," [n.p.] (11 Feb. 1910); DMS, *Records*, DA-3, Box 12:5, DCA, where the letter was copied into the minutes of the faculty meeting.

58. Meeting Minutes, Vol. V, p. 464 (17 Apr. 1908); DC Trustees, *Records*, Vault Mss., DCA.

59. "Records of the faculty of medicine in Dartmouth College, 1863–1925," p. [345] (15 Feb. 1910); DMS, *Records*, DA-3, Box 12:5, DCA.

60. John H. Nichols, Henry M. Christian, and Edward H. Nichols (a typed note in the file giving the name as "Weabels" appears to be an error) to E. J. Bartlett, 21 Feb., 21 Feb., and 24 Feb. 1910, respectively; DC Office of the President, *Records*, DP-10 (Nichols), Box 2:12, DCA.

61. Abraham Flexner to Ernest Fox Nichols, 4 May 1910; DC Office of the President, *Records*, DP-10 (Nichols), Box 2:12, DCA.

62. John M. Gile, "The Dartmouth Medical School," *DAM* 3, no. 9 (Aug. 1911): [302].

63. For further discussion of this point, see Kenneth M. Ludmerer, "The Plight of Clinical Teaching," *Bull. Hist. Med.* 57 (1983): 218–29.

64. "Records of the faculty of medicine in Dartmouth College, 1863–1925," pp. [354–58] (10 Oct. 1910); DMS, *Records*, DA-3, Box 12:5, DCA.

65. John M. Gile, "The Dartmouth Medical School," *DAM* 3, no. 9 (Aug. 1911): [302].

66. "Records of the faculty of medicine in Dartmouth College, 1863–1925," [n.p.] (25 Sept. 1912); DMS, *Records*, DA-3, Box 12:5, DCA.

67. "Records of the faculty of medicine in Dartmouth College, 1863–1925," [n.p.] (10 Jan. 1913); DMS, *Records*, DA-3, Box 12:5, DCA.

68. Dartmouth would much later undertake a joint program somewhat akin to this, with Brown University. See ch. 11.

69. The letter was copied in full into the faculty minutes. See "Records of the faculty of medicine in Dartmouth College, 1863–1925," [n.p.] (19 Jan. 1913); DMS, *Records*, DA-3, Box 12:5, DCA.

70. DC Office of the President, *Records*, DP-10 (Nichols), Box 2:12, DCA.

71. [Unsigned], "Report drawn up for use of the Special Trustee Committee and of the President"; DMS, *Records*, DA-3, Box 14:5, DCA. The following several quotations are all taken from this report.

72. "Records of the faculty of medicine in Dartmouth College, 1863–1925," [n.p.] (19 Jan. 1913); DMS, *Records*, DA-3, Box 12:5, DCA.

73. [Editorial], "The Influence of the Carnegie Foundation on Medical Education," *JAMA* 53, no. 7 (14 Aug. 1909): 512–14 and 559–60, at 559.

74. "Records of the faculty of medicine in Dartmouth College, 1863–1925," [n.p.] (10 Mar. 1913); DMS, *Records*, DA-3, Box 12:5, DCA. A typed (carbon) copy of this report is in DC Trustees, *Records*, DA-1, Box 32:25, DCA.

75. Graham's letter to nonresident faculty was transcribed in full into the faculty minutes. See "Records of the faculty of medicine in Dartmouth College, 1863–1925," [n.p.] (17 Mar. 1913); DMS, *Records*, DA-3, Box 12:5, DCA. Stewart's letter, from which the several quotations in the following paragraphs come, appears in the same meeting's minutes.

76. "Records of the faculty of medicine in Dartmouth College, 1863–1925," [n.p.] (19 Apr. 1913); DMS, *Records*, DA-3, Box 12:5, DCA.

77. George Sellers Graham, "The Medical School," *DAM* 4, no. 9 (Aug. 1912): [332].

78. DC Trustees, "Committee to Consider the Present Status of Medical Education and the Medical School" [1913]; Special Collections, Ms. DA-517, DCA.

79. Letter to resident faculty members, 22 Apr. 1913; DC Office of the President, *Records*, DP-10 (Nichols), Box 15:39, DCA.

80. Meeting Minutes, Vol. VI, p. 160 (26 Apr. 1913); DC Trustees, *Records*, Vault Mss., DCA. Nichols's committee report on which this vote was based—from which these quotations were taken—gives a thoughtful account of each alternative to dropping the two final years (and the attendant problems) that had been considered. DC Trustees, "Committee to Consider the Present Status of Medical Education and the Medical School" [1913]; Special Collections, Ms. DA-517, DCA.

81. Memorandum from the President "To the Alumni of the Dartmouth Medical School" (30 Apr. 1913); DC Office of the President, *Records*, DP-10 (Nichols), Box 15:39, DCA. for full text, see Appendix C, p. 298.

82. "Records of the faculty of medicine in Dartmouth College, 1863–1925," [n.p.] (12 May and 14 June 1913); DMS, *Records*, DA-3, Box 12:5, DCA.

83. John Martin Gile, "The Medical School," *DAM* 5, no. 9 (Aug. 1913): 271–72.

84. "Associated Schools Hold Commencement," *DAM* 6, no. 8 (June 1914): 295.

85. Frederic Pomeroy Lord, "Dartmouth Medical School, Its Present Status and Its Possibilities," *DAM* 6, no. 9 (Aug. 1914): 333–34.

86. N. P. Colwell to Ernest Fox Nichols, 30 Sept. 1914, and the CME's pamphlet No. 85, p. 18; DC Office of the President, *Records*, DP-10 (Nichols), Box 29:39, DCA.

87. Colin C. Stewart, "Dartmouth Medical School," *DAM* 7, no. 9 (Aug. 1915): 344.

88. Shryock, "Medical Licensure," [3].

Chapter 7. Reassessing the School's Identity

1. Robert Frost, "To the Thawing Wind," *The Poetry of Robert Frost* (Edward Connery Lathem, ed.), (New York: Holt, Rinehart and Winston, 1969), 11.

2. Meeting Minutes, Vol. VII, p. 64 (27 Oct. 1922); DC Trustees, *Records*, Vault Mss., DCA.

3. DMS Faculty, "Report of Committee of Dartmouth Medical School Faculty on Future Status of Dartmouth Medical School" (Hanover, N. H.: 20 Apr. 1923), p. 4; DCA.

4. DMS Faculty, "Report on Future Status," pp. 7, 12; DCA.

5. DMS Faculty, "Report on Future Status," pp. 18, 21; DCA. Against this backdrop the Hitchcock Clinic was founded four years later, as we shall see; it does not stretch credulity to suggest that this is also where the first foundation stones were laid for the Dartmouth-Hitchcock Medical Center of today.

6. DMS Faculty, "Report on Future Status," pp. 9, 22, and 13 respectively; DCA.

7. Meeting Minutes, Vol. VII, p. 80 (4 May 1923); DC Trustees, *Records*, Vault Mss., DCA.

8. "Records of the faculty of medicine in Dartmouth College, 1863–1925"; DMS, *Records*, DA-3, Box 12:5, DCA.

9. "Medical Alumni Association" *DAM* 20, no. 9 (Aug. 1928): 871.

10. Carleton B. Chapman, *Dartmouth Medical School: The First 175 Years* (Hanover, N.H.: UPNE, 1973), 51–52.

11. The first meeting of the Hitchcock Clinic took place on 13 June 1927. See "Reports of Clinic Meetings, [etc.]," in a loose-leaf binder among the Bowler papers currently in the hands of his daughter Janet Bowler FitzGibbons.

12. See the unsigned draft of a letter ("Spring 1926" handwritten in the margin) clearly written by Bowler to the trustees of the Mary Hitchcock Memorial Hospital. From the Bowler papers mentioned earlier.

13. F. P. Lord, "Fifty Years of Teaching" (22 July 1948), p. 18; Mss. 948422, DCA.

14. This and the next several quotations are from John F. Gile, "Staff Organization," presented on behalf of the Hitchcock Clinic to members of the Hospital Corporation at its annual meeting on 30 July 1931; offprint, 6 pp. From the Bowler papers.

15. Bill Cunningham, "Dr. Gile A Saint In North Country," *Boston Herald* (1 Feb. 1955): 25.

16. "Records of the faculty of medicine in Dartmouth College, 1863–1925," [n.p.] (17 June 1923, 7 June 1924, 30 Sept. 1924, and 3 Feb. 1925); DMS, *Records*, DA-3, Box 12:5, DCA.

17. "Dartmouth College Medical School, Minutes of the Committee of the Faculty, July 8, 1927–March 26, 1936," [n.p.] (14 Sept. 1927); DMS, *Records*, DA-3, Box 12:7, DCA.

18. Confidentiality was in play; no names are mentioned.

19. College records show the class of 1924 was twenty-one strong, all but two of whom were from Dartmouth College; see *Dartmouth College and Associated Schools General Catalog, 1769–1940* (Hanover, N.H.: Dartmouth College Pubs., 1940), 887.

20. See "Records of the faculty of medicine in Dartmouth College, 1863–1925," [n.p.] (25 Jan. 1925 and 29 Sept. 1927); DMS, *Records*, DA-3, Box 12: 5, DCA.

21. He did not bother to mention that he himself was one of those who had "completed the two-year course" but was not (yet) a candidate for an M.D. degree. "Dartmouth College Medical School, Minutes of the Faculty Meetings, October 4, 1927–March 24, 1936," [n.p.] (4 Oct. 1927); DMS, *Records*, DA-3, Box 12:6, DCA.

22. "Dartmouth College Medical School, Minutes of Faculty Meetings, October 4, 1927–March 24, 1936," [n.p.] (1 Oct. 1935); DMS, *Records*, DA-3, Box 12:6, DCA.

23. "Dartmouth College Medical School, Minutes of the Faculty Meetings, October 4, 1927–March 24, 1936," [n.p.] (3 May 1928); DMS, *Records*, DA-3, Box 12:6, DCA.

24. "Dartmouth College Medical School, Minutes of the Faculty Meetings, October 4, 1927–March 24, 1936," [n.p.] (12 Nov. 1929); DMS, *Records*, DA-3, Box 12:6, DCA.

25. "Dartmouth College Medical School, Minutes of the Faculty Meetings,

October 4, 1927–March 24, 1936," [n.p.] (21 Oct. 1930); DMS, *Records*, DA-3, Box 12:6, DCA.

26. "Dartmouth College Medical School, Minutes of the Faculty Meetings, October 4, 1927–March 24, 1936," [n.p.] (15 June 1932 and 4 Oct. 1932); DMS, *Records*, DA-3, Box 12:6, DCA.

27. "Dartmouth College Medical School, Minutes of the Faculty Meetings, October 4, 1927–March 24, 1936," [n.p.] (25 Sept. 1934 and 1 Oct. 1935); DMS, *Records*, DA-3, Box 12:6, DCA.

28. "Dartmouth College Medical School, Minutes of the Faculty Meetings, October 4, 1927–March 24, 1936," [n.p.] (3 May 1928, 23 May 1928, and 29 Aug. 1928); DMS, *Records*, DA-3, Box 12:6, DCA.

29. "Dartmouth College Medical School, Minutes of the Faculty Meetings, October 4, 1927–March 24, 1936," [n.p.] (21 Oct. 1930 and 4 Feb. 1932); DMS, *Records*, DA-3, Box 12:6, DCA.

30. William D. Cutter to Ernest M. Hopkins, 26 Dec. 1935; DC Office of the President, *Records*, DP-11 (Hopkins), Box 229: DMS, 1935–36.

31. "Dartmouth College Medical School, Minutes of the Faculty Meetings, October 4, 1927–March 24, 1936," [n.p.] (10 Oct. 1935); DMS, *Records*, DA-3, Box 12:6, DCA.

32. Whether Bowler had yet seen the abstract that Cutter had sent the day before to President Hopkins is not clear; if he had, it would help explain the heights of annoyance to which he allowed himself to rise in this letter to the alumni.

33. "Dartmouth College Medical School, Minutes of the Faculty Meetings, October 4, 1927–March 24, 1936," [n.p.] (19 Nov. 1935); DMS, *Records*, DA-3, Box 12:6, DCA.

34. JPB to [DMS Alumni], 27 Dec. 1935; DMS, *Records*, DA-3, Box 14:4, DCA.

35. H. G. Weiskotten and Harold Rypins, "Dartmouth Medical School"; DMS, *Records*, DA-3, 1935–36 Folder. The summary of the report was transcribed into the minutes: "Dartmouth College Medical School, Minutes of the Faculty Meetings, October 4, 1927–March 24, 1936," [n.p.] (4 Feb. 1936); DMS, *Records*, DA-3, Box 12:6, DCA. The full "Weiskotten Report" (as it came to be called) did not appear for several years: Herman B. Weiskotten, Alphonse M. Schwitalla, William D. Cutter, and Hamilton H. Anderson, *Medical Education in the United States: 1934–1939* (Chicago: AMA, 1940). Relevant though it was to affairs at Dartmouth, it does not seem to have made any impression on the Board of Trustees; there are no references to it in the trustees' records. See Meeting Minutes, Vol. VIII (for the years 1940–1942); DC Trustees, *Records*, Vault Mss., DCA.

36. "Dartmouth College Medical School, Minutes of the Committee of the Faculty, October 4, 1927–March 24, 1936," [n.p.] (19 Sept 1927); DMS, *Records*, DA-3, Box 12:7, DCA.

37. "Dartmouth College Medical School, Committee of the Faculty Minutes, July 8, 1927–March 26, 1936," [n.p.] (21 June 1934); DMS, *Records*, DA-3, Box 12:7, DCA.

38. "Dartmouth College Medical School, Minutes of the Faculty Meetings, October 4, 1927–March 24, 1936," [n.p.] (24 Mar. 1936); DMS, *Records*, DA-3, Box 12:6, DCA.

39. "Dartmouth College Medical School, Minutes of the Faculty Meeting,

October 4, 1927–March 24, 1936," [n.p.] (21 Oct. 1930); DMS, *Records*, DA-3, Box 12:6, DCA.

40. "Dartmouth College Medical School, Committee of the Faculty Minutes, July 8, 1927–March 26, 1936," [n.p.] (13 July and 26 July 1927); DMS, *Records*, DA-3, Box 12:7, DCA.

41. In fairness, it should be pointed out that although one student from the Syvertsen years I interviewed was explicit and detailed in his allegation that Syvertsen imposed a strict quota for Jews (no more than one each year), another student from later in Syvertsen's tenure as dean insisted just as firmly that he never saw discrimination of any sort from Syvertsen toward any of the Jews. There is evidence that President Hopkins himself was unabashed about having a quota for Jewish students at the College in 1945; for a brief discussion of this, see David C. Bisno, *Eyes in the Storm* (Norwich, Vt.: Norwich Publ., 1994), 149–50. But Hopkins was by no means alone among Ivy League presidents in taking such a stand, nor was it only students who faced quotas. "Medical faculties, like faculties throughout the university, established formal or informal quotas for Jews, particularly to senior positions." Kenneth M. Ludmerer, *Time to Heal* (New York: OUP, 1999), 47.

42. "Dartmouth College Medical School, Committee of the Faculty Minutes, July 8, 1927–March 26, 1936," [n.p.] (14 and 19 Sept. 1927); DMS, *Records*, DA-3, Box 12:7, DCA.

43. "Dartmouth College Medical School, Committee of the Faculty Minutes, July 8, 1927–March 26, 1936," [n.p.] (22 Mar. 1929); DMS, *Records*, DA-3, Box 12:7, DCA.

44. "Dartmouth College Medical School, Committee of the Faculty Minutes, July 8, 1927–March 26, 1936," [n.p.] (23 Mar. 1931); DMS, *Records*, DA-3, Box 12:7. DCA.

45. "Dartmouth College Medical School, Committee of the Faculty Minutes, July 8, 1927–March 26, 1936," [n.p.] (15 Mar. 1934); DMS, *Records*, DA-3, Box 12:7, DCA.

46. "Dartmouth College Medical School, Committee of the Faculty Minutes, July 8, 1927–March 26, 1936," [n.p.] (17 Apr. and 21 June 1934); DMS, *Records*, DA-3, Box 12:7, DCA.

47. See *Dartmouth . . . General Catalog*, 733, 742.

48. "Dartmouth College Medical School, Committee of the Faculty Minutes, July 8, 1927–March 26, 1936," [n.p.] (1 and 12 Mar. 1935; also 26 Mar. 1936); DMS, *Records*, DA-3, Box 12:7, DCA.

49. See *Dartmouth . . . General Catalog*, 759, 761.

50. Rolf Syvertsen to Harry French, 25 Mar. 1938; DMS, *Records*, DA-3, Box 10:45, DCA.

51. *Dartmouth . . . General Catalog*, 818; see also, *Dartmouth '39* (Albany, N.Y.: Argus-Greenwood, Inc., [1964]), 211.

52. "Dartmouth College Medical School, Committee of the Faculty Minutes, July 8, 1927–March 26, 1936," [n.p.] (16 May 1931); DMS, *Records*, DA-3, Box 12:7, DCA. Recall the related discussion from the nineteenth century concerning Dempsey Rollo Fletcher, Isaac H. Snowden, Alexander Lang, and Daniel Laing in ch. 4.

53. DC Office of the President, *Records*, DP-11 (Hopkins), Box 12:39, DCA.

54. Meeting Minutes, Vol. VI, p. 343 (19 Oct. 1917); DC Trustees, *Records*, Vault Mss., DCA.

55. DC Office of the President, *Records*, DP-11 (Hopkins), Box 12:39, DCA.

56. See "Class of 1914" obituary notice, *DMSAM* 1, no. 1 (Fall 1976): 36.

57. John M. Gile to Frederic P. Lord, 19 June 1919; Mss. 919219, DCA.

58. *DAM* 58, no. 3 (Dec. 1965): 80. Two pages had also been devoted to Lord in the *DMSQ* (Autumn 1965): [8–9].

59. Arthur Ecker, "Alumni Notes," *DM* 16, no. 1 (Fall 1991): 56. More generally, the "Alumni Notes" in this particular issue of *DM* constitute a rich source of recollections from class secretaries of 1924 through 1991. The impetus behind the editorial request for the correspondents to "wax nostalgic" instead of soliciting the latest news from classmates was the opening of the new medical center—a look back to the old in the midst great enthusiasm over the new.

60. Joseph Placak, "Once upon a time . . . ," *DMSAM* (Spring/Summer 1982): 32.

61. DMS, *Records*, DA-3, Box 11:6 (Faculty Biographical Records), DCA.

62. "Furnace Gas Kills Nine at Theta Chi House," *DAM* 26, no. 6 (Mar. 1934): 18.

63. A recent account of the accident and the massive rescue effort is John Morton, "Unforgiving Forests," *DM* 25, no. 2 (Winter 2000): 28–35.

64. The recollections from Lyle (DC 1934, DMS 1935), Kramer (DC 1932, DMS 1933), and Chipman (DMS 1941) come from "Alumni Notes," *DM* 16, no. 1 (Fall 1991): 58, 57, and 59 respectively.

65. For this quotation and much of the other information on Miller, see DMS, *Records*, DA-3, Box 11:15 (Faculty Biographical Records), DCA. See also Miller (1924) Alumni Folder, DCA.

66. All of the documents cited and quoted in these three paragraphs are in DMS, *Records*, DA-3, Box 14:4 ("DMS letters from 1920s–1930s"), DCA.

67. L. B. Howe to "Dear Doctor [Frost (presumably)]," 14 Mar. 1878; DMS, *Records*, DA-3, Box 9:3, DCA. Emphasis in the original.

68. Frederick C. Waite, "The Development of Anatomical Laws in the States of New England," *NEJM* 233, no. 24 (13 Dec. 1945): 725.

69. Edward Mortimer, 20 Jan. 2000, personal communication. See also accompanying copy of Edward Mortimer to Robert Lindsay, 24 Oct. 1999, personal communication. For more on the Sextons, see *Rolf Christian Syvertsen: A Tribute to a Mentor* (Lebanon, N.H.: DMS Office of Development, 2000), 14; also the untitled and unsigned, two-page, typed account (plus photo) in the Medical School Vertical File, Anatomy Dept., DCA.

70. *Dartmouth . . . General Catalog*, 452, lists Syvertsen as a member of the class of 1918 whose B.S. degree was conferred in 1921 (two years after he had returned to Dartmouth following his army service in France).

71. *Syvertsen: A Tribute*, 3.

72. *Syvertsen: A Tribute*, 8, 9.

73. *Syvertsen: A Tribute*, 12, 13.

74. Robert Fairchild (DC 1929, DMS 1931), 17 Nov. 1998, personal communication.

75. See, for example, entries in "Dartmouth College Medical School, Minutes of the Committee of the Faculty, July 8, 1927–March 26, 1936" (27 Oct. 1930, 23 Mar. 1931, 16 May 1931, 20 June 1933, 25 Aug. 1933, and 21 Sept. 1933); DMS, *Records*, DA-3, Box 12:7, DCA.

76. *Syvertsen: A Tribute*, 15.

Chapter 8. Fading Fortunes, Facing Facts

1. Edna St. Vincent Millay, *Mine the Harvest* (New York: Harper & Bros., 1954), 129.

2. Kenneth M. Ludmerer, *Time to Heal* (New York: OUP, 1999), 27.

3. The AMA's Council on Medical Education had been expanded to include hospitals as part of its mandate and was thus the Council on Medical Education and Hospitals (CME&H); I shall continue to refer to it as the CME, since the hospital was not under review at the time.

4. SMT, "Dartmouth Medical School, The Years of Refounding (1955–1963): A Memoir" [unpubl. ms., 1995], p. 14; Tenney, Stephen Marsh, Papers, MS-901, DCA.

5. Joseph Placak, "Once upon a time . . . ," *DMSAM* (Spring/Summer 1982): 22.

6. This "Combined Academic & Medical Course" continued to be popular at DMS for some time; see, for instance, its description in the discussion of Dartmouth Medical School (for the 1952–1953 year) that appeared in the *Dartmouth College Bulletin* 17, no. 8 (June 1952): 17–19; DC Hist. R 747.D37.

7. For a brief discussion of this and an excerpt from Hopkins's letter to Cutter, see Carleton B. Chapman, *Dartmouth Medical School: The First 175 Years* (Hanover, N. H.: UPNE, 1973), 52, 54.

8. "History Repeats in American Medical Education," and "Incomplete Schools," *JAMA* 105, no. 9 (31 Aug. 1935): 723.

9. D. G. Anderson and Anne Tipner, "Medical Education in the United States and Canada," *JAMA* 141 (3 Sept. 1949): 31, 37.

10. Franklin H. West (DC 1943, DMS 1943), "Alumni Notes," *DM* 16, no. 1 (Fall 1991): 60.

11. John Mahoney (DC 1948, DMS 1949), "Alumni Notes," *DM* 16, no. 1 (Fall 1991): 62.

12. These recollections are from the edited excerpt of Robert Giles's *Conscience is Good Medicine* (Austin, Texas: Nortex Press, 2000) that appeared in see *DMSAN&N* (Winter 2001): 13.

13. Bob Joy (DC 1945, DMS 1949), quoted by John Mahoney, "Alumni Notes," *DM* 16, no. 1 (Fall 1991): 63.

14. Bruce LaFollette (DC 1954, DMS 1955), *DM* 16, no. 1 (Fall 1991): 65.

15. John Mahoney, "Alumni Notes," *DM* 16, no. 1 (Fall 1991): 62.

16. James G. Schneider, *The Navy V-12 Program: Leadership for a Lifetime* (Boston: Houghton, Mifflin, 1987), 376.

17. Dan Wise, "The Hanover Home Front," *DM* 19, no. 4 (Summer 1995): 23.

18. "Converted Faculty" and "Degrees for Medics," *DAM* 35, no. 9 (June 1943): 25.

19. *DAM* 35, no. 8 (May 1943): 20.

20. "Letters from Dartmouth Men in the Armed Forces," *DAM* 36, no. 2 (Nov. 1943), 17. The photo had been taken on 23 Oct. 1943.

21. William R. Schillhammer, Jr., "Alumni Notes," *DM* 16, no. 1 (Fall 1991): 61, 62.

22. J. Robert Lindsay (DC 1944, DMS 1944), "Alumni Notes," *DM* 16, no. (Fall 1991): 61.

23. John Grindlay to JPB, 7 Feb. 1943. This and other letters quoted in what

follows in the text are among the papers that Bowler's daughter Janet Fitzgibbons and her sister Patsy Leggat generously loaned to me. For more on this remarkable correspondence, see Constance E. Putnam, "Between the Front and Doctor Bowler," *DM* 27, no. 2 (Winter 2002): 52–55, 62.

24. Henry Heyl to JPB, 7 Oct. 1943.

25. *DAM* 38, no. 4 (Jan. 1946): 39.

26. Ralph Hunter to JPB, 27 Mar. 1943.

27. Gile suffered from both pneumonia and a heart attack in 1943; his death twelve years later was a result of long-standing heart disease (which many males in his family had).

28. Ralph Hunter to JPB, 12 Jan. 1944 (postmarked 26 Feb. 1944).

29. G. Bruce Lemmon, "Reflections on D plus 6 Day." The original of this memoir remains in private hands. A condensed version appeared—under the title "Pacific Reflections on a Time of Trial"—in *DMSAN&N* (Winter 1999): 15.

30. John Feltner to JPB, 8 May 1943.

31. Megan McAndrew Cooper, *A History of the Mary Hitchcock Memorial Hospital* (Lebanon, N.H.: MHMH, 1991), 31, 32, 33.

32. Wise, "Home Front," 24.

33. David C. Bisno, *Eyes in the Storm—President Hopkins's Dilemma: The Dartmouth Eye Institute* (Norwich, Vt.: Norwich Press Books, 1994). The account that follows in the text is based largely on that source. See also Bisno, "Masters of Vision," *DM* 18, no. 4 (Summer 1994): 30–39, 68.

34. Bisno, *Eyes*, 27; xii, 66, 67, 144.

35. Bisno, *Eyes*, 171, 176.

36. Bisno, *Eyes*, 144, 151.

37. For a brief account of the matter, see William L. McLaughlin, "A happy Hobson's choice," *DM* 17, no. 4 (Summer 1993): 13. What follows in the text relies heavily on McLaughlin's summary. I am indebted to Howard Green for some of the language used to describe how DMS became involved with the VA.

38. *Dartmouth College Bulletin* 17, no. 8 (June 1952): 30; DC Hist. R 747.D37.

39. McLaughlin, "Hobson's choice," 13, quoting from Paul Hawley's address before the AMA House of Delegates. See *JAMA* 129, no. 17 (22 Dec. 1945): 1192–94.

40. McLaughlin, "Hobson's choice," 13.

41. Walter B. Crandell, "White River Junction Veterans Administration Hospital"; DC Trustees, *Records*, DA-1, Box 12:3 (Dartmouth Medical School [11/61–4/ 64]), DCA.

42. McLaughlin, "Hobson's choice," 13.

43. For more on this period at the VA Hospital, see "Engineer of success at the White River VA," *DM* 16, no. 1 (Fall 1991): 6–7.

44. John Milne, "A Short History of the Hitchcock Foundation" (Dec. 1988): 1. For more on the Foundation's history, see also "The Hitchcock Foundation" (a Hitchcock Foundation brochure dated 1947–1948) and a document of the same title dated 1981.

45. Gerald O'Connor and Michael Shoob, "A golden arch," *DM* 21, no. 3 (Spring 1997): 20.

46. Two points of particular interest emerge from this unpublished talk. Barker was particularly interested in the extent to which Smith's putative atheism,

or at least "unorthodox beliefs," affected his (non)acceptance into New Haven society; he also stressed Smith's relative poverty, by pointing out that his grave is in the "College Plot" in the Grove Street Cemetery in New Haven, reserved largely for indigent students who died while at Yale. He further mentioned that "Yale has named for Nathan Smith a building converted into a dormitory and used by the School of Nursing." Creighton Barker, "Some Notes on Nathan Smith and His Encounter with Yale Orthodoxy." Creighton Barker Papers. M&A, YUL.

47. The newspaper clippings and program are in the DMS Sesquicentennial 1947 Vertical File, DCA; see also Harry Savage, "Medical School Celebrates Its 150th Year" (with photos), *DAM* 41, no. 1 (Oct. 1948): 22–23.

48. SMT, "Memoir," p. 13.

49. Chapman, *175 Years*, 54–55.

Chapter 9. Rising to a New Challenge

1. Franklin Donaldson (trans.), *The Maxims of Humankind's Earliest Wisdom Literature* (New York: Vantage, 1990), 21.

2. Charles E. Widmayer, *John Sloan Dickey: A Chronicle of his Presidency of Dartmouth College* (Hanover, N.H.: UPNE, 1991), 124. Widmayer's brief account of this period in DMS's history, in his ten-page chapter "A Medical 'Refounding,'" though not accurate in all details, summarizes well what transpired.

3. Carleton B. Chapman, *Dartmouth Medical School: The First 175 Years* (Hanover, N. H.: UPNE, 1973), 55.

4. One TPC report noted that there had been "no formally constituted TPC subcommittee on the Medical School comparable to the other survey subcommittees. Dean Donald H. Morrison and others investigated the situation for the TPC and rendered informal reports to it during the period 1954–1957." TPC Report: Basis for Decision to "Refound" DMS (February 1960); DC Trustees, *Records*, DA-1, DCA.

5. Mary Daubenspeck, in the draft of a piece that appeared in condensed form as "Dining, dancing, and deans' toasts at evening gala," *DM* 22, no. 1 (Summer–Fall 1997): 15–17, put this remark into writing as Tenney was offering his tribute to Morrison.

6. "Initial Report" and "Second Report of the Schedule Committee" (Feb. 1955); DC Office of the Provost, *Records*, DA-7, Box 24:1, DCA.

7. DHM, "Dartmouth College Hitchcock Medical Center" (6 Jan. 1955), p. 3; DC Office of the President, *Records*, DP-12 (Dickey), 89:2, DCA.

8. Yet one more indication of John Bowler's importance to the medical school: It was later stated that the "views developed by Dr. Bowler in this meeting proved to be in large agreement with those expressed by Dr. Gregg at the conclusion of his investigations here." TPC Memorandum (18 Apr. 1955), DC Trustees, *Records*, DA-1, TPC (Medical School Study), DCA.

9. The erstwhile student's memories on the latter point are substantiated in the so-called Gregg report (see n 10), which included the following: "The Medical School gets exceptional students. (This impression was strengthened and documented during Dr. Gregg's visit.)"

10. "Memorandum for the Medical School Study File" (the "Gregg Report")

and DHM, "Memorandum of Dr. Alan Gregg's Views on the Dartmouth Medical School" (15 Jan. 1955); DC Office of the Provost, *Records*, DA-7, Box 22: 32, DCA.

11. "Views of Dr. Alan Gregg on the Dartmouth Medical School" (the "Gregg Report," 21 Jan. 1955, attached to the Report of June 7, 1957); DC Office of the Provost, *Records*, DA-7, Box 24:1, DCA. Chapman, in his *175 Years*, ix, identified this unpublished memorandum as the "only record" of Gregg's views on the situation at Dartmouth. But see the letter quoted and discussed in the next paragraph as well as the two memoranda just mentioned.

12. Years later, in 1996, DMS's Dean Andrew Wallace (in the course of delivering the annual Alan Gregg Lecture at the AAMC's 1996 annual meeting) went so far as to say that "Dartmouth has a medical school today in no small measure as a consequence of Alan Gregg."

13. Gregg to JSD, 12 Feb. 1955, attached as Exh. B to TPC Memorandum, 18 Apr. 1955; DC Trustees, *Records*, TPC (Medical School Study), DA-1, DCA.

14. TPC Memorandum (18 Apr. 1955); DC Trustees, *Records*, TPC (Medical School Study), DA-1, DCA.

15. SMT, "Alan Gregg," in David C. Bisno, *Eyes in the Storm—President Hopkins's Dilemma: The Dartmouth Eye Institute* (Norwich, Vt.: Norwich Press Books, 1994), 233.

16. SMT, "Dartmouth Medical School, The Years of Refounding (1955–1963): A Memoir" [unpubl. ms., 1995], p. 10; Tenney, Stephen Marsh, Papers, MS-901, DCA. Tenney's 41-page memoir is rich in detail and personal recollection. I have relied heavily on it for the particulars of Tenney's position on various points in these early years of the refounding project especially; unless otherwise indicated, quotations in the pages that follow are from Tenney's "Memoir."

17. The emphasis here has to have been on "develop" and "first-rate," since a two-year school existed; improvements were what Morrison was calling for.

18. DHM to SMT (25 Feb. 1955); DC Office of the Provost, *Records*, DA-7, Box 24:8, DCA.

19. DHM, "Ad Hoc Committee on Proposed Medical Science Building" (13 July 1955); DC Office of the Provost, *Records*, DA-7, Box 23:5, DCA.

20. SMT to DHM, 29 Nov. 1955; DC Office of the Provost, *Records*, DA-7, Box 24:4, DCA.

21. "Study of Medical School Organization" (25 Nov. 1955); DC Office of the Provost, *Records*, DA-7, Box 24:7; DCA.

22. The overture from Dartmouth College to the Rockefeller Foundation on 8 Feb. 1956, which contained a general prospectus of the Medical School, appears to be where the term "refounding" was first used outside the College. JSD to Dean Rusk [Rockefeller Foundation], 8 Feb. 1956; DC Office of the President, *Records*, DP-12 (Dickey), Box 46: Development Council, H-Z, DCA. (Tenney credits Morrison with having introduced the term. SMT, "Memoir," p. 25.) Dickey used the word in another letter—JSD to Philip S. Broughton, 18 Sept. 1956—and, in a "Memorandum on the Dartmouth Medical School" (20 Dec. 1956), Morrison referred to the "refounding" of the school; DC Office of the Provost, *Records*, DA-7, Box 23:5 and Box 22:25 (respectively), DCA. Thereafter the term appears with growing frequency.

23. William McCann to Alan Gregg, 14 Feb. 1955; DC Office of the Provost, *Records*, DA-3, Box 24:8, DCA.

24. SMT, "Memoir," pp. 14–15.

25. Dean Smiley and Edward Turner to JSD, 22 June 1956; DC Office of the Provost, *Records*, DA-7, Box 22:8, DCA.

26. The Medical School was not alone. Throughout the College and its graduate professional schools, Dartmouth—unlike other academic institutions—did not use the rank of Associate Professor.

27. SMT, "Memoir," p. 12.

28. This summary of Morrison's take on the situation is derived from (and all of the quotations in what follows are taken from) DHM, "Memorandum of Comments on the 1956 Report of the Survey Liaison Team on Dartmouth Medical School" (7 Sept. 1956); Office of the Provost, *Records*, DA-7, Box 22:8, DCA. This had been preceded by an unsigned, undated memo headed "Comments on the Survey Report," also in Box 22:8.

29. JSD to Philip S. Broughton, 18 Sept. 1956; DC Office of the Provost, *Records*, DA-7, Box 23:5, DCA.

30. Status of Medical School Planning, 25 Oct. 1956; DC Trustees, *Records*, DA-1, Box 37:49, DCA.

31. Meeting Minutes, Vol. XI, pp. 68–69 (26 Oct. 1956); DC Trustees, *Records*, DA-1, DCA.

32. SMT, "Memoir," pp. 17–18.

33. "Dartmouth Medical School" (5 Mar. 1957); DC Office of the Provost, *Records*, DA-7, Box 22:32, DCA.

34. JPB, "The Two-Year Medical School—Its Role in the Doctor Production Problem," *Jrnl. of the Maine Med. Assoc.* (Nov. 1957). Copy in DC Office of the Provost, *Records*, DA-7, Box 23:5, DCA.

35. "Report of Committee to Study the Premedical Curriculum"; DC Premedical Committee, *Records*, DA-294, Box 1:4, DCA.

36. Thomas E. O'Connell to JSD and DHM, 13 Feb. 1957; DC Office of the Provost, *Records*, DA-7, Box 24:10, DCA. Emphases in original.

37. This view was corroborated a month later in "Medicine Is Asked To Add 25 Schools: Yale Dean Says New Units Will Be Required by 1975 to Meet U.S. Needs," *NYT* (4 June 1957): 37.

38. This and the preceding several quotations are taken from Dudley Orr, "Memorandum on the Medical School" (6 May 1957); DC Office of the Provost, *Records*, DA-7, Box 23:5, DCA.

39. "Report on the Medical School" (7 June 1957), Meeting Minutes, Vol. XI, pp. 166–67; DC Trustees, *Records*, DA-1, DCA. The supporting documents were inserted in the trustees' minutes just following these pages.

40. SMT, "Memoir," pp. 19–22.

41. JSD to Henry Heald, 2 July 1957; DC Office of the Provost, *Records*, DA-7, Box 22:25, DCA.

42. JSD, "Internal Memorandum: Reorganization of Dartmouth Medical Education and Research Activities" (16 Aug. 1957); DC Office of the Provost, *Records*, DA-7, 23:5, DCA.

43. JSD, "Internal Memorandum: Reorganization of Dartmouth Medical Education and Research Activities" (16 Aug. 1957); DC Office of the Provost, *Records*, DA-7, 23:5, DCA.

44. SMT, "Memoir," pp. 18–19.

45. For the story of how the new physiology department came into being, see S. Marsh Tenney, "The Department of Physiology," *DMSQ* 5, no. 4 (Spring 1969): 97–102.

46. SMT, "Progress Report on the Dartmouth Medical School" (20 Sept. 1957): 2, 4; DC Hist. R747.D22 P76, DCA.

47. SMT, "Memoir," p. 24.

48. The powerhouse created by this influx of faculty oriented toward science research would later be offset by the decision to grant faculty voting privileges to all the part-time clinical faculty. This would increasingly be an issue in the 1960s.

49. SMT, "Second Progress Report on the Dartmouth Medical School, 1957–1959" (27 Dec. 1959), pp. 4, 5, 8; DC Hist. R747.D22 P76, DCA.

50. "Dartmouth's Medical Metamorphosis," *DAM* 52, no. 3 (Dec. 1959): [5 pp.]. Copy in DMS, *Records*, DA-3, Box 14:7, DCA. A 32-page booklet titled "Medical Education and Dartmouth" spelled out the reasons for the campaign; the "National Leadership"—all those listed were either DMS graduates or faculty—was an impressive group.

51. SMT, "Memoir," p. 31.

52. Darley Ward, "Dartmouth's Medical Opportunity"; Dartmouth Convocation on Great Issues of Conscience in Modern Medicine; *Records*, DA-17, Box 1: "Complete transcriptions, original and file copy," DCA.

53. SMT, "Third Progress Report on the Dartmouth Medical School, 1959–1961" (12 Feb. 1962); DC Hist. R747.D22 P76, DCA.

54. SMT, "Memoir," pp. 32, 33.

Chapter 10. A Question of Balance

1. Virgil, *The Aeneid*, Lib. 1, l. 204. Robert Fitzgerald, trans., *The Aeneid: Virgil* (New York: Random House, 1981), 10.

2. DC Office of the Provost, *Records*, DA-7, Box 22:31, DCA. Various proposals for Ph.D. programs with dates in late 1959 or early 1960 are filed in the same box, with comparative data from other institutions. The idea was more revolutionary than is now obvious. Dartmouth had no Ph.D. programs at the time; molecular biology would prove the opening wedge. Soon after the inauguration of that program, John Kemeny (later president of Dartmouth) was instrumental in starting a mathematics Ph.D.

3. Leonard Rieser, "Summary of Meeting with Dr. Tenney and Mr. Masland" (30 Sept. 1959); DC Trustees, *Records*, DA-1, Box 37:50, DCA.

4. SMT to RCF, 8 May 1961; DC Office of the Provost, *Records*, DA-7, Box 23:8, DCA.

5. "Dr. Gilbert Horton Mudge Named Dean of Medical School," *DAM* 54, no. 4 (Jan. 1962): 19. See also "Associated School News, Medical School," p. 73.

6. Mahlon Hoagland, *Toward the Habit of Truth* (New York: Norton, 1990), 54.

7. Carleton B. Chapman, *Dartmouth Medical School: The First 175 Years* (Hanover, N.H.: UPNE, 1973), 62.

8. One example of how faculty supportive of the molecular biology program tried to fit into the medical-school teaching is the course created by Peter von Hippel and Arnold Wishnia (biochemistry), Allan Munck (physiology), and Joseph Harris (physics) on physicochemical principles, to be taught to first-year medical students. It may have been too idealistic—it didn't last more than a

couple of years—but it was a case of science faculty taking initiative in the mission of the Medical School.

9. Statement by the Policy Committee, Dartmouth Medical School, 1 Jan. 1958; DC Office of the Provost, *Records*, DA-7, Box 22:32, DCA.

10. Philip Denenfeld to File, 8 May 1967. From the AAUP files.

11. Some members of the faculty escape the negative language altogether. Lafayette Noda and Peter von Hippel in particular have been singled out by more than one of their (erstwhile) colleagues for praise of their efforts to serve as peacemakers.

12. SMT, "Second Progress Report on the Dartmouth Medical School, 1957–1959" (27 Dec. 1959): 3; DC Hist. R747.D22 P76, DCA.

13. SMT, "Third Progress Report on the Dartmouth Medical School, 1959–1961" (12 Feb. 1962): i, 6; DC Hist. R747.D22 P76, DCA.

14. GHM to SMT, 8 Dec. 1961. From the Mudge papers (loaned by and currently in the hands of the Mudge family).

15. JSD to John Meck and John Masland, 3 Jan. 1962; DMS, *Records*, DA-3, Box 24: 13, DCA.

16. RCF to JSD, 15 Nov. 1961; DC Office of the Present, *Records*, DP-12 (Dickey), Box 73: Molecular Biology, DCA.

17. RCF to GHM, 30 Nov. 1961. From the Mudge papers.

18. GHM to Tisdale, 9 May 1962. From the Mudge papers.

19. SMT, "Third Progress Report on the Dartmouth Medical School, 1959–1961" (12 Feb. 1962): 2; DC Hist. R747.D22 P76, DCA.

20. SMT, "Dartmouth Medical School, The Years of Refounding (1955–1963): A Memoir" [unpubl. ms., 1995], p. 34; Tenney, Stephen Marsh, Papers, MS-901, DCA.

21. The name change seems to have been initiated by Mudge, who thought "Medical Advisory Group of the Dartmouth Medical School" more clearly identified the group as serving on invitation of the trustees. See GHM to JSD, 25 July 1962; DC Office of the Provost, *Records*, DA-7, Box 23:32, DCA.

22. Minutes of Advisory Board meeting (1 Oct. 1962), pp. 11–12; DC Office of the Provost, *Records*, DA-7, Box 22:3, DCA.

23. RCF to GHM, 28 Dec. 1962. Emphasis in the original. From the Mudge papers.

24. LN to GHM, 18 Jan. 1963. From the Mudge papers.

25. RCF to GHM, [?] Jan. 1963. Emphasis in the original. From the Mudge papers.

26. SMT, "Memoir," p. 34.

27. The unpleasant possibility exists that anti-Asian prejudice was at play throughout the affair. But the views of those who have speculated (or *insisted*) that such prejudice existed are offset by at least as many observers, including some who would have been most affected, who say nothing of the sort was true. One former faculty member with a "foreign" name has explicitly suggested that what today would be considered a welcome sign of diversity—a faculty of people with names like Morales, Watanabe, Noda, Inoué, Sato, von Hippel, Szent-Györgyi, Conti, Englander, Gellert—was part of the problem for at least some of those in charge. No one will ever know for sure.

28. JSD to Masland and GHM, 28 Feb. 1963. Emphasis in the original. From the Mudge papers.

29. JSD to Medical School Faculty (26 Apr. 1963), Master File: Medical School 11/61–4/64; DC Trustees, *Records*, DA-1 (74), Box 12:3, DCA.

30. JSD to GHM, "Letter of July 10, 1963"; DC Office of the President, *Records*, DP-12 (Dickey), Box 89:37, DCA.

31. JSD to GHM, 11 July 1963. From the Mudge papers.

32. [Unsigned, untitled], ten-point memorandum on the plan to establish departments of medicine and surgery, 4 Mar. 1964; SI to Dept. of Cytology, 24 Mar. 1964; [unsigned, undated] response to SI. From the Mudge papers.

33. SI to Leonard Rieser, 31 Mar. 1964. From the Mudge papers.

34. GHM, "Report on the Dartmouth Medical School to the Trustees of Dartmouth College, 1962–1964" (April 1964), pp. 9, 3, 6, 8 respectively. Emphasis in the original. From the Mudge papers.

35. GHM to JSD, "Proposal to Establish Departments of Medicine and Surgery" (14 Sept. 1964). From the Mudge papers.

36. GHM to Leonard Rieser, "The Medical School and Graduate Education" (20 Apr. 1964). From the Mudge papers.

37. RCF, et al., "Current Status and Space and Financial Needs of the Molecular Biology Graduate Program" (9 June 1964); DC Office of the Provost, *Records*, DA-7, Box 23:8, DCA.

38. SMT, "Memoir," p. 37.

39. "Med School Begins Doctoral Studies In Physics, Physiology-Pharmacology," *The Dartmouth* (4 Jan. 1965): 1.

40. GHM to JSD, 24 Mar. 1965; DC Office of the President, *Records*, DP-12 (Dickey), 89:40 "Medical School Personnel—Mudge Resignation," DCA. Copies of Mudge's handwritten notes to Barry Wood, Robert Loeb, and George Berry are in the Mudge papers.

41. "Report of the Trustees Planning Committee Subcommittee on Dartmouth Medical School" (15 May 1965). Emphasis in the original. Also Philip O. Nice to Dudley Orr (same date); DC Trustees, *Records*, DA-1, Box 70:5, DCA.

42. SMT, "Memoir," p. 35.

43. SMT to JSD, 26 Aug. 1964; DC Office of the Provost, *Records*, DA-7, Box 22:4, DCA. Emphases in the original.

44. Minutes of Advisory Board Meeting (16 Sept. 1964), pp. 3, 4; DC Office of the Provost, *Records*, DA-7, Box 22:4, DCA.

45. Peter von Hippel and Andrew Szent-Györgyi, "Added comments" appended (pp. 13–14) to the Report of the Trustees Planning Committee Subcommittee on Dartmouth Medical School; DC Trustees, *Records*, DA-1, Box 70:5, DCA.

46. SMT to DHM, 26 July 1955; DC Office of the Provost, *Records*, DA-3, Box 26:8, DCA.

47. See "Remarks of John W. Masland to the faculty of the Dartmouth Medical School, May 21, 1965," prepared from notes by James W. Stevens; DC Office of the Provost, *Records*, DA-7, Box 22:4, DCA.

48. Hoagland, *Truth*, 133.

49. John Masland to JSD, 26 May 1965; DC Office of the Provost, *Records*, DA-7, Box 22:4, DCA.

50. GHM, "A Chronology of Recent events relating to Dartmouth Medical School, with a few comments" (31 May 1965). From the Mudge papers.

51. "Remarks of Dr. Mudge at Advisory Board" (6 June 1965). From the Mudge papers.

52. Meeting Minutes, Vol. XIII, pp. 468–69 (9 Oct. 1965); DC Trustees, *Records*, DA-1, DCA. See also *DMSQ* 3, no. 1 (Summer 1966): 13, for the text of the resolutions.

53. SMT, "Memoir," p. 34.

54. "Tenney Named Acting Dean Of Med School," *The Dartmouth* (3 Dec. 1965): 1.

55. LN, SI, RCF, et al. to W. P. Fidler (AAUP), 16 Dec. 1965. From the AAUP files. A covering note (on the same date), over Inoué's signature, makes explicit that there had been prior discussion with Bentley Glass, then president of the AAUP. According to Kenneth Cooper, one of the fourteen signatories, he and Lafayette Noda wrote and signed the first letter to the AAUP, though its date and addressee are no longer clear. Kenneth W. Cooper, 16 Apr. 2003, personal communication.

56. Henry Payson to PD, 7 Feb. 1966. From the AAUP files.

57. These quotations and that in the next paragraph are from PD to GHM, Robert Weiss, and others who had written to the AAUP, 14 Feb. 1966. From the AAUP files.

58. "11 Med School Profs Resign" and "Resigned Profs Explain Position," *VN* (8 and 9 Apr. 1966, respectively): 1 (in both cases), and "Eleven Professors Quit . . . ," *The Dartmouth* (8 Apr. 1966): 1. The *Valley News* had a further story three days later. "The Lid Clamps Shut On Med School Hassle," *VN* (12 Apr. 1966): 1.

59. Carl M. Cobb, "11 Quit Dartmouth Med Staff," *BG* (9 Apr. 1966): 1; "Claims Dartmouth Resignations 'Timed,' " *NH Sunday News* (10 Apr. 1966): 3–4.

60. M. A. Farber, "Angry Biologists Quit Dartmouth," *NYT* (15 Apr. 1966): 41, 50.

61. Yet at least with respect to the *Sunday News* story in which it was claimed that the news was "timed" to coincide with a major national meeting of scientists, Inoué and eight others signed an affidavit denying responsibility for the statement and further certifying that it was false. Statement to the Trustees, 11 Apr. 1966; DC Office of the President, *Records*, DP-12 (Dickey), Box 94: "Medical School Controversy," DCA.

62. GHM to John Masland, 21 Apr. 1966; Barry Wood to GHM, 3 May 1966; DeWitt Stetten to GHM, 4 May 1966; Robert Loeb to GHM, 13 May 1966; Francis Dieuaide to GHM, 18 May 1966. The president of the Dartmouth AAUP chapter, Harry Thomas Schultz (though not on the distribution list), likewise thanked Mudge for sending a copy. "I also appreciate your having taken the trouble of writing out a detailed statement of fact. So far as I know you are the only person involved in this sad business to have done so." Schultz to GHM, 13 May 1966. All these documents are from the Mudge papers.

63. Schultz had also received a letter from Tenney, countering some of Mudge's position. SMT to Harry Schultz, 11 May 1966; DC Office of the Provost, *Records*, DA-7, Box 22:6, DCA.

64. [Charles Widmayer], "Dissension at the Medical School," *DAM* 58, no. 8 (May 1966): 19. The medical school readership was treated to a parallel piece: Philip O. Nice, "Editorial," *DMSQ* 3, no. 1 (Summer 1966): 1.

65. PD to JSD, 9 May 1966, and JSD to PD, 17 May 1966; DC Office of the Provost, *Records*, DA-7, Box 22:6, DCA. In contrast, a few weeks later Carleton B. Chapman (who had just been named dean) was quoted saying he would be "very willing to work with" an AAUP consultant. A. D. Ghiselin, "Medical Dean Could Favor Mediation Bid," *VN* (10 June 1966): 1. Obviously he changed his mind; it never happened. See PD to AAUP Staff, 14 Dec. 1966, p. 4. From the AAUP files.

66. GHM to PD, 2 June 1966. From the Mudge papers.

67. Further reports from Dartmouth had been received by the AAUP indicating that the situation was not improving: A formal request from a large group of Dartmouth faculty members for the services of an AAUP consultant had been received; Dickey had been asked to honor that request. It did not appear that any real progress had been made, and Denenfeld was not going to pretend it had. PD to GHM, 6 June 1966. From the Mudge papers.

68. GHM to SI, 15 June and 5 July, 1966; GHM to LN, 30 June 1966. From the Mudge papers.

69. "Dartmouth Names Medical Dean," *NYT* (19 May 1966): 30.

70. Cooper, LN, and RCF to PD, 28 and 29 July 1966. From the AAUP files.

71. See, e.g., *NH Sunday News* (10 Apr. 1966): 4.

72. PD to Committee T File (DMS), 23 Aug. 1966, and John Masland to PD, 26 Aug. 1966. From the AAUP files. Emphasis in the original.

73. PD to File, 10 Oct. 1966, and Kenneth Cooper to PD, 12 Oct. 1966. From the AAUP files.

74. CBC, "Statement to the Faculty of Dartmouth Medical School" (31 Oct. 1966): 2, 5, 9, 10. Copy in C. Putnam's files.

75. PD to AAUP Staff, 14 Dec. 1966. From the AAUP files.

76. PD to CBC, 5 Jan. 1967. From the AAUP files.

77. CBC to PD, 11 Jan. 1967. From the AAUP files.

78. Cooper (and LN) to PD, 17 Feb. 1967. From the AAUP files.

79. PD to Cooper, 3 Mar. 1967. From the AAUP files.

80. Kenneth Cooper to PD, 7 Mar. 1967; PD to Cooper, 14 Mar. 1967. From the AAUP files.

81. PD to File, 8 May 1967. From the AAUP files. For the record, "surveillance" is "not a term used by AAUP to assign a specific status to a problem." Jordan E. Kurland (AAUP), 10 Apr. 2003, personal communication.

82. PD to CBC, [late June 1967], and CBC to PD, 5 July 1967. From the AAUP files.

83. PD to CBC, 5 Jan. 1967. From the AAUP files.

84. Hoagland, *Truth*, 25. Hoagland devotes little space to Dartmouth in his book, despite having been on the DMS faculty as chair of the biochemistry department (1967–1970) in the immediate aftermath of the upheaval.

85. Hoagland, *Truth*, 82–83.

86. SMT, "Third Progress Report on the Dartmouth Medical School, 1959–1961" (12 Feb. 1962): 6–7; DC Hist. R747.D22 P76, DCA.

87. In 1995, DMS and Dartmouth College inaugurated a joint molecular and cellular biology graduate program, in what must have been a bittersweet development for some outside observers—and perhaps some of the participants as well.

Chapter 11. Tradition and Innovation

1. Galway Kinnell, "Where the Track Vanishes," *What a Kingdom it Was* (Boston: Houghton Mifflin, 1960), 57.

2. Tenney joked in his memoir that on "the downtown streets of Hanover" he learned he "had been christened the 're-acting dean.'" SMT, "Dartmouth Medical School, The Years of Refounding (1955–1963): A Memoir" [unpubl. ms., 1995], p. 39; Tenney, Stephen Marsh, Papers, MS-901, DCA.

3. Kenneth M. Ludmerer, *Time to Heal* (New York: OUP, 1999), 157.

4. "Report of the Trustees Planning Committee Subcommittee on Dartmouth Medical School" (15 May 1965), p. 5; DC Trustees, *Records*, DA-1, Box 70:5, DCA.

5. Dudley W. Orr, "Draft of Proposed Charge to the TPC Subcommittee on the Medical School" [1963], Master File: Medical School, 11/61–4/64; DC Trustees, *Records*, DA-1 (74), Box 12:3, DCA.

6. JSD, "Remarks . . ." (14 Nov. 1960), DC Office of the President, *Records*, DP-12 (Dickey), Box 62: Speech—National Fund for Medical Education Dinner.

7. "A Case for More Two-Year Schools," *Medical World News* (Sept. 15, 1961): 23.

8. GHM, Kurt Benirschke, and Robert Weiss, "Role of Clinical Investigation in the Dartmouth Medical School" (18 Sept. 1962); DC Office of the Provost, *Records*, DA-7, Box 23:3, DCA.

9. Henry L. Heyl, "Editorial," *DMSQ* 1, no. 2 (Autumn 1964): [n.p.].

10. "Undergraduate Medical Education," *JAMA* 202, no. 8 (Nov. 20, 1967): 729.

11. Minutes of Executive Committee (25 Feb. 1966); DC Office of the Provost, *Records*, DA-7, Box 22:26, DCA.

12. F. P. Lord to JPB, 4 Jan. 1936. From the Bowler papers.

13. GHM to Allan Tisdale, 4 Jan. 1966. From the Mudge papers.

14. SMT, "A Memoir," p. 39.

15. See, e.g., William Green, "Med School Faculty Ponders Expansion to Four-Year Plan," *The Dartmouth* (4 May 1966): 1; John Lannan, "Dartmouth Expands Its Medical School," *Boston Sunday Herald* (1 May 1966).

16. SMT, "Memoir," p. 39.

17. Charles E. Widmayer, *John Sloan Dickey: A Chronicle of His Presidency of Dartmouth College* (Hanover, N.H.: UPNE, 1991), 133. See also Meeting Minutes, Vol. XIII, pp. 468–69 (9 Oct. 1965); DC Trustees, *Records*, DA-1, DCA.

18. GHM to Robert Loeb, 26 July 1966. From the Mudge papers.

19. "The Dartmouth Medical School" (Hanover, N.H., DMS; [?/1974]): 8; DC Trustees, *Records*, DA-1, Box 23:67, DCA. For a reasonably full account of how the three-year curriculum worked, see Carleton B. Chapman, *Report of the Dean: Dartmouth Medical School 1966–67 to 1971–72* (Hanover, N.H.: Reporter Press, Oct. 1972), 44–51; DC Trustees, *Records*, DA-1, Box 23:56, DCA. For excerpts from this report, see Appendix D, p. 300. See also, e.g., "Medical School to Revive M.D. Degree," *DAM* 60, no. 6 (June 1968): 15.

20. Carleton B. Chapman, *Dartmouth Medical School: The First 175 Years* (Hanover, N.H.: UPNE, 1973), 67. Chapman says the retreats were in May 1969; this is clearly a typographical error. The trustees' vote was in April 1968; the revised "Basic Science Curriculum" had been introduced in September 1968.

21. William Green, "Med School Faculty Ponders Expansion to Four-Year Plan," *The Daily Dartmouth* (4 May 1966): 1.

22. Barbara Blough and Dana Cook Grossman, "Two Hundred Years of Medicine at Dartmouth," in Dana Cook Grossman and Heinz Valtin, eds., *Great Issues for Medicine in the Twenty-First Century: Ethical and Social Issues Arising out of Advances in the Biomedical Sciences, Ann. N.Y. Acad. Sci.* 882 (1999), xviii.

23. Press release (27 Feb. 1970), DC Office of the Provost, *Records*, DA-7, Box 22:26, DCA.

24. SMT, "Memoir," pp. 25, 26.

25. The correspondence between John Meck and JPB, Mar./Apr. 1962, and a copy of the press release, are in the Bowler papers. Also, SMT, 3 Apr. 1998, personal communication.

26. "Farewell, Nathan Smith," *DM* 15, no. 1 (Fall 1990): 11; see also photo (and caption) of "Medical North," *DM* 16, no. 1 (Fall 1991): 66. The first residence for the female medical students had been President Lord's former home, at 41 College Street.

27. Chapman, *175 Years* (Hanover, N.H.: UPNE, 1973), 74. Evidence that Chapman was wrong is easy to find. See, e.g.: "A committee under the chairmanship of Dr. Gilbert H. Mudge, Professor and Chairman of the Department of Medicine. . . . ," "Departmental News," *DMSQ* 3, no. 1 (Summer 1966): 15. Copies of the testy exchange of letters between Chapman and Mudge in January 1967 are in the Mudge papers.

28. See "A towering figure in international health," *DM* 26, no. 3 (Spring 2002): 13.

29. Thomas P. Almy, "The Role of Graduate Medical Education in Dartmouth's Expanding Program," *DMSQ* 5, no. 2 (Autumn 1968): 53, 54.

30. Among the department's noteworthy achievements is its outstanding record in bringing in research money. See "Fount of funding," *DM* 16, no. 1 (Fall 1991): 45.

31. John G. Kemeny, "Remarks before the Dartmouth Alumni Council" (15 June 1973); DC Trustees, *Records*, Box 23:73, DCA.

32. JCS, "From the Dean," *DMSAM* 13, no. 4 (Spring 1977): 2 and *DMSAM* 14, no. 4 (Spring 1978): 2.

33. John G. Kemeny, "Medical School Long Range Plan: Progress Report" (2 Oct 1978); DC Trustees, *Records*, DA-1, Box 23:71, DCA.

34. Stanley M. Aronson, 10 Aug. 1999, personal communication.

35. "Second Thoughts at the Medical School," *DAM* 70, no. 5 (Jan./Feb. 1978): 23. The intensity of the program was considerable; students who earned an M.D. in three years felt they had been put through the mill. George P. Butterworth (DC 1972, DMS 1975), personal communication.

36. See the summary of the findings of the Tucker Committee (chaired by Gary Tucker) in JCS, "The Dartmouth Medical School" (May 1978 Report); DC Office of the President, *Records*, DP-13 (Kemeny), Box 60: Medical School—Dean, p. 5.

37. *Dartmouth Medical School* (Hanover, N.H.: DMS, 1980): 20.

38. The dramatic increase in the number of applicants enabled DMS to begin being more selective. Philip O. Nice, "The Dartmouth Medical Student," *DMSQ* 1, no. 4 (Spring 1965): [n.p.].

39. Joseph F. O'Donnell, "Alumni Notes" (1971), *DM* 16, no. 1 (Fall 1991): 71. This issue of *DM* is particularly rich in recollections of student life in the past on the occasion of the dramatic changes being brought about by the move to the new DHMC campus.

40. Eric K. Larson, "Alumni Notes" (1981), *DM* 16, no. 1 (Fall 1991): 73.

41. "10 Questions," *DMSAM* (Winter 1985): 12–17, 27.

42. Andrew G. Wallace, "Pardonable pride" and "National award for community service at DMS," *DM* 19, no. 4 (Summer 1995): 2 and 4.

43. Nancy Roberts Trott, "Art, Literature—And Medicine?" *VN* (18 Nov. 1996): A2.

44. *Dartmouth Medical School* (Hanover, N.H.: DMS, 1978), 29; "Ever More Role Models," *DM* 22, no. 4 (Summer 1998): 3.

45. "Year 1s: A class with class," *DMSAM* 12, no. 2 (Winter 1987/88): 2.

46. "Let us now praise the DMS Class of 2001," *DM* 22, no. 2 (Winter 1997): 5.

47. Robert E. Nye, Jr., "Women and Medicine at Dartmouth," *DMSAM* (Spring 1979): 13–17, 34.

48. RWMcC, "Making a difference," *DMSAM* 13, no. 2 (Winter 1988): 9.

49. French had her own impressive Dartmouth connections. She was the daughter of Harry T. J. French, one of the Clinic founders; her two brothers were also physicians, Dartmouth College and DMS graduates. (She was preceded at DMS by anesthesiologist Marina Bosien, who practiced at the VA Hospital from 1953 to 1955.) "Elizabeth French Chair is established by an anonymous donor," *DM* 25, no. 4 (Summer 2001): 12–13.

50. Frances McCann, " 'The one less traveled,' " *DM* 22, no. 1 (Summer/Fall 1997): 86–87.

51. Lucile Smith, " 'The Old Days,' " in "Women in Medicine," *DMSAM* 13, no. 3 (Spring 1989): 22; "Active emerita," *DM* 16, no. 1 (Fall 1991): 45. "Women in Medicine" includes pieces by eight other women as well.

52. Robert E. Nye, Jr., "Women and Medicine at Dartmouth," *DMSAM* 3, no. 2 (Spring 1979): 13, 14, 15.

53. Now a successful surgeon, with past slights largely forgiven, she preferred not to give details about her Dartmouth experience or be identified. Personal communication.

54. Kristina Rosbe, "A tale of two surgery rotations," *DM* 16, no. 2 (Winter 1991): 13.

55. Rosemary Lunardini, "Navajo surgeon becomes dean of student affairs," *DM* 21, no. 2 (Winter 1997): 4–5.

56. Alvord is quoted in Laura Stephenson Carter, "Once and future medicine," *DM* 24, no. 3 (Spring 2000): 43. See also Lori Arviso Alvord and Elizabeth Cohen van Pelt, *The Scalpel and the Silver Bear* (New York: Bantam, 1999).

57. Rosemary Lunardini, "A Place on the Plain," *DM* 20, no. 1(Fall 1995): 25, 26, 69.

58. See *DM* 21, no. 2 (Winter 1997): 5, and *DM* 22, no. 1 (Summer/Fall 1997): 19.

59. "Kudos for Cancer Center," *DM* 15, no. 1 (Fall 1990): 6–7.

60. Katherine Phillips, "The Norris Cotton Cancer Center: Linking Basic and Clinical Science," *DMSAM* 6, no. 1 (Fall 1981): 14–19, 43–44.

61. "NIH's Sporn named to DMS's Oscar Cohn Chair," *DM* 20, no. 1 (Fall 1995): 13; Rosemary Lunardini, "Michael Sporn: Father of chemoprevention," *DM* 23, no. 1 (Fall 1998): 42–43.

62. S. Marsh Tenney, "The Department of Physiology," *DMSQ* 5, no. 4 (Spring 1969): 98.

63. "A valuable strain," *DM* 16, no. 1 (Fall 1991): 25.

64. "Researchers from 3 Continents to Gather . . ." (13 Aug. 1981); DC Trustees, *Records*, DA-1, Box 23–66, DCA.

65. Rosemary Lunardini, "Hot Property," *DM* 16, no. 3 (Spring 1992): 22.

66. "Joint biotechnology firm to market DMS research," *DMSAM* 12, no. 2 (Winter 1987/88): 6, 7.

67. "Anonymous allegations of misconduct recur," *DM* 19, no. 4 (Summer 1995): 16.

68. Steven C. Swett, "Medarex Charges Declared Baseless," *VN* (5 Feb. 1993): 1, 6; "Investigation finds no merit to charges," *DM* 17, no. 3 (Spring 1993): 9. See also "Anonymous allegations," 16.

69. Bob Hookway, "A Question of Degrees," *DM* 21, no. 2 (Winter 1996): 41. In general on the work of CECS, see Rosemary Lunardini, "Center for the Evaluative Clinical Sciences" (Hanover, N.H.: Dartmouth College, 2001).

70. John Wennberg and Alan Gittelsohn, "Variations in Medical Care among Small Areas," *Scientific American* 246, no. 4 (Apr. 1982): 120–34.

71. Susan Dentzer, "Doctor Wennberg's Uncertainty Principle," *DAM* 83, no. 8 (May 1991): 18.

72. See, e.g., "Dr. Wennberg on Outcomes Research: What Does It Really Mean?" *Managed Medicine* 2, no. 1 (1991): 7–11; and John E. Wennberg, "Outcomes Research, Cost Containment, and the Real of Health Care Rationing," *NEJM* 323, no. 17 (25 Oct. 1990): 1201–4.

73. "Viewing the aged with new eyes," *DM* 17, no. 4 (Summer 1992): 6–7; "Joanne Lynn: The truth about 'wasted' costs," *DM* 20, no. 3 (Spring 1995): 6; Rosemary Lunardini, "Neurosurgeon: Outcomes up and costs down," *DM* 21, no. 3 (Spring 1996): 10; Catherine Tudish, "The Making of a Medical Skeptic," *DM* 23, no. 4 (Summer 1999): 24.

74. Stephen K. Plume, 15 Oct. 2002, personal communication.

75. Rosemary Lunardini, "The Mapmakers," *DM* 24, no. 3 (Spring 1996): 23, 24, 26–27.

Chapter 12. Education for the Future

1. Henry R. Viets, "The Full Flood of Overtones," *Medical History, Humanism, and the Student of Medicine* (Hanover, N.H.: Dartmouth Pubs., 1960), 31.

2. DMS Overseers Annual Report, pp. 16, 20; DC Trustees, *Records*, DA-1, Box 34:8 [1983–4 (n.d.)], DCA.

3. Agnar Pytte, "Background Paper on Professional Schools and Graduate Programs at Dartmouth College" [1984], pp. 3, 4, 5, 8–9, 10, 13; DC Trustees, *Records*, DA-1, Box 59:12, DCA.

4. Taken from the "Valedictory Charge" Smith is reported to have given to the graduates at DMS in 1806. Recorded by William C. Ellsworth, "Chemical Lectures As Delivered in a Course of Lectures at Dartmouth College . . . ," [29–31], in Smith, Nathan, "William C. Ellsworth . . ."; Vault Mss., DCA.

5. James O. Freedman, 29 Oct. 1998, personal communication.

6. Peter von Hippel, 14 Apr. 2001, personal communication.

7. William L. McLaughlin, "A happy Hobson's choice," *DM* 17, no. 4 (Summer 1993): 13, quoting from the Hitchcock Clinic's 1955 Annual Report on the Veterans Administration Hospital Affiliation (14 Feb. 1956), p. 2.

8. Carleton B. Chapman, *Dartmouth Medical School: The First 175 Years* (Hanover, N. H.: UPNE, 1973), 37, 38.

9. Don Penfield, 27 Jan. 2000, personal communication.

10. "The Hitchcock Foundation," 1947–1948 brochure, courtesy of Michael Shoob.

11. "Dartmouth Medical School" (5 March 1957); DC Office of the Provost, *Records*, DA-7, Box 22:32, DCA.

12. "Graduate Medical Education" [?/1959]; DC Office of the Provost, *Records*, DA-7, Box 22:31, DCA.

13. GHM to Jarrett H. Folley, 9 Feb. 1969. From the Mudge papers.

14. Edward Cavaney to John Masland, 10 Dec. 1963; DC Office of the Provost, *Records*, DA-7, Box 23:2, DCA.

15. Heinz Valtin, "Why A Medical School?" *Supplement to the Valley News* (8 June 1997): 2.

16. Joint Medical Affairs Committee, Summary of Meeting, 14 July 1966; DC Office of the Provost, *Records*, DA-7, Box 23:1, DCA.

17. GHM to Jarrett H. Folley, 9 Feb. 1969. From the Mudge papers.

18. GHM to Jarrett Folley, 28 Dec. 1965 and 6 July 1966. From the Mudge papers.

19. Harry C. Bird, 17 Dec. 1999, personal communication.

20. It will be recalled that this had been a sore point during the molecular biology upheaval.

21. [CBC], "Report on Dartmouth Medical School to the AAMC-AMA Liaison Committee on Medical Education," [1972]. DC Hist. R/747/D22/D32/1972/oversize.

22. Liaison CME, "Report of the Survey of Dartmouth Medical School (14–16 Feb. 1972). From the Mudge papers.

23. CBC to medical school faculty, 16 June 1972. From the Mudge papers.

24. Don Penfield, 27 Jan. 2000, personal communication.

25. GHM to CBC, 13 July 1972. From the Mudge papers.

26. DMS has been the subject of surveys since 1914. In each of the years 1934, 1956, 1957, 1960, 1968, and 1972, accreditation of the two-year program was renewed. In 1972, the new three-year program was given "provisional accreditation," which was followed by full accreditation in 1973. The most recent survey—1975—had noted improvements but still found nine categories of issues about which to be concerned. Ad Hoc Survey Team of the LCME, "Report of the Survey of Dartmouth Medical School," 21–25 May 1979; DC Office of the Trustees, *Records*, DA-1, Box 34:80, DCA.

27. Walsh McDermott, "Statement on Dartmouth Medical College," 1 Oct. 1978. From the Mudge papers.

28. Ad Hoc Survey Team of the LCME, "Report of the Survey of Dartmouth Medical School," 21–25 May 1979; DC Office of the Trustees, *Records*, DA-1, Box 34:80, DCA.

29. SMT, "Dartmouth Medical School, The Years of Refounding (1955–1963): A Memoir" [unpubl. ms., 1995], p. 41; Tenney, Stephen Marsh, Papers, MS-901, DCA.

30. John G. Kemeny, "Remarks before the Dartmouth Alumni Council" (15 June 1973); DC Trustees, *Records*, DA-1, Box 23:73, DCA.

31. Rosemary Lunardini, "Auspicious Assessment," *DM* 14, no. 3 (Spring 1990): 25.

32. *Dartmouth Medical School* (Hanover, N.H.: DMS, 1980): 14, 15.

33. Some of the text immediately before this (as well as of what follows) about the Clinic is taken, or adapted, from Constance E. Putnam, "A Long-Running Hit," *DM* 27, no. 2 (Winter 2002): 28–39.

34. All VA hospital staff members would, however, continue to be full members of the DMS faculty.

35. Megan McAndrew Cooper, *Mary Hitchcock Memorial Hospital, 1893–1991* (Hanover, N.H.: MHMH, 1991), 61–62, 62.

36. Rosemary Lunardini, "Auspicious Assessment," *DM* 14, no. 3 (Spring 1990): 28. The lopsidedly affirmative vote was a reflection of faculty members believing a promise had been made *not* to divide the school. Disappointment and frustration (or worse) set in for some, later, as the reality unfolded

37. "Memorandum of Understanding," 19 Dec. 1985; DC Office of the President, *Records*, DP-14 (McLaughlin), Box 82: Mary Hitchcock Memorial Hospital, DCA.

38. "Statement of the Board of Trustees," 8 June 1986; DC Office of the President, *Records*, DP-14 (McLaughlin), Box 76: Dartmouth Medical School.

39. Megan McAndrew Cooper, *Mary Hitchcock Memorial Hospital, 1893–1991* (Hanover, N.H.: MHMH, 1991), 65.

40. Ralph Jimenez, "New Hospital Has Different Look, Attitude," *BG* (29 Sept. 1991): 7.

41. James W. Varnum to MHMH and HC staff, 14 Oct. 1991. Accompanying the letter was a copy for each addressee of Megan McAndrew Cooper's commemorative book (see *supra*, n35).

42. Ralph Jimenez, "Mammoth Moving Job Goes Smoothly," *BG* (6 Oct. 1991): 30.

43. "Dedicating the new DHMC," *DM* 16, no. 1 (Fall 1991): 3–6.

44. Andrew G. Wallace, 12 Aug. 1997, personal communication; also, "Parting thoughts," *DM* 22, no. 4 (Summer 1998): 2.

45. Andrea R. Williams (quoting Marsha Borling of Baird/Borling Associates), "Dartmouth-Hitchcock Medical Center, Physician/Staff Satisfaction Survey," *CenterView* 4, no. 11 (Sept. 2002).

46. Today, the "Dartmouth-Hitchcock Clinic" ("Dartmouth" was added to the name in 1999, following the dissolution of the two-year-old merger between the Hitchcock and the Lahey clinics) has practice sites scattered across New Hampshire and Vermont. Physicians in these clinics have the full support of all the Lebanon campus represents, but they remain local doctors serving local patients. They are not required to refer their patients to the DHMC. This represents a new level of commitment at DHMC to community service and quality care.

47. Andrew G. Wallace, "Educating Tomorrow's Doctors," *Supplement to the Valley News* (8 June 1997): 5.

48. "Proposal [to Spaulding-Potter Charitable Trusts in Concord, N.H.] for Development of a Program in Community Medicine at [DMS]," 25 June 1968); DC Office of the Provost, *Records*, DA-7, Box 22:8, DCA.

49. "Final Report of the Medical School Survey Committee to the Trustees of Dartmouth College," 1 April 1973; DC Trustees, *Records*, DA-1, Box 23:70, DCA.

50. "The Dartmouth Medical School" (Hanover, N.H.: DMS, [?/1974]): 8; DC Trustees, *Records*, DA-1, Box 23:67, DCA.

51. Press release, "Mellon Foundation Awards Dartmouth Medical School

$450,000 for 'Rural Outreach' Clinical Education," 13 Oct. 1977; DC Hist. R/747/D3/D85.

52. Rosemary Lunardini, "Thomas Almy: Primary care a primary concern," *DM* 22, no. 4 (Winter 1997): 44.

53. Jerome Nolan, DHMC Housestaff 1952–1954, 1 Aug. 1999, personal communication.

54. Donald Catino, "The Challenge of Rural Primary Care: Its Teaching and Practice," *DM* (Fall 1979): 20.

55. "The Hitchcock Foundation," information sheet, 1981.

56. Press release, 19 Oct. 1976; DC Trustees, *Records*, DA-1, Box 23:64, DCA.

57. Press release, 3 Apr. 1981; DC Trustees, *Records*, DA-1, Box 23:66, DCA.

58. Lee McDavid, "DHART proves its mettle, is made permanent," *DM* 23, no. 3 (Winter 1998): 8.

59. Martha G. Regan-Smith, "An out-and-out overhaul of the clinical curriculum," *DMSAM* 14, no. 2 (Winter 1989): 10–11.

60. Andrew G. Wallace, "A lifelong process of education," *DM* 16, no. 2 (Winter 1991: 2. Emphases in the original.

61. Office of Admissions, "Dartmouth Medical School," September 1994; Medical School Vertical File VII, DCA.

62. Nancy Serrell, "Former Director: Koop Institute Still Just an Intriguing Idea," *VN* (12 Jan. 1994): A1.

63. Marsha F. Goldsmith, "Dartmouth Medical School Bicentennial," *JAMA* 278, no. 6 (13 Aug. 1997): 458.

64. C. Everett Koop, 3 Jan. 2000, personal communication.

65. Andrew G. Wallace, "Parting thoughts," *DM* 22, no. 4 (Summer 1998): 2. Emphases in the original.

66. "Research Income is up 36 percent," *DM* 15, no. 1 (Fall 1990): 2. Funding increases had, by the following year, made Dartmouth College the "fifth-fastest-growing research university in the country." See "Dartmouth: Fifth fastest in research growth," *DM* 16, no. 1 (Fall 1991): 7. (By 1997, research income had risen to $53 million, and since the figure has climbed to $112 million.)

67. James A. Spalding, "Dixi Crosby," *Surgery, Gynecology and Obstetrics* (Oct. 1926): 541.

68. Peter K. Spiegel, "The First Clinical X-ray Made in America—100 Years," *Amer. Jrnl. Roentgenology* 164 (Jan. 1995): 241–43. The story of the story, so to speak, appears in Rosemary Lunardini, "X Marks the Spot," *DM* 20, no. 2 (Winter 1995): 38–43, 73.

69. On 27 Jan. 1896, Arthur W. Wright—a physicist at Yale—"made the first X-ray in the United States"—but it was not a *clinical* x-ray. [Photo caption], *Yale Medicine* 32, no. 1 (Winter/Spring 1998): 29.

70. Radford Tanzer, 12 Dec. 2000, personal communication.

71. Worham L. Fitch, "Extracts From Lectures on Surgery Delivered at the Medical Institution at New Haven by Nathan Smith 1824," p. 74. Yale course lectures collection (RU 159). M&A, YUL.

72. The descriptions of these several events relies in part on Jonathan Douglas, "Claims to Fame," *DM* 16, no. 1 (Fall 1991): 22–27.

73. Press release, 3 Apr. 1981; DC Trustees, *Records*, DA-1, Box 23:66, DCA.

74. [Photo caption,] *DM* 14, no. 3 (Spring 1990): 25.

75. Lee McDavid, "The Dartmouth Difference," *DM* 22, no. 1 (Summer/Fall 1997): 80–91, at 91.

76. James O. Freedman, "Medical Education and the American Future," in Dana Cook Grossman and Heinz Valtin, eds., *Great Issues for Medicine in the Twenty-First Century: Ethical and Social Issues Arising out of Advances in the Biomedical Sciences*, *Ann. N.Y. Acad. Sci.* 882 (1999), 4, 7.

77. Quoted in Rosemary Lunardini, "The New Dean," *DM* 15, no. 1 (Fall 1990): 16.

78. Andrew G. Wallace, "Educating Tomorrow's Doctors: The Thing That Really Matters Is That We Care," *Academic Medicine* 72, no. 4 (Apr. 1997): 253–58, at 254. (The quotation is taken from the oral version of the talk; some of the language was altered when the paper was published.) See also James O. Freedman, *Idealism and Liberal Education* (Ann Arbor: Univ. of Michigan Press, 1996.

79. Andrew G. Wallace, "Letter from the Dean" (Hanover, N.H.: DMS, Winter 1997).

Index

Library of Congress Cataloging-in-Publication Data

Putnam, Constance E., 1943–
The science we have loved and taught : Dartmouth Medical School's first two centuries / Constance E. Putnam ; foreword by James E. Wright.
p. cm.
Includes bibliographical references and index.
ISBN 1–58465–370–1 (cloth : alk. paper)
1. Dartmouth Medical School—History. 2. Medical colleges—New Hampshire—History. 3. Medical education—New Hampshire—History. I. Title.
R747.D22P88 2004
610'.71'17423—dc22 2004002176